Case Files™

Physiology

Second Edition

EUGENE C. TOY, MD
The John S. Dunn Senior Academic Chief and Program
  Director
Obstetrics and Gynecology Residency
The Methodist Hospital, Houston
Clerkship Director and Clinical Associate Professor
Department of Obstetrics and Gynecology
University of Texas Medical School at Houston
Houston, Texas

NORMAN WEISBRODT, PhD
Professor and Interim Chairman
Department of Integrative Biology and Pharmacology
University of Texas Medical School at Houston
Houston, Texas

WILLIAM P. DUBINSKY, JR., PhD
Professor of Integrative Biology and Pharmacology
University of Texas Medical School at Houston
Houston, Texas

ROGER G. O'NEIL, PhD
Professor of Integrative Biology and Pharmacology
University of Texas Medical School at Houston
Houston, Texas

EDGAR T. WALTERS, PhD
Professor of Integrative Biology and Pharmacology
University of Texas Medical School at Houston
Houston, Texas

KONRAD P. HARMS, MD
Associate Program Director
Obstetrics and Gynecology Residency
The Methodist Hospital, Houston
Assistant Clinical Professor
Weill Cornell College of Medicine
Houston, Texas

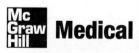

New York Chicago San Francisco
Lisbon London Madrid Mexico City
Milan New Delhi San Juan Seoul
Singapore Sydney Toronto

The *McGraw·Hill* Companies

Case Files™: Physiology, Second Edition

1 2 3 4 5 6 7 8 9 0   DOC/DOC   12 11 10 9 8

ISBN 978-0-07-149374-1
MHID 0-07-149374-3

Notice

Medicine is an ever-changing science. As new research and clinical experience broaden our knowledge, changes in treatment and drug therapy are required. The authors and the publisher of this work have checked with sources believed to be reliable in their efforts to provide information that is complete and generally in accord with the standard accepted at the time of publication. However, in view of the possibility of human error or changes in medical sciences, neither the editors nor the publisher nor any other party who has been involved in the preparation or publication of this work warrants that the information contained herein is in every respect accurate or complete, and they disclaim all responsibility for any errors or omissions or for the results obtained from use of the information contained in this work. Readers are encouraged to confirm the information contained herein with other sources. For example, and in particular, readers are advised to check the product information sheet included in the package of each drug they plan to administer to be certain that the information contained in this work is accurate and that changes have not been made in the recommended dose or in the contraindications for administration. This recommendation is of particular importance in connection with new or infrequently used drugs.

This book was set in Times Roman by International Typesetting and Composition.
The editor was Catherine A. Johnson.
The production supervisor was Catherine H. Saggese.
Project management was provided by Gita Raman, International Typesetting and Composition.
The cover designer was Thomas De Pierro.
RR Donnelly was printer and binder.

This book is printed on acid-free paper.

Library of Congress Cataloging-in-Publication Data

Case files. Physiology / Eugene C. Toy [et al.].—2nd ed.
    p. ; cm.
  Includes index.
  ISBN-13: 978-0-07-149374-1 (pbk. : alk. paper)
  ISBN-10: 0-07-149374-3 (pbk. : alk. paper)
    1. Human physiology—Problems, exercises, etc.   2. Human physiology—Case studies.
  I. Toy, Eugene C.   II. Title: Physiology.
  [DNLM: 1. Physiological Processes—Case Reports.   2. Physiological Processes—
  Examination Questions.   QT 18.2 C337 2009]
  QP40.C37 2009
  612—dc22   2008018251

❖ DEDICATION

*To my outstanding obstetrics and gynecology residents who
exemplify excellence and make coming to work each day a joy:
Erica, Amber, Brad, Tara, Barrett, Kelli, Jennifer, Tametra,
Stephen, Kristin, Tina, Lauren, Jessica, Vian,
Kathryn, and Stan.*

—ECT

*To our many medical students over the past 25 years who
have taught us so much.*

—NW, WPD, RGO, ETW

*To my wife, Heidi, and sons, Koen and Kort, for their many sacrifices
on my behalf and their unwavering love and support.
To my parents, Paul and Lois, for their guidance
and love throughout my life.
To my brother, Kent, for being a great role model and
my best friend.*

—KPH

❖ CONTENTS

❖ CONTRIBUTORS

Paul G. Harms, PhD
Professor
Faculty of Reproductive Biology
Departments of Animal Science & Veterinary Integrated Biosciences
Texas A&M University
College Station, Texas
Female Reproductive Biology
Physiology of Pregnancy

Alaina Johnson
Class of 2008
University of Texas Medical School at Houston
Houston, Texas
Basal Ganglia
Electrical Activity of the Heart
Oxygen-Carbon Dioxide Transport

❖ ACKNOWLEDGMENTS

The inspiration for this basic science series occurred at an educational retreat led by Dr. L. Maximilian Buja, who at the time was the Dean of the University of Texas Medical School at Houston and is currently Executive Vice President for Academic Affairs. It has been such a joy to work together with Drs. Weisbrodt, Dubinsky, O'Neil, and Walters, who are accomplished scientists and teachers. It has been rewarding to collaborate with Dr. Konrad Harms, a friend, a scholar, and an excellent teacher. Dr. Harms found collaborating with his father, Dr. Paul Harms, a neuroendocrinologist and reproductive physiologist at Texas A&M University, to be a true privilege, joy, and honor. I appreciate the many hours and talent of Alaina Johnson, who reviewed the entire manuscript and served as a major consultant. I would like to thank McGraw-Hill for believing in the concept of teaching by clinical cases. I owe a great debt to Catherine Johnson, who has been a fantastically encouraging and enthusiastic editor. At the University of Texas Medical School at Houston, I would like to recognize the bright and enthusiastic medical students who have inspired us to find better ways to teach. At Methodist Hospital, I appreciate Drs. Mark Boom, Alan L. Kaplan, Karin Pollock-Larsen, H. Dirk Sostman, and Judy Paukert, and Mr. Reggie Abraham. At St. Joseph Medical Center, I would like to recognize our outstanding administrators: Phil Robinson, Pat Mathews, Laura Fortin, Dori Upton, and Drs. John Bertini and Thomas V. Taylor. I appreciate Marla Buffington's advice and assistance. Without the help from my colleagues, Drs. Simmons, Schachel, and McBride, this book could not have been written. Most important, I am humbled by the love, affection, and encouragement from my lovely wife, Terri, and our four children, Andy, Michael, Allison, and Christina.

Eugene C. Toy

❖ INTRODUCTION

Often, the medical student will cringe at the "drudgery" of the basic science courses and see little connection between a field such as physiology and clinical situations. Clinicians, however, often wish they knew more about the basic sciences, because it is through the science that we can begin to understand the complexities of the human body and thus have rational methods of diagnosis and treatment.

Mastering the knowledge in a discipline such as physiology is a formidable task. It is even more difficult to retain this information and to recall it when the clinical setting is encountered. To accomplish this synthesis, physiology is optimally taught in the context of medical situations, and this is reinforced later during the clinical rotations. The gulf between the basic sciences and the patient arena is wide. Perhaps one way to bridge this gulf is with carefully constructed clinical cases that ask basic science-oriented questions. In an attempt to achieve this goal, we have designed a collection of patient cases to teach physiology-related points. More important, the explanations for these cases emphasize the underlying mechanisms and relate the clinical setting to the basic science data. We explore the principles rather than emphasize rote memorization.

This book is organized for versatility: to allow the student "in a rush" to go quickly through the scenarios and check the corresponding answers and to provide more detailed information for the student who wants thought-provoking explanations. The answers are arranged from simple to complex: a summary of the pertinent points, the bare answers, a clinical correlation, an approach to the physiology topic, a comprehension test at the end for reinforcement or emphasis, and a list of references for further reading. The clinical cases are arranged by system to better reflect the organization within the basic science. Finally, to encourage thinking about mechanisms and relationships, we intentionally used open-ended questions in the cases. Nevertheless, several multiple-choice questions are included at the end of each scenario to reinforce concepts or introduce related topics.

We appreciate the good feedback from the various medical students from across the country. We have adopted many of these suggestions. In this second edition, there have been 30 cases that were substantially rewritten and 16 new figures to improve the readability and explanations. We think this second edition is an even better product.

HOW TO GET THE MOST OUT OF THIS BOOK

Each case is designed to introduce a clinically related issue and includes open-ended questions usually asking a basic science question, but at times, to break up the monotony, there will be a clinical question. The answers are organized into four different parts:

PART I

1. **Summary**
2. A **straightforward answer** is given for each open-ended question.
3. **Clinical Correlation**—A discussion of the relevant points relating the basic science to the clinical manifestations, and perhaps introducing the student to issues such as diagnosis and treatment.

PART II

An approach to the basic science concept consisting of two parts
1. **Objectives**—A listing of the two to four main principles that are critical for understanding the underlying physiology to answer the question and relate to the clinical situation.
2. **Discussion** of the physiologic principles.

PART III

Comprehension Questions—Each case includes several multiple-choice questions that reinforce the material or introduce new and related concepts. Questions about the material not found in the text are explained in the answers.

PART IV

Physiology Pearls—A listing of several important points, many clinically relevant, reiterated as a summation of the text and to allow for easy review, such as before an examination.

Applying the Basic Sciences to Clinical Medicine

PART 1. APPROACH TO LEARNING PHYSIOLOGY

Physiology is best learned through a systematic approach, by understanding the cellular and macroscopic processes of the body. Rather than memorizing the individual relationships, the student should strive to learn the underlying rationale, such as: "The cell membrane allows passage of some molecules and not others based on lipid solubility, size of the molecule, concentration gradient, and electrical charge. Because the cell membrane is formed by a lipid bilayer, molecules that are lipid-soluble pass through more easily. Smaller molecules and those without an electrical charge also transfer more easily. Finally, the concentration gradient 'drives' the molecular transport, with the larger gradient providing a greater 'force'."

PART 2. APPROACH TO DISEASE

Physicians usually tackle clinical situations by taking a history (asking questions), performing a physical examination, obtaining selective laboratory and imaging tests, and then formulating a diagnosis. The synthesis of the history, physical examination, and imaging/laboratory tests is called the **clinical database.** After a diagnosis has been reached, a treatment plan usually is initiated, and the patient is followed for a clinical response. Rational understanding of disease and plans for treatment are best acquired by learning about the normal human processes on a basic science level; similarly, being aware of how disease alters the normal physiologic processes is best understood on a scientific level. Physiology also requires the ability to appreciate the normal workings of the human body, whereas pathophysiology focuses on how disease or disruption of the normal state affects the same mechanisms. The student should strive to learn the reason a disease manifests as certain symptoms or signs.

PART 3. APPROACH TO READING

There are six key questions that help stimulate the application of basic science information to the clinical setting:

1. **What is the likely mechanism for the clinical finding(s)?**
2. **What is the likely cellular response to a certain change in environment?**
3. **With the biochemical findings noted, what clinical processes are expected?**
4. **Given physiologic readings (hemodynamic, pulmonary, etc.), what is the likely disease process?**
5. **What is the likely cellular mechanism for the medication effect?**
6. **What graphic data best depict the physiologic principle?**

1. **What is the likely mechanism for the clinical finding(s)?**

The student of physiology should try to place the understanding of
the body in the context of molecular interactions, cellular adaptation,
and responses by organ system. The physician must elicit data by asking questions and performing a physical examination. Through this
process, the clinician forms a differential diagnosis of possible causes
for the patient's symptoms. An understanding of the mechanisms by
which physiological events give rise to the clinical manifestations
allows for rational therapy and prognosis and directs future research.
The student is advised to "think through" the mechanisms rather than
memorize them. For instance, a pituitary adenoma may affect peripheral vision. Instead of memorizing this fact, the student should recall
that the medial (nasal) aspects of both ocular retinas are innervated by
optic nerves, which travel close to the midline and cross at the optic
chiasm near the pituitary gland. Thus, an enlarging pituitary adenoma
will impinge first on the nerve fibers at the optic chiasm, leading to a
loss of visual acuity in the bitemporal regions, so-called bitemporal
hemianopia. The clinician can screen for this by testing the patient's
visual fields through testing peripheral vision on the lateral aspects.

2. **What is the likely cellular response to a certain change in
    environment?**

The study of physiology must be approached on different levels. The
macroscopic as well as the microscopic responses are important. When
a change in the environment occurs (a stressor), individual cells adapt
so that the organ adjusts, and ultimately the entire organism adapts. For
instance, during an overnight fast, when serum glucose levels fall,
leading to hypoglycemia, the body adapts. In the short term, the effects
of insulin and glucagon on several key regulatory reactions in intermediary metabolism are directly opposed. During the fasting state, insulin
levels fall and glucagon levels rise; these hormones act on glycogen
synthesis or breakdown. Net production or breakdown of glycogen is
dependent on the relative rates of the two reactions. These facts illustrate the hormonal responses.

In regard to biochemical factors, often these reactions are controlled
by phosphorylation-dephosphorylation cycles, and sometimes, these
effects can be attributed to one common factor: in this case, cyclic
adenosine monophosphate (cAMP). Glucagon activates *adenyl
cyclase*, causing an increase in cellular cAMP levels and *protein kinase
A* (PKA) activity. Insulin binding to its receptor, a *tyrosine kinase*, activates a signaling pathway that activates *protein kinase B* (PKB) and
protein phosphatase-1. An example of the regulatory effects of these
two hormones is the glycogen synthetic pathway. Glycogen levels are
controlled by the relative rates of glycogen synthesis and glycogenolysis. *Glycogen synthase* activity is regulated by a phosphorylation-
dephosphorylation cycle. In the absence of insulin, glycogen synthase

is phosphorylated by a specific protein kinase. That kinase is inactivated in the presence of insulin, reducing the phosphorylation of glycogen synthase. The reaction is reinforced by an insulin-dependent activation of protein phosphatase-1 that dephosphorylates and activates glycogen synthase. Protein phosphatase-1 has multiple substrate proteins within the cell, one of which is phosphorylase. Phosphorylase catalyzes the breakdown of glycogen and is activated by phosphorylation with PKA and inactivated by dephosphorylation.

Thus, after the ingestion of a carbohydrate-containing meal, the rise in plasma insulin levels will cause an activation of glycogen synthase and an inhibition of phosphorylase. A fall in the plasma glucose reduces secretion of pancreatic insulin and stimulates secretion of glucagon. The hepatocyte responds to these changes with a decrease in protein phosphatase activity (as a result of decreased insulin levels) and an increase in PKA activity (as a result of elevated glucagon levels). The overall effect is an increase in glycogenolysis with the production of glucose.

3. **With the biochemical findings noted, what clinical processes are expected?**

This is the converse of explaining clinical findings by reference to cellular or biochemical mechanisms. An understanding of the underlying molecular biology allows an extrapolation to the clinical findings. The student is encouraged to explore relationships between microscopic function and clinical symptoms or signs. The patient is aware only of overt manifestations such as pain, fatigue, and bleeding. Usually, substantial subclinical changes are present. The student's understanding of these relationships, as depicted below, provides opportunities to detect disease before it is clinically evident or to disrupt the disease process before it becomes advanced.

Biochemical → Cellular → Subclinical changes → Clinical symptoms

One example is the understanding of the development of cervical cancer. It is known that human papillomavirus (HPV) is the primary oncogenic stimulus in the majority of cases of cervical intraepithelial neoplasia (CIN) and cervical cancer. HPV, particularly in the virulent subtypes, such as 16 and 18, incorporates its DNA into the host cervical epithelium cells, leading some women to develop CIN. Over years, the CIN progresses to cervical cancer; when this becomes advanced, it becomes evident by the patient's development of abnormal vaginal bleeding, lower abdominal pain, or back pain if metastasis has occurred. Awareness of this sequence of events allows for the possible development of an HPV vaccine, assays for HPV subtypes to assess the risk of CIN or cancer, and cytologic analysis of CIN when it is still asymptomatic (Pap smear), with appropriate treatment before cancer arises. The result is a 90% decrease in mortality from cervical cancer compared with the situation before the advent of the Pap smear.

4. **Given physiologic readings (hemodynamic, pulmonary, etc.), what is the likely disease process?**

The clinician's ability to interpret data relative to the physiologic and pathophysiologic processes is fundamental to rational therapy. For instance, a pulmonary artery catheter may be used to approximate the measure of a patient's left atrial pressure. In an instance of severe hypoxemia and diffuse pulmonary infiltrates on a chest radiograph, a common diagnostic dilemma is whether the patient has fluid overload and is in congestive heart failure or whether this represents acute respiratory distress syndrome (ARDS). In volume overload, the increased hydrostatic pressure drives fluid from the pulmonary capillaries into the pulmonary interstitium, leading to inefficient gas exchange between the alveoli and the capillary. The treatment for this condition would be diuresis, such as with furosemide, to remove fluid. In contrast, with ARDS, the pathophysiology is leaky capillaries, and the pulmonary capillary pressure is normal to slightly low. The therapy in this case is supportive and entails waiting for repair; diuresis may lead to hypovolemia and hypotension. In essence, the question is whether the patient is "wet" or "leaky," and the wrong therapy may be harmful. The pulmonary artery wedge pressure catheter is helpful in this case, because high pressures would suggest volume overload whereas normal-to-low pressures would suggest ARDS with leaky capillaries.

5. **What is the likely cellular mechanism for the medication effect?**

The student is best served by understanding the cellular mechanisms for not only physiologic responses but also responses to medications. For instance, an awareness of the behavior of digoxin allows one to understand its effect on the heart. Digoxin is a cardiac glycoside that acts indirectly to increase intracellular calcium. Digitalis binds to a specific site on the outside of Na^+-K^+-ATPase, reducing the activity of that enzyme. All cells express Na^+-K^+-ATPase, but they express different isoforms of the enzyme; the isoforms expressed by cardiac myocytes and vagal neurons are the most susceptible to digitalis. Inhibition of the enzyme by digitalis causes an increase in intracellular Na^+ and decreases the Na^+ concentration gradient across the plasma membrane. This Na^+ concentration provides the driving force for the Na^+-Ca^{2+} antiporter. The rate of transport of Ca^{2+} out of the cell is reduced, and this leads to an increase in intracellular Ca^{2+} and greater activation of contractile elements and an increase in the force and velocity of contraction of the heart. The electric characteristics of myocardial cells also are altered by the cardiac glycosides. The most important effect is a shortening of the action potential that produces a shortening of both atrial and ventricular refractoriness. There is also an

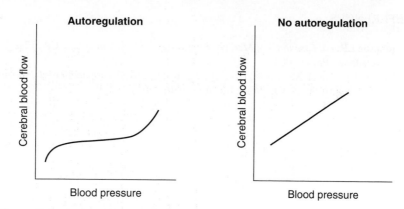

Figure I-1. Cerebral blood flow versus peripheral blood pressure.

increase in the automaticity of the heart both within the atrioventricular (AV) node and in the cardiac myocytes.

6. **What graphic data best depict the physiologic principle?**

The basic scientist must be able to interpret data in various forms and propose explanations and theories that are then tested. Data in long lists of numbers are often inconvenient and untenable to analyze. Thus, graphic representation to allow for the determination of relationships and trends is critical. The student also should be skilled in the interpretation of graphic data and the correlation of those data to physiologic processes. For instance, the brain has a well-developed autoregulatory capacity to maintain a constant cerebral blood flow despite the fact that the systemic blood pressure is variable. In other words, with hypotension, the cerebral vessels dilate to allow for brain perfusion, whereas with hypertension, the cerebral vessels constrict. Of course, there are limits to this adaptation at the extremes of blood pressures (see Figure I-1).

PHYSIOLOGY PEARLS

❖ There are six key questions to stimulate the application of basic science information to the clinical arena.

❖ The student should strive to understand physiology from the molecular, cellular, organ, and entire organism viewpoints.

❖ Understanding the physiology allows for rational diagnostic and therapeutic interventions.

REFERENCES

Johnson LR, ed. *Essentials of Medical Physiology*. 3rd ed. San Diego, CA: Elsevier Academic Press; 2003.

Kasper DL, Fauci AS, Longo DL, et al., eds. *Harrison's Principles of Internal Medicine*. 16th ed. New York: McGraw-Hill; 2004.

SECTION II
Clinical Cases

❖ CASE 1

A 43-year-old man presents to the physician's clinic with complaints of epigastric pain. After a thorough workup, the patient is diagnosed with peptic ulcer disease. He is started on a medication that inhibits the "proton pump" of the stomach.

◆ **What is the "proton pump" that is referred to above?**

◆ **What type of cell membrane transport would this medication be blocking?**

◆ **What are four other types of transport across a cell membrane?**

ANSWERS TO CASE 1: MEMBRANE PHYSIOLOGY

Summary: A 43-year-old man with peptic ulcer disease is prescribed a proton pump inhibitor.

 Proton pump: H^+-K^+-ATPase (adenosine triphosphatase) pump.

 Type of cell membrane transport: Primary active transport.

 Other types of transport: Simple diffusion, restricted diffusion, facilitated diffusion, secondary active transport (cotransport and countertransport [exchange]).

CLINICAL CORRELATION

Peptic ulcer disease is seen commonly in a primary care physician's office. Patients often complain of a gnawing or burning midepigastric pain that is worse several hours after meals and is relieved with food or antacids. Some patients with ulcerative disease may present only with an upper gastrointestinal (GI) bleed. Risk factors for peptic ulcer disease include alcohol, nonsteroidal anti-inflammatory drugs (NSAIDs), tobacco, and physiologic stress (sepsis, trauma). Infection with *Helicobacter pylori* has been proven to play a significant role in ulcer formation and must be treated when identified. Controlling acidity within the stomach also is important in the treatment of patients with peptic ulcer disease. One such medication is omeprazole, which blocks the H^+-K^+-ATPase proton pump within the parietal cells in the stomach. When the proton pump is inhibited, the H^+ cannot be transported into the lumen of the stomach against its electrochemical gradient. This decrease in stomach acidity will give a patient relief from symptoms caused by the defective intestinal mucosal lining. Treatment for 6 to 8 weeks will allow for healing of the peptic ulcers.

APPROACH TO MEMBRANE PHYSIOLOGY

Objectives

1. Know the components and structure of a cell membrane (lipid bilayer).
2. Understand the different types and examples of transport across a cell membrane.
3. Understand the concept of diffusion and equilibrium potentials.

Definitions

Diffusion: The movement of molecules across membranes as a result of a concentration gradient (uncharged molecules) or electrochemical gradient (charged molecules) across the membranes.

Active transport: The movement of molecules across membranes against a chemical or electrochemical gradient. This type of transfer requires the input of energy.

DISCUSSION

Intracellular membranes allow for the compartmentalization of cell components and the maintenance of the concentration gradients required for cell metabolism. Cell membranes mark cell boundaries and allow for the maintenance of an intracellular composition that differs from the extracellular composition. However, for a cell to function, inorganic and organic molecules must be able to pass through the cell membrane, often in a regulated manner. The current understanding is that the **cell membrane** consists mainly of a **bilayer of phospholipids** positioned so that their **hydrophilic components face the aqueous intracellular** and **extracellular fluids** and their **hydrophobic portions interact to form a lipid core.** Within and/or associated with this bilayer are cholesterol and many proteins. The proteins may span the width of the bilayer (integral proteins) or may adhere to one surface or the other (peripheral proteins). The number and types of proteins differ from one cell type to another, and in polarized cells such as those found in epithelia, proteins in the basolateral cell membrane differ from those in the apical membrane. These membrane-bound proteins serve many functions, including the transport of molecules, especially those which are water soluble, across the cell membrane.

Transport across membranes mainly occurs through **diffusion** and **active transport**. Diffusion, in turn, can be by **simple diffusion, restricted diffusion, and/or facilitated diffusion.** Each of these processes is described below.

Many molecules move across membranes as a result of a difference in the concentration of the molecules inside and outside the cell. Such movement is called diffusion. The force inducing the net diffusion is provided by the molecular movement and greater repulsion of the molecules in the more concentrated solution. The **rate of movement (J)** can be described by the equation:

$$J = P\Delta C$$

where P is the **permeability coefficient** of the membrane in question and ΔC is the **concentration gradient** across the membrane. The rate of diffusion of lipid-soluble substances depends on **concentration** and **lipid solubility.** The size of the molecule does not seem to matter. Such diffusion is called **simple diffusion** and may result from simple dissolution in lipid portions of the membrane and appearance on the other side. For many water-soluble solutes that can permeate a membrane, both their concentration and their hydrated size are important. Such diffusion is called **restricted diffusion** and occurs through proteinaceous pores or channels in the membrane.

If the solute is uncharged (eg, urea, glucose, water, lipids), this relation, considering only the chemical gradient and the permeability, will suffice. However, **if the solute is charged** (eg, ions such as sodium and chloride), the **rate of diffusion** will depend on the **electrochemical gradient,** which is the difference between the actual membrane potential and the **equilibrium potential (E)** for any specific set of intracellular and extracellular concentrations. In millivolts, E can be calculated by using the **Nernst equation:**

$$E = [60/z] \log C_o/C_i$$

where z is the valence of the solute and C_o and C_i are its concentrations on the outside and the inside of the membrane, respectively. The membrane potential (V) can be measured, and then the rate of diffusion (J) can be expressed as

$$J = G \ (V - E)$$

where G is the conductance of the membrane to the ion. When V is equal to E, there will be no net movement of the ion if its movement is by passive diffusion; however, changes in concentrations and/or changes in V will result in diffusion until electrochemical equilibrium is reestablished. Also, for the restricted diffusion of ions, the charge of the amino acids lining the channel, as well as the size of the channel, determines selectivity.

The diffusion of **larger water-soluble solutes** such as **glucose** depends not only on **size** but also on **structure.** Such diffusion is called **facilitated diffusion** and involves proteins called **carriers.** Facilitated diffusion differs from restricted diffusion in that facilitated diffusion displays a high degree of structural specificity and exhibits saturation kinetics. That is, the rate of diffusion will reach a plateau as the concentration gradient is increased.

Although diffusion can account for the movement of many solutes across cell membranes, many other solutes are **transferred against a chemical or electrochemical gradient.** This type of transfer **requires the input of energy** and is called **active transport.** Active transport is accomplished by complex integral membrane proteins that utilize adenosine triphosphate (ATP) to bring about conformational changes that result in the transport of a solute from a lower chemical/electrochemical concentration to a higher one. If the protein complex involved in the transport also is involved in the splitting of ATP, the transport is called primary active transport. There are not many examples of primary active transport processes, but the one that transports sodium out of the cell and potassium into the cell (the sodium pump) is common to almost all cells. It is responsible for maintaining **intracellular low sodium and high potassium concentration** with respect to the extracellular fluid. Others include the ones that transport calcium out of most cells, and that transport **hydrogen ion** out of parietal cells into the gastric lumen (see Figure 1-1).

In many cells, especially many specialized epithelial cells, the carrier involved in the active transport is **not** the one with the **ATPase activity.** Instead, the ability of the carrier to transport one solute against a chemical/electrochemical gradient is **coupled** to the transport of another solute, usually **sodium,** down its electrochemical gradient. The sodium gradient in turn is maintained by the "sodium pump." The coupling can be such that the entry of sodium powers the entry of a solute against a gradient. Such cotransport is the way **glucose** is absorbed by cells of the intestinal and renal proximal tubule epithelia (see Figure 1-2). In contrast, the entry of sodium can power the extrusion of another solute. Such countertransport is responsible for the removal of calcium from myocardial cells.

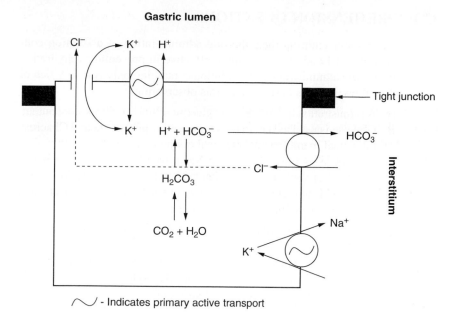

Gastric lumen

$\curvearrowright$ - Indicates primary active transport

Figure 1-1. Gastric parietal cell. H^+ is actively pumped out at the apical membrane by the H^+-K^+-ATPase. Cl^- follows down its electrochemical gradient.

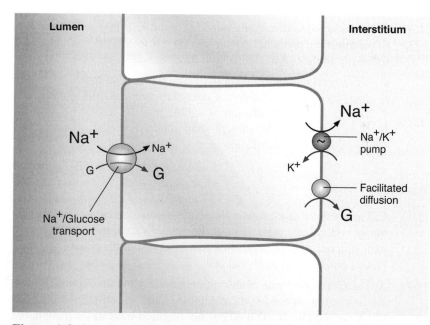

Figure 1-2. Renal proximal tubule cell. Glucose is tightly associated with sodium transport.

COMPREHENSION QUESTIONS

[1.1]   In a patient with diarrhea, the oral administration of a solution containing NaCl and glucose is more effective in preventing dehydration than is the administration of a solution containing only NaCl. Which of the following facts best explains this observation?

A. Administration of the NaCl and glucose solution reduces stool output.
B. Glucose is used as fuel to effect the cotransport of Na and Cl across the apical membrane of intestinal epithelial cells.
C. The cotransport of glucose and Na across the apical membrane of intestinal epithelial cells facilitates Na and water absorption.
D. The NaCl and glucose solution empties from the stomach at a faster rate than does a solution containing NaCl alone.

[1.2]   The rate of absorption of a drug taken orally is found to increase as the dose ingested is increased up to a point where further increases in dose result in no further increases in the rate of absorption. Absorption does not appear to result in the splitting of ATP. Which of the following processes best describes the drug absorption?

A. Facilitated diffusion
B. Primary active transport
C. Restricted diffusion
D. Secondary active transport
E. Simple diffusion

[1.3]   A drug is noted to cause only a change in the resting membrane potential of intestinal epithelial cells from −60 mV to −50 mV. Which of the following findings is most likely to be observed?

A. Decreased rate of diffusion of potassium into the cells
B. Increased rate of diffusion of potassium into the cells
C. Decreased rate of diffusion of sodium into the cells
D. Increased rate of diffusion of sodium into the cells
E. Decreased rate of diffusion of urea into the cells

Answers

[1.1]   **C.** The presence of glucose in the solution greatly increases the absorption of sodium and water. This occurs because sodium is cotransported with glucose and because there are many sodium-glucose cotransporters on intestinal epithelial cells.

[1.2]   **A.** The fact that the rate of absorption reaches a maximum even though the concentration outside the membrane is increased indicates saturation kinetics. The fact that ATP is not required indicates diffusion, not active transport. Therefore, facilitated diffusion best describes the transport process.

[1.3]   **C.** A lower inside negative membrane potential in nonexcitable cells such as intestinal epithelial cells would decrease the diffusion of sodium into the cell down its electrochemical gradient, which now would be lower. It would increase the diffusion of potassium out of the cell down its electrochemical gradient, which now would be greater. The rate of diffusion of urea, an uncharged solute, would not be altered.

PHYSIOLOGY PEARLS

❖ Lipid-soluble molecules pass through membranes down their concentration gradients by passive diffusion.

❖ Small water-soluble molecules and ions diffuse through membranes down their electrochemical gradients by restricted diffusion.

❖ Large water-soluble molecules diffuse through membranes down their concentration gradients by facilitated diffusion.

❖ Certain water-soluble molecules and ions also can pass through membranes against their electrochemical gradients by an active transport process that requires the splitting of ATP.

REFERENCES

Kutchai HC. Cell physiology. In: Levy MN, Koeppen BM, Stanton BA, eds. *Berne & Levy, Principles of Physiology*. 4th ed. Philadelphia, PA: Mosby; 2006:3-26.

Schultz SG. Membrane transport. In: Johnson LR, ed. *Essential Medical Physiology*. 3rd ed. San Diego, CA: Elsevier Academic Press; 2003:37-70.

❖ CASE 2

A 27-year-old woman presents to her gynecologist for contraception. The patient has tried various forms of barrier methods and wants to try the "pill" or an "injection." During the history and physical examination, the patient states that she often forgets to take her prescribed antibiotics and travels frequently. After discussing all options, the patient decides to try medroxyprogesterone (Depo-Provera), a progesterone hormone. She is given the injection and instructed to follow up in 3 months for the next injection.

◆ **How do injectable hormones or hormone pills provide contraception?**

◆ **At a cellular level, where is the receptor for progesterone located?**

◆ **What is exocytosis?**

ANSWERS TO CASE 2: PHYSIOLOGIC SIGNALS

Summary: A 27-year-old woman desires hormonal contraception.

◆ **Mechanism of action of hormone contraception:** Increased circulating progesterone causes negative feedback at the level of the anterior pituitary, causing inhibition of the follicle-stimulating hormone (FSH), luteinizing hormone (LH) surge, and hence follicular development and ovulation.

◆ **Location of progesterone receptor:** Nucleus of cell.

◆ **Exocytosis:** Process by which contents within the secretory vesicles are delivered to extracellular fluid.

CLINICAL CORRELATION

A good fund of knowledge about the coordination of cellular activity with the changing external and internal environment is critical for understanding the pathophysiology and making the diagnosis of many diseases as well as understanding the mechanism of action of many medications. Graves disease (hyperthyroidism) is caused by circulating thyroid-stimulating immunoglobulins that bind to the thyroid-stimulating hormone (TSH) receptors on the thyroid gland, stimulating the release of T_3 and T_4 and causing clinical symptoms of hyperthyroidism. Diagnosis of hyperthyroidism is made with measurement of the TSH level, which is low because of the negative feedback on the anterior pituitary from the increased T_3 and T_4 levels. Certain medications may bind to a particular cellular receptor with more affinity and prolonged duration, providing the necessary treatment for many conditions. Hormonal contraception is an example of the way medications can interact with cellular activity to cause the desired outcome; in this case anovulation.

APPROACH TO PHYSIOLOGIC SIGNALS

Objectives

1. Understand the basics of physiologic signals.
2. Understand the types, storage, and secretion of chemical signals.
3. Know the responses of target cells (positive and negative feedback).
4. Describe the types of cellular receptors and their locations.

Definitions

Hormone: A chemical substance that is produced and released from one tissue or organ and carried by the blood to a target tissue or organ, where it acts to produce a specific response.

Chemical signal or signaling molecule: Any chemical substance, including hormones, that can act as a communication signal within and between cells.

Receptor: Cellular receptors are specialized molecules or a complex of molecules (proteins or glycoproteins) on the cell surface or within the cell that specifically bind a signaling molecule or ligand.

Endocrine gland: A group of cells that produce and secrete a hormone.

Transducer: A biochemical pathway (signal transduction pathway) within the cell that is activated upon the binding of a ligand to a receptor and modulates a downstream effector molecule (enzyme, ion channel, etc.).

DISCUSSION

The development and survival of multicellular organisms require that cells sense and respond in a coordinated manner to physical and chemical environmental "signals." Two major systems have evolved to communicate and coordinate organ and cellular functions. These systems are the nervous system, which integrates responses between tissues and organs through electrical (action potentials) and chemical (synaptic transmission) signals, and the endocrine system, which integrates tissue and organ functions through **chemical signals (hormones)** secreted from **endocrine glands.** However, it is known that all cells, even those outside the two "classical" communications systems, normally can sense and respond to physical and chemical signals in the microenvironment surrounding the cells.

By far, the most common form of communication between cells is through chemical signals. **Chemical signals** may be as diverse as **ions, amino acids, fatty acids, peptides, proteins,** and **steroids.** For a cell to sense and respond to changes in these signals, **receptors** must reside in or on the "sensing" cells that sense the chemical change (specifically bind the chemical) and then respond by activating biochemical pathways (signal transduction pathways) within the cell that can lead to a defined response by the cell. These receptors may reside on the surface of the cell, within the cytoplasm, or in the nucleus. The cellular molecular messages linked to the activation of the receptor underlie the response of the cell to changes in the intracellular and extracellular environments, which in turn lead to regulation of diverse cellular activities such as growth and proliferation, cell motility, reproduction, and gene expression, among many others. The mechanisms underlying these molecular messages often have similar patterns or biochemical components that form the bases of cellular communication in physiologic systems.

Early views of chemical signaling and signal transduction came from studies of the endocrine system and the role of hormones as chemical signals. A **hormone** is a chemical substance that is produced in and released from one tissue or organ and is carried by the blood to a target tissue or organ, where it acts to produce a specific response. An **endocrine gland** is a group of cells that produce and secrete a hormone. It is generally considered that chemical communication can involve the production of a hormone or chemical signal by one cell type that in turn can act in one of three ways: on distant tissues or cells (**endocrine**), on neighboring cells in the same tissue or organ (**paracrine**), and on the same cell that released the signaling molecule (**autocrine**).

Chemical substances that can act as chemical signals within and between cells can be grouped as follows: **peptides and proteins,** such as vasopressin, somatostatin, growth hormone, and insulin; **amines,** such as dopamine and epinephrine; **steroids,** such as estradiol, progesterone, testosterone, and aldosterone; and other **small molecules,** such as amino acids, nucleotides, gases (eg, nitric oxide), and ions (eg, calcium, magnesium). Some chemical signals initially are synthesized and stored within secretory vesicles in a cell until a signal induces the release of the signaling molecule from the cell. Peptide, protein, and amine hormones typically are handled in this manner. In contrast, steroid hormones are not stored but are produced when they are needed. For small chemical molecules, most are not stored but are produced as needed, as has been observed for nitric oxide.

For a molecule to act as a signal, it first must bind to a cellular receptor. Cellular **receptors** are specialized molecules or a complex of molecules (proteins or glycoproteins) on the cell surface or within the cell that specifically bind a signaling molecule or ligand. Typically, the receptor, when activated (when it binds a ligand), initiates an intracellular cascade of biochemical events that act as a **transducer (signal transduction pathway)** that ultimately impinges on an **effector** molecule, such as an enzyme, ion channel, or transcription factor, that initiates a **cellular response** (eg, cell division, gene expression, contraction, secretion). The response of one cell or tissue may induce a feedback loop to shut down (**negative feedback**) or enhance (**positive feedback**) the initial signal and response. The feedback effect may be on the signal, receptor, transducer (transduction pathway), or effector (see Figure 2-1).

Plasma membrane receptors represent the cells frontline system for responding to alterations in chemical signals in the extracellular environment. Cell surface receptors can be grouped according to the structure of the receptor and its linkage to the underlying signal transduction pathways. **G protein–coupled receptors (GPCRs)** are a superfamily of receptors that work indirectly through a heterotrimeric guanosine triphosphate-binding protein, or G protein, which links the receptor to an effector molecule such as an enzyme or an ion channel. These receptors are integral membrane proteins or glycoproteins with seven transmembrane segments (often called seven-transmembrane receptors). The extracellular domains cluster together to form a binding pocket for a specific agonist or ligand (peptide, protein, and amine hormones such as vasopressin, angiotensin II, and epinephrine).

The intracellular domains have a number of regulatory binding sites, including sites for the binding of G proteins (see the references at the end of this case for details). G proteins typically provide the link between the first chemical signal at the cell surface (**first messenger**) and the subsequent intermediate chemical signals within the cell, the so-called **second messengers.** Second messenger systems have the potential to amplify the original signal

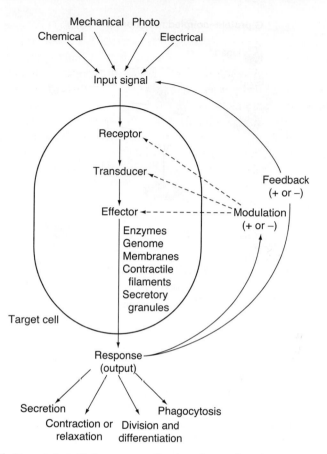

Figure 2-1. Events in cellular communication. Input signals are recognized by a receptor and translated into a biochemical change by a transducer mechanism. The biochemical signal then acts on the cellular apparatus or effector to produce a physiologic response or output. The output may feed back directly or indirectly to affect the source of the input signal and increase or decrease its intensity. The output also may act directly or indirectly to modulate the cellular response to a signal by augmenting or damping events at the level of the receptor, the transducer, or the effector apparatus.

because the binding of a ligand to its receptor can generate hundreds of second messenger molecules. Second messenger systems also can provide specificity and diversity in the cellular response (see the references at the end of this case). Although there are a wide variety of extracellular chemical signals and receptors (GPCRs), there are only a few substances that act as second messengers. The heterotrimeric G proteins can link (inhibit or activate) to adenylyl cyclase to generate cyclic adenosine monophosphate (cAMP), the initial second

G protein–coupled receptors (GPCR)

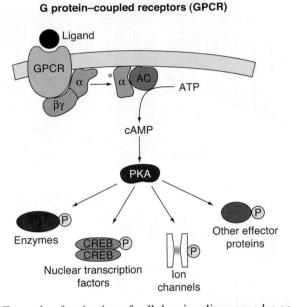

Figure 2-2. Example of activation of cellular signaling cascades and associated processes by G protein–coupled receptors (GPCR). Several specific steps lead to activation of the receptor and downstream effector molecules. (1) Binding of a ligand (eg, epinephrine, vasopressin) to its receptor activates the specific GPCR. (2) The activated receptor interacts with a heterotrimeric G protein (a GTP-binding protein made up of α, β, and γ subunits), leading to exchange of GDP with GTP on the α subunit (activated G protein). (3) The activated G protein dissociates from the receptor into a GTP-bound α subunit (*) and a separate βγ subunit complex, both of which can regulate downstream effectors. (4) In the example, the activated α subunit is a stimulator subunit (as opposed to an inhibitory subunit) which associates with adenylate cyclase to activate the enzyme leading to production of cAMP. (5) cAMP, in turn, binds to the regulatory subunit of its downstream effector, protein kinase A (PKA), leading to dissociation of PKA into catalytic and regulatory subunits. (6) The catalytic subunit of PKA is then free to catalyze the phosphorylation of a range of downstream effector proteins, including glycogen phosphorylase kinase, glycogen synthase, phosphodiesterases, phosphoprotein phosphatases, ion channels, and certain nuclear transcription factors (eg, CREB), thereby controlling downstream cellular process associated with the phosphorylated proteins.

messenger to be identified, which in turn activates its primary effector, protein kinase A (cAMP-dependent protein kinase), or other effectors. Figure 2-2 shows an example of the signaling cascade associated with a typical GPCR that is coupled through a stimulatory G protein linked to activation of adenylyl cyclase and production of cAMP, a major second messenger present in all cells (see below).

The catecholamines epinephrine and norepinephrine exert their effects by binding to adrenergic receptors (α- and β-adrenergic receptors) and generating cAMP, leading to a response (eg, arteriole constriction, glycogenolysis). GPCRs also can link through G proteins to guanylyl cyclase to generate cGMP as a second messenger, such as for photoreceptor responses, or link to phospholipase C (PLC) to generate diacylglycerol (DAG) and inositol 1,4,5-triphosphate (IP_3), as is observed for a broad array of calcium-dependent responses. In addition, GPCRs can also link to phospholipase A_2 to generate arachidonic acid, leading to the production of the eicosanoids that underlie inflammatory responses and gastric acid secretion.

Tyrosine kinase-dependent receptors are a second major type of cell membrane receptor and include receptors for growth factors, cytokines, and many hormones. These receptors belong to several families of receptors, but all typically signal through activated tyrosine kinases. These receptors have only one transmembrane-spanning domain where the extracellular portion contains a ligand-binding domain. A major family of this type of receptor is the **receptor tyrosine kinases (RTK),** which include receptors for insulin, fibroblast growth factor (FGF), epidermal growth factor (EGF), and nerve growth factor (NGF). Binding of an agonist such as FGF to its receptor induces a conformational change that facilitates **dimerization** of two receptor molecules.

Dimerization induces a close association of the cytoplasmic portions of the subunits, allowing the tyrosine kinase activity of each subunit to phosphorylate tyrosine residues on the opposing subunit, a process called **autophosphorylation,** thus activating the receptor complex. This process also may activate the phosphorylation of tyrosine residues on other cytoplasmic proteins, leading to diverse responses. The phosphorylated sites serve as high-affinity binding sites for intracellular signaling molecules, most notably to the **src homology (SH) domains** SH2 and SH3 of cytoplasmic proteins such as growth factor receptor-bound protein-2 (GRB2) and phospholipase Cγ (PLCγ). These activated proteins in turn activate downstream signaling pathways such as **mitogen-activated protein (MAP) kinase** cascades that in turn regulate a multitude of processes, including gene transcription. An example of a signaling pathway regulated by RTK is shown in Figure 2-3.

A separate receptor family grouped under the tyrosine kinase-dependent receptors consists of the **tyrosine kinase-associated receptors.** Receptors in this family bind cytokines such as interleukin 2 (IL-2), IL-3, and IL-4 and interferon alpha (IFN-α), IFN-β, and IFN-γ, along with some growth factors, such as leukemia inhibitory factor, and prolactin (PRL). These receptors do not have intrinsic tyrosine kinase activity but interact with other cytoplasmic molecules that do have tyrosine kinase activity. Ligand binding to a receptor subunit induces dimerization/trimerization which leads to association of proteins with tyrosine kinase activity, such as the **src family** of receptor-associated

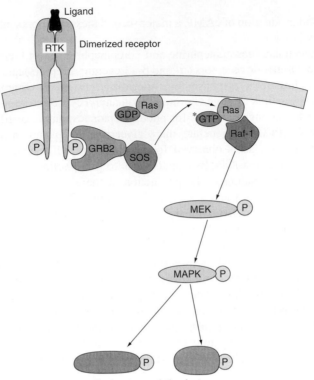

Receptor tyrosine kinases (RTK)

Figure 2-3. Example of activation of cellular signaling cascades and associated processes by RTK. Several specific steps lead to activation of the receptor which, in turn, activates specific nuclear transcription factors through a Ras-dependent signaling pathway (Ras is a small GTP-binding protein different from the heterotrimeric G proteins activated by GPCR). (1) Binding of a ligand (eg, EGF, platelet-derived growth factor, insulin, FGF) to the extracellular domain of a specific RTK leads to dimerization of two receptor monomers to activate the receptor. (2) The activated RTK undergoes autophosphorylation of itself on tyrosine residues in the cytoplasmic domain. (3) A growth factor receptor-bound protein-2 (GRB2), containing a Src homology domain-2 (SH2), recognizes and binds to the specific phosphotyrosine residues on RTK which, in turn, recruit a guanine nucleotide exchange protein, SOS (son of sevenless). (4) SOS activates membrane-bound Ras by inducing an exchange of GDP for GTP on Ras. (5) The activated Ras-GTP (*) complex recruits other signaling proteins, such as Raf-1 (a serine-threonine kinase also known as mitogen-activated protein, MAP) that initiates a cascade of protein kinases: Raf-1 phosphorylates and activates MEK (MAP kinase kinase, MAPKK) followed by MEK-induced phosphorylation and activation of MAPK (MAP kinase, also called ERK1/2 or extracellular signal-regulated kinase). (6) MAPK subsequently phosphorylates a variety of cytoplasmic proteins or, as shown in the example, translocates to the nucleus where it phosphorylates a number of nuclear transcription factors which can activate or inhibit the transcription of a wide range of genes.

proteins and the **Janus family** (JAKs) of receptor-associated proteins. Activation of these proteins activates signaling cascades that control multitude of processes related to inflammation and gene transcription.

A third family of cell membrane receptors consists of receptors that are themselves ion channels, the **receptor channels (receptor-operated channels).** These are ligand-gated ion channels that are activated (channel opening) upon the binding of a ligand. These receptors also have been called **inotropic receptors** to distinguish them from **metabotropic receptors,** which act via metabolic pathways. These receptors are characterized by rapid responses because intermediary biochemical pathways are not used. The receptor channels typically are localized to a synapse or neuromuscular junction where rapid communication is imperative. The receptors represent a larger group of ligand-gated channels and include receptors for acetylcholine, α-aminobutyric acid (GABA), serotonin, and glutamate. Many other channels also are thought to function as receptor channels.

Intracellular receptors (nuclear receptors) represent a separate class of receptors that bind ligands that can diffuse readily across the cell membrane; that is, the ligands are lipophilic. This class includes **steroid hormones** (eg, estrogen, progesterone, testosterone, aldosterone, corticosteroid), **vitamin D, retinoic acid (vitamin A),** and **thyroid hormone.** When these ligands diffuse into a cell and bind to their intracellular receptors, the complex becomes an activated **transcription factor** that enhances or represses the expression of various target genes by binding to specific DNA sequences called **hormone responsive elements.** These DNA sequences may be located in the immediate vicinity of the gene's promoters or at a considerable distance from them. The various nuclear receptors display specific cell and tissue distributions so that considerable diversity may exist in the response of one cell and that of another in regard to what gene is enhanced or repressed. Typical cellular responses include inflammatory responses, proliferation, and differentiation.

COMPREHENSION QUESTIONS

[2.1] NGF is a critical first messenger that controls the development and survival of certain neurons, such as sensory neurons of the dorsal root ganglia. Upon the binding of NGF to its receptor, an early step required for transduction involves the TrkA receptor tyrosine kinase. Which of the following processes most likely occurs?

A. Coupling of TrkA to a G protein
B. Autophosphorylation of TrkA
C. Protein kinase A phosphorylation of TrkA serine residues
D. Protease cleavage of the extracellular *N*-terminal domain of TrkA
E. Dissociation of dimeric TrkA isoforms to a monomeric form

[2.2]   A fasting person is noted to have a nearly normal rate of muscle metabolism. This can occur through the actions of epinephrine that induces glycogen breakdown. In muscle cells, this effect of epinephrine is mediated via the binding to a β_2-adrenergic receptor that is coupled via G proteins to an effector enzyme as part of the transduction pathway that controls glycogen breakdown. What effector enzyme is coupled to the β_2 receptor to induce this response?

   A. Phospholipase C
   B. Phospholipase A_2
   C. Phospholipase D
   D. Adenylyl cyclase
   E. Guanylyl cyclase

[2.3]   A 45-year-old scientist is diagnosed with type II diabetes mellitus. It is explained to him that the mechanism of this type of diabetes is a postreceptor issue, with the hormone being insulin. Which of the following is most accurate in describing type II diabetes?

   A. Serum insulin deficiency
   B. Counterregulatory hormone excess
   C. Insulin receptor is involved
   D. Secondary messenger is involved

Answers

[2.1]   **B.** Binding of NGF to TrkA monomers causes dimerization. The dimer form rapidly induces transautophosphorylation of each monomer to activate the receptor.

[2.2]   **D.** The muscle β_2-adrenergic receptor is G_s protein coupled via the G_s subunit to adenylyl cyclase, leading to the generation of cAMP. The elevation in cAMP leads to the activation of protein kinase A and the induction of phosphorylase kinase to the active form, which in turn activates glycogen phosphorylase, leading to the breakdown of glycogen (increasing production of glucose 6-phosphate and glucose metabolism). Simultaneously, protein kinase A leads to the inhibition of glycogen synthase, thereby inhibiting the conversion of glucose to glycogen.

[2.3]   **D.** Type II diabetes is a postreceptor problem that affects the secondary messenger. There is sufficient insulin and a normal insulin receptor; however, the signal of the hormone-receptor complex is altered, leading to the observed insulin resistance.

PHYSIOLOGY PEARLS

❖ G protein–coupled receptors are cell membrane receptors that upon binding of a ligand (angiotensin II, vasopressin, epinephrine, etc.) couple through G proteins to activate downstream effectors such as adenylyl cyclase, phospholipase C, and phospholipase A_2, which in turn control a broad range of physiologic processes.

❖ Tyrosine kinase-dependent receptors are cell membrane receptors that upon the binding of a ligand (EGF, FGF, interleukin 2, etc.) dimerize to activate tyrosine kinase domains to regulate downstream signaling cascades that control inflammation, gastric secretion, and gene expression.

❖ Receptor channels, or receptor-operated channels, are cell membrane receptors that are also ion channels. Binding of a ligand (acetylcholine, glutamate, etc.) directly activates the channel (opening) without intermediary biochemical pathways or cascades, leading to a rapid response. Such channels are highly expressed at synapses and at the neuromuscular junction.

❖ Intracellular receptors, or nuclear receptors, are activated by the binding of a lipophilic hormone (ligand) that diffuses across the cell membranes. Once these receptors are activated, they bind to specific DNA sequences in the hormone-responsive element of a target gene to activate or repress DNA transcription, leading to inflammatory responses, proliferation, and differentiation.

REFERENCES

Goodman HM. Control of cell function. In: Johnson LR, ed. *Essential Medical Physiology*. 3rd ed. San Diego, CA: Elsevier Academic Press; 2003:Chap 2.

Roman LM. Signal transduction. In: Boron WF, Boulpaep EL, eds. *Medical Physiology*. Philadelphia, PA: Elsevier Science; 2003:Chap 4.

❖ CASE 3

A 6-year-old boy is brought to the family physician after his parents noticed that he had difficulty moving his arms and legs after a soccer game. About 10 minutes after leaving the field, the boy became so weak that he could not stand for about 30 minutes. Questioning revealed that he had complained of weakness after eating bananas, had frequent muscle spasms, and occasionally had myotonia, which was expressed as difficulty in releasing his grip or difficulty opening his eyes after squinting into the sun. After a thorough physical examination, the boy was diagnosed with hyperkalemic periodic paralysis. The family was advised to feed the boy carbohydrate-rich, low-potassium foods, give him glucose-containing drinks during attacks, and have him avoid strenuous exercise and fasting.

◆ **What is the effect of hyperkalemia on cell membrane potential?**

◆ **What is responsible for the repolarizing phase of an action potential?**

◆ **What is the effect of prolonged depolarization on the skeletal muscle Na^+ channel?**

ANSWERS TO CASE 3: ACTION POTENTIAL

Summary: A 6-year-old boy who experiences profound weakness after exercise is diagnosed with hyperkalemic periodic paralysis.

 Effect of hyperkalemia on membrane potential: Depolarization.

 Repolarization mechanisms: Activation of voltage-gated K^+ conductance and inactivation of Na^+ conductance.

 Effect of prolonged depolarization: Inactivation of Na^+ channels.

CLINICAL CORRELATION

Hyperkalemic periodic paralysis (HyperPP) is a dominant inherited trait caused by a mutation in the α subunit of the skeletal muscle Na^+ channel. It occurs in approximately 1 in 100,000 people and is more common and more severe in males. The onset of HyperPP generally occurs in the first or second decade of life. HyperPP is neither painful nor life-threatening but can be disruptive to normal activities. Symptoms are muscle weakness and paralysis, sometimes preceded by myotonia, fasciculations, or spasms. Fortunately, significant paralysis almost never occurs in intercostals or diaphragm muscles, and so breathing is not impaired. Attacks can occur spontaneously but often are triggered by exercise, stress, fasting, or the ingestion of large quantities of K^+ (eg, in bananas). For unknown reasons, exercise-induced paralysis always follows exercise—it does not occur during exercise. Because exercise can produce hyperkalemia and hyperkalemia triggers HyperPP attacks, there must be an additional mechanism that protects skeletal muscle during but not after intense activity. The mechanisms that underlie the effects of HyperPP result from several known mutations in the α subunit of the skeletal muscle Na^+ channel that prevent it from closing effectively. Ineffective closing results in a small, persistent inward current that continuously depolarizes the muscle membrane; this lowers the action potential threshold, producing the hyperexcitability that results in fasciculations (spontaneous twitches) and spasms under resting conditions. If the depolarization increases further, as occurs when extracellular $[K^+]$ is elevated, the Na^+ channels inactivate and remain inactivated until repolarization occurs. This inactivation blocks action potential initiation in the muscle and produces paralysis. When extracellular $[K^+]$ decreases, the depolarization is reduced, inactivation is removed, and the paralysis is relieved. Amelioration of HyperPP attacks is attempted by reducing plasma K^+ levels. Insulin promotes the transport of extracellular K^+ into intracellular compartments by activating the Na-K pump. Eating high-carbohydrate diets or pure glucose increases insulin secretion and thus decreases extracellular $[K^+]$. Conversely, fasting decreases insulin secretion and can elevate extracellular $[K^+]$, increasing the chances of myotonia and paralysis in HyperPP patients.

APPROACH TO ACTION POTENTIAL PHYSIOLOGY

Objectives

1. Know the mechanisms of the resting potential.
2. Understand the mechanisms of the action potential in axons and skeletal muscle.

Definitions

Action potential: A rapid, depolarizing change in membrane potential (often overshooting, so that the potential transiently reverses) that is used by excitable cells to convey all-or-none electrical signals quickly from one point on the cell to the remainder of the cell.

Electrotonic conduction: The passive, exponentially falling, spread of a difference in membrane potential between different membrane regions, which occurs with potentials subthreshold for an action potential or with perturbations of membrane potential in inexcitable membrane regions.

Nernst equilibrium potential: The membrane potential at which, for a given ion, there is no net flow of the ion across the membrane, which corresponds to the electrical force that exactly offsets the driving force of the concentration gradient acting on that ion.

Resting potential: The electrical potential difference across the plasma membrane in the absence of action potentials or synaptic potentials.

Voltage-gated channel: Pore-forming protein complexes that allow ions to flow across a membrane, and which can be opened (or, in some cases, closed) by a change in membrane potential.

DISCUSSION

The mechanisms that underlie the action potential cannot be understood without an understanding of how a **resting membrane potential** is generated. The resting potential in nearly all mammalian cells is produced primarily by **diffusion of K^+ down its concentration gradient from inside to outside the cell,** whereas the membrane remains relatively impermeable to other ions. The **intracellular concentration of K^+ is very high compared with the outside concentration** because K^+ **is pumped into the cell by the Na^+-K^+-ATPase (adenosine triphosphatase)** (see Figure 3-1). Because the membrane is effectively impermeable to intracellular anions, as K^+ **flows down its concentration gradient, it leaves behind anions.** A transmembrane potential (V_m) develops as the K^+ efflux brings a positive charge to the region just outside the membrane, leaving an equal amount of negative charge just inside the membrane. This process is self-limiting because as soon as a membrane becomes permeable to K^+ and K^+ efflux begins, the resulting separation of the charge generates an electrical driving force on the ions, and the electrical driving

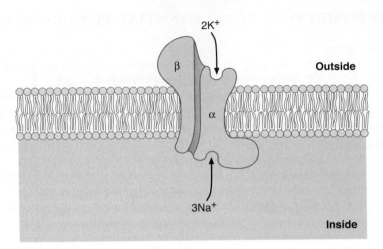

Figure 3-1. Na⁺-K⁺-ATPase pump. The α subunit is the catalytic subunit, which uses adenosine triphosphate (ATP) for energy to drive the extrusion of three Na⁺ ions for every two K⁺ ions taken into the cell. The β subunit is important for assembly and membrane targeting of the Na⁺-K⁺-ATPase. Pump activity can be blocked by cardiac glycosides, such as ouabain.

force soon equals the opposing chemical driving force (the K⁺ concentration gradient). For K⁺ or any ion X, this equilibrium occurs at a V_m called the **Nernst equilibrium potential,** which is defined as the electrical driving force (E_X) that exactly offsets the chemical driving force. The electrical driving force is represented by the left side and the chemical driving force is represented by the right side of the Nernst equation:

$$E_X = \frac{RT}{zF} \ln \frac{[X]_o}{[X]_i}$$

R is the gas constant, T is the temperature in degrees Kelvin, z is the valence of the ion, F is the Faraday constant, and $[X]_o$ and $[X]_i$ are the ion's extracellular and intracellular concentrations. In the case of K⁺ at 37°C and converting to $\log_{10}$, the equation becomes

$$E_k = 60 \log \frac{[K^+]_o}{[K^+]_i}$$

It is important to note that a given ion X is at equilibrium across the membrane only when $V_m = E_X$. Because of the relatively high intracellular concentrations of K^+ in mammalian cells, E_K **is always quite negative** (eg, ~ −90 mV). Because of the pumping action of the Na^+-K^+-ATPase, the concentration gradient for Na^+ is in the opposite direction (ie, $[Na^+]_o$ >> $[Na^+]_i$), and thus E_{Na} = ~ +55 mV. However, in cells, such as glia, in which there is no significant permeability to Na^+, Na^+ influx makes almost no contribution to V_m.

In most cells, including all excitable cells, $V_m \neq E_K$, although the values are often close. This is the case because the membrane is also permeable to other ions, and it is the net effect of all ion permeability across the membrane that determines V_m. In many axons, V_m is determined almost entirely by opposing fluxes (or, in electrical terms, currents) carried by K^+ and Na^+. These can be described, in terms of the ratio of permeabilities ($\alpha = P_{Na}/P_K$) and ionic concentrations, by the **Goldman-Hodgkin-Katz equation,** which is closely related to the Nernst equation:

$$V_m = 60 \log \frac{[K^+]_o + \alpha[Na^+]_o}{[K^+]_i + \alpha[Na^+]_o}$$

In an axon at rest, α = approximately 0.01, and so the contributions of the Na^+ concentrations in the expression are slight, and V_m is close to E_K (~ −90 mV). In many neuronal cell bodies or dendrites, P_{Na} is somewhat greater than this when the cell is at rest and V_m is more depolarized (eg, ~ −65 mV). Permeabilities (P) often are referred to by their electrical equivalents, conductances (g). Note that an increase in extracellular K^+, that is, **hyperkalemia, will depolarize cells, whereas hypokalemia will hyperpolarize cells.**

An all-or-none action potential is generated in an axon when membrane depolarization reaches a level at **which voltage-gated Na^+ channels open,** increasing P_{Na}. This results in an inward current of Na^+, which causes further depolarization, which then opens additional Na^+ channels. This regenerative (positive feedback) cycle quickly produces an overshooting action potential. In terms of the Goldman-Hodgkin-Katz equation, α quickly goes from approximately 0.01 to 100, V_m becomes dominated by the Na^+ concentration gradient, and thus V_m approaches E_{Na} at the peak of the action potential. Axonal action potentials last only a few milliseconds because two mechanisms rapidly **repolarize** the membrane. One is the activation of **voltage-gated K^+ channels** that open with a slight delay compared with the Na^+ channels, resulting in the delayed rectifier outward current carried by K^+ ions. Although this reduces α by increasing P_K, a second depolarization-triggered mechanism, **Na^+ channel inactivation,** reduces α by decreasing P_{Na}. Thus, depolarization initially opens Na^+ channels (activation) but then closes Na^+ channels (inactivation), and the channels remain closed until the membrane repolarizes to a level close to the normal resting potential. This means that prolonged depolarization produced for example, by hyperkalemia, can make excitable cells inexcitable.

The changes in permeability, expressed in terms of conductance (g), that underlie the action potential in axons are shown in Figure 3-2. The mechanisms

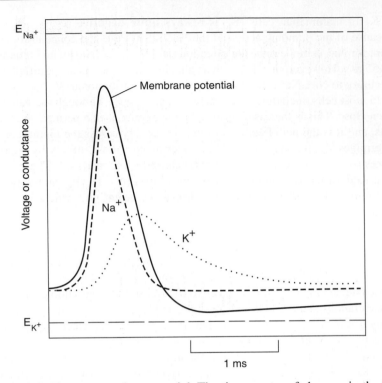

Figure 3-2. The nerve action potential. The time course of changes in the Na⁺ and K⁺ conductance is depicted.

for repolarizing the membrane after each action potential (which is critical for preventing summation of action potentials and permitting firing at high frequencies) are also responsible for the biphasic **refractory period** that follows each action potential. Inactivation of Na⁺ channels completely prevents action potential initiation, causing the **absolute refractory period.** After Na⁺ inactivation is removed by repolarization, the membrane remains less excitable than normal during the **relative refractory period,** during which the delayed rectifier K⁺ channels are transiently open.

The action potential **propagates** because the depolarization and overshoot in an active region (where voltage-gated Na⁺ channels are open) spread passively by **electrotonic conduction** to adjacent regions, depolarizing those regions and triggering the same regenerative sequence when the neighboring Na⁺ channels are opened by the electrotonically conducted depolarization. Electrotonic conduction occurs because the positive Na⁺ ions entering the cell in the active region are attracted to the net negative charge inside neighboring membrane that is hyperpolarized, and neighboring anions are attracted to the positive region inside the active membrane. The opposite current flow occurs outside the membrane. These intracellular and extracellular currents combine in a local circuit that quickly depolarizes membrane adjacent to an active region.

Current density underlying **electrotonic propagation** of depolarization (or hyperpolarization) **declines exponentially with distance.** The effectiveness of electrotonic propagation often is compared by using the space or length constant λ, which varies with the square root of the diameter of the axon. This means that electrotonic propagation of current in front of an active region projects farther in axons with larger diameters and therefore that **conduction of action potentials is faster in larger axons.** The velocity of action potential conduction also depends on how much time it takes for a region of membrane to depolarize. This is characterized by the time constant τ, which varies directly with membrane resistance R_m and membrane capacitance C_m. If R_m or C_m is large, the rate with which a region of membrane can depolarize (or hyperpolarize) is slow, and this reduces the velocity of action potential conduction. Mammals have increased action potential velocity by myelinating many axons, which in effect reduces C_m. The **most rapidly conducting axons are both myelinated and have large diameters** (ie, have small τ and large λ). Demyelinating diseases such as multiple sclerosis profoundly decrease conduction velocity and cause serious neurologic problems.

COMPREHENSION QUESTIONS

[3.1] The resting transmembrane potential (V_m) of a nerve axon is essential for signal generation. Instantaneous elimination of which of the following would most rapidly bring V_m close to 0 mV?

A. Active transport of K^+ out of the cell
B. Active transport of Na^+ out of the cell
C. Concentration gradient for Na^+
D. High membrane permeability to K^+
E. High membrane permeability to Na^+

[3.2] Hyperkalemia reduces the excitability of neurons and muscle cells. Which of the following best describes the effect of increased extracellular potassium $[K^+]_o$?

A. Depolarizes the cell, thus reducing action potential amplitude
B. Depolarizes the cell, thus inactivating voltage-gated Na^+ channels
C. Hyperpolarizes the cell, which increases the action potential threshold
D. Increases the activity of the Na-K-ATPase, which hyperpolarizes the cell
E. Stimulates endocytosis of Na^+ channels

[3.3] The velocity of action potential conduction is noted to be affected by various parameters. If the conduction velocity were found to be augmented, which of the following characteristics would most likely be decreased?

A. Action potential amplitude
B. Effective membrane capacitance
C. The concentration gradient for Na^+
D. The rate at which Na^+ channels open in response to depolarization
E. Na^+ channel density uniformly along a fiber

Answers

[3.1] **D.** The immediate cause of the resting potential is the high membrane permeability to K^+ compared with other ions; if this permeability were to be eliminated, V_m would instantly depolarize to within several mV of 0 mV. It would not quite reach 0 mV because of the electrogenic effect of the Na^+-K^+-ATPase (which pumps three Na^+ ions out for every two K^+ ions pumped in). The diffusion of K^+ down its concentration gradient in the absence of diffusion of anions out of the cell or diffusion of other cations into the cell causes a slight separation of charge across the membrane that generates most of the resting potential. The active transport of K^+ into the cell (not, as in answer A, out of the cell) is necessary for setting up the concentration gradient that results in the diffusion of K^+ out of the cell. This gradient (and therefore V_m) would take a long time to dissipate if active transport were stopped. Because the membrane is effectively impermeable to Na^+ at rest, the transport and concentration gradient for Na^+ has very little effect on the resting potential (answers B, C, and E).

[3.2] **B.** Sustained depolarization, as occurs with hyperkalemia, inactivates voltage-gated Na^+ channels, which remain inactivated until the membrane repolarizes, thus blocking action potential generation. If action potentials are generated, their amplitude will be reduced (answer A), but this is a consequence rather than a cause of reduced excitability. Hyperpolarization also can reduce excitability by increasing the depolarization needed to reach action potential threshold (answers C and D), but this would be produced by hypokalemia, not by hyperkalemia. There is no evidence that prolonged hyperkalemia decreases the number of Na^+ channels in the membrane (answer E).

[3.3] **B.** Effective membrane capacitance is decreased in many mammalian axons by myelination—the tight wrapping of many glial membranes around the axon, which is functionally equivalent to increasing the thickness of the membrane. Because conduction velocity is inversely related to membrane capacitance, which is related inversely to effective membrane thickness, a decrease in membrane capacitance increases conduction velocity. Decreasing action potential amplitude (answer A) will decrease rather than increase action potential velocity (see Case 8), as will decreasing the concentration gradient for Na^+ (because this will reduce action potential amplitude). In addition, decreases in the opening rate or density of Na^+ channels will decrease conduction velocity.

PHYSIOLOGY PEARLS

❖ The resting potential is generated by the high permeability of the membrane to K^+ compared with other ions, which allows a very small amount of K^+ to diffuse out of the cell in the absence of net diffusion of other ions, causing a charge separation across the membrane.

❖ The resting potential and action potential in simple excitable systems, such as axons, that are permeable only to K^+ and Na^+, can be described by the Goldman-Hodgkin-Katz equation, which states that V_m is determined by opposing currents carried by K^+ and Na^+, which are determined entirely by (1) the ratio of permeabilities to K^+ and Na^+ and (2) their concentration gradients across the cell membrane.

❖ An action potential is generated when membrane depolarization reaches a level at which voltage-gated Na^+ channels open, increasing P_{Na} (or, in electrical terms, g_{Na}), which results in an inward current of Na^+, which causes further depolarization, opening additional Na^+ channels in a positive feedback cycle.

❖ Inactivation of Na^+ channels during an action potential prevents subsequent action potential initiation during the brief absolute refractory period, whereas the relative refractory period continues shortly thereafter because the delayed rectifier K^+ channels remain open for a somewhat longer period.

❖ The spread of depolarization in front of an active region of membrane during an action potential occurs by electrotonic propagation, which is characterized by an exponential decay of the depolarization with distance along the fiber.

❖ The velocity of action potential conduction is increased by myelinating axons, which decreases their effective membrane capacitance, and by increasing the fiber diameter, which decreases the intracellular resistance.

REFERENCES

Byrne JH. Resting potentials and action potentials in excitable cells. In: Johnson LR, ed. *Essential Medical Physiology*. San Diego, CA: Elsevier Academic Press; 2003:71-96.

Moczydlowski EG. Electrical excitability and action potentials. In: Boron WF, Boulpaep EL. *Medical Physiology*. Philadelphia, PA: Elsevier Science; 2003:172-203.

A 32-year-old woman presents to her primary care physician's office with difficulty chewing food. She states that when she eats certain foods that require a significant amount of chewing (meat), her jaw muscles become weak and "tired." After a period of rest, her jaw muscles regain their strength until she eats again. The patient is diagnosed with myasthenia gravis and is started on neostigmine, an acetylcholinesterase (AChE) inhibitor.

◆ **What effect would an AChE inhibitor have at the neuromuscular junction?**

◆ **How would a large reduction in extracellular [Ca^{2+}] affect synaptic transmission at the neuromuscular junction?**

◆ **What is the ionic mechanism that underlies the endplate potential (EPP) produced by acetylcholine (ACh) release?**

ANSWERS TO CASE 4: SYNAPTIC POTENTIALS

Summary: A 32-year-old woman is diagnosed with myasthenia gravis and is being treated with neostigmine.

◆ **Effect of AChE inhibitor:** Blocks the degradation of ACh, causing an increase in the endplate potential, and prolongs the action of ACh at the motor endplate.

◆ **Effect of reducing $[Ca^{2+}]_o$:** Reduces Ca^{2+}-dependent exocytosis of ACh from vesicles in the presynaptic terminal.

◆ **Ionic mechanism of EPP:** ACh opens ligand-gated channels that are equally permeable to Na^+ and K^+. The net effect is depolarization that reaches action potential threshold in the muscle cell.

CLINICAL CORRELATION

Myasthenia gravis is a neuromuscular disease with classic symptoms of weakness and fatigue of skeletal muscles. Myasthenia gravis is seen more commonly in females, with peak incidence at 20 to 30 years of age. Men have a peak of incidence at around 50 to 60 years of age. The underlying pathophysiology is the development of antibodies to peripheral ACh receptors. The release of ACh remains normal, but because of the reduction in the number of receptors, the EPP is reduced and may fail to reach threshold for muscle action potentials. This is most likely to occur during repetitive firing and twitch summation because ACh release decreases during repetitive activity, and if the EPP is reduced to begin with, it will fall below the action potential threshold more rapidly. This reduces twitch summation, causing weakness and fatigue, and explains the classic symptoms of myasthenia gravis: muscle weakness that increases with repetitive muscle use (eg, chewing) and partially recovers with rest. Treatment with AChE inhibitors decreases the degradation of ACh, thus enhancing and prolonging each EPP, increasing twitch summation and reducing weakness.

APPROACH TO SYNAPTIC POTENTIALS

Objectives

1. Understand the physiology of the neuromuscular junction.
2. Understand the synaptic physiology within the nervous system.

Definitions

Endplate potential (EPP): The excitatory postsynaptic potential (EPSP) at the neuromuscular junction caused by the opening by ACh of nicotinic ACh receptors in the muscle endplate.

Inhibitory synapses: Synapses in which neurotransmitter release produces an inhibitory postsynaptic potential (IPSP) that reduces the ability of the postsynaptic cell to fire action potentials.

Ionotropic receptor: A receptor that is also an ion channel and therefore produces a change in membrane potential when binding of a neurotransmitter opens (or, in some cases, closes) the channel.

Metabotropic receptor: A receptor that is linked by signal transduction pathways to potentially diverse cellular responses, including effects on ion channels (not directly linked to the receptor), neurotransmitter release, and gene transcription.

DISCUSSION

The **neuromuscular junction** is the synapse between a **motor neuron** and a **skeletal muscle cell.** Although it shares basic functions with other chemical synapses, the neuromuscular junction has unique features that ensure that each **EPP is large** enough to exceed the action potential threshold in the muscle cell. At the **endplate,** the **motor neuron** axon arborizes into **numerous terminal boutons** that contain **large numbers of ACh-filled vesicles.** ACh is synthesized in the boutons from choline and acetyl-coenzyme A by choline acetyltransferase. ACh then is pumped into the vesicles by a specific ACh-H^+ exchanger. The boutons lie over junctional folds in the postsynaptic membrane that contain nicotinic ACh receptors closely apposed to presynaptic active zones. The basal lamina between the presynaptic and postsynaptic membranes contains a high concentration of the degradative enzyme **AChE.**

Synaptic transmission begins when an action potential propagates from the main axon into the endplate. Consequent **depolarization** of the bouton opens **voltage-gated Ca^{2+} channels,** producing an **influx of Ca^{2+}** that then **binds to specific proteins that cause fusion of vesicles with the plasma membrane and exocytosis of ACh.** The ACh diffuses across the synaptic cleft. Binding of ACh to nicotinic ACh receptors on the junctional folds causes the ligand-gated channels to open in an **all-or-none** fashion. The channels are equally permeable to Na^+, **which flows into the cell,** and to K^+, **which flows out of the cell.** The combined Na^+ and K^+ current depolarizes the muscle cell from its resting potential (~ -80 mV) to the threshold for the action potential (~ -50 mV), with the resulting action potential propagating across the entire muscle cell. Because both Na^+ (which has a very positive equilibrium potential, E_{Na}) and K^+ (which has a very negative equilibrium potential, E_K) flow through the ACh-gated channels at the endplate, the **reversal potential** (defined as the potential where the sum of the inward Na^+ and outward K^+ current through the open channels is 0) is close to 0 mV, which is approximately halfway between E_{Na} and E_K. If resting membrane potential is more negative than the reversal potential, ACh produces a **depolarizing** change in membrane potential, becoming less negative. If resting membrane potential is more positive than the reversal potential, ACh produces a **hyperpolarizing** change in membrane potential, becoming more negative. The **nicotinic ACh receptor is an ionotropic receptor:** a receptor protein that is itself an ion channel. Postsynaptic potentials mediated by a ligand, such as ACh, binding to an inotropic receptor have very brief durations (tens of milliseconds). The duration of the EPP is limited by rapid hydrolysis of ACh by AChE and by diffusion of ACh away from the active zones. At other synapses, such as those utilizing glutamate, dopamine, norepinephrine (NE), serotonin, γ-aminobutyric acid (GABA), or glycine as a neurotransmitter, active reuptake by high-affinity systems involving Na^+ cotransport is also important for removing the neurotransmitter rapidly.

Chemical transmission at other synapses also involves Ca^{2+}-**dependent exocytosis** of neurotransmitters but can differ in the neurotransmitter released, the receptors bound by the neurotransmitter, the ions involved in mediating the postsynaptic response, and whether metabolic responses are involved. Within the **central nervous system (CNS),** excitatory synapses often utilize **glutamate** as a neurotransmitter, and this opens channels like those in the neuromuscular junction that are permeable to both Na^+ and K^+. The reversal potential of these synapses is also close to 0 mV. However, individual excitatory postsynaptic potentials (EPSPs) at central synapses are much smaller than the EPP (<1 mV vs. >40 mV) because each action potential releases only one or a few vesicles rather than the 100 or so vesicles released at the endplate. Activation of neurons depends on **temporal summation** of many small EPSPs arriving at a high frequency from the same presynaptic neuron and on **spatial summation** of small EPSPs arriving simultaneously from many presynaptic neurons. In contrast, only a single presynaptic neuron synapses with each muscle cell, every EPP reaches action potential threshold (producing a twitch), and temporal summation of EPPs does not occur (instead, temporal summation of twitches is important).

The **nervous system** has numerous **inhibitory** synapses, most of which utilize **GABA** or **glycine** as a neurotransmitter. Inhibitory ligand-gated channels often are **selectively permeable to Cl^-,** which usually has an equilibrium potential slightly negative to the resting potential of the neuron. Opening Cl^- channels at inhibitory synapses produces an inhibitory postsynaptic potential (IPSP) that opposes the depolarizing effects of simultaneously released excitatory neurotransmitters. The nervous system also has **modulatory synapses** in which a neurotransmitter such as **glutamate, ACh, dopamine, NE, serotonin, or a neuropeptide** binds to metabotropic receptors that can be coupled by G proteins to enzymes, such as adenylyl cyclase or phospholipase C, that activate cell signaling cascades, which then may alter neuronal function in various ways for periods that can range from seconds to weeks or longer and may contribute to the formation and storage of memories.

COMPREHENSION QUESTIONS

[4.1]   Which of the following enzymes catalyzes the synthesis of ACh?

   A. Acetyl-coenzyme A
   B. Acetylcholinesterase (AChE)
   C. Acetylcholine-H$^+$ (ACh-H$^+$) exchanger
   D. Amino acid decarboxylase
   E. Choline acetyltransferase

[4.2]   Which of the following is the most common action of γ-aminobutyric acid (GABA):

   A. Opening channels permeable to Cl$^-$
   B. Opening channels permeable to Ca^{2+}
   C. Opening channels permeable to Na$^+$ and K$^+$
   D. Closing channels permeable to Na$^+$
   E. Closing channels permeable to Cl$^-$ and K$^+$

[4.3]   Which of the following statements distinguishes excitatory chemical synapses in the brain from the neuromuscular junction?

   A. Excitation is produced by ligand-gated channels.
   B. Ligand-gated channels increase permeability to both Na$^+$ and K$^+$.
   C. Postsynaptic action potentials are triggered when a sufficient number of voltage-gated Na$^+$ channels are opened by an EPP or by summating EPSPs.
   D. Temporal summation and spatial summation onto the postsynaptic cell increase the likelihood that a postsynaptic action potential will be evoked.
   E. The synaptic reversal potential is close to 0 mV.

Answers

[4.1]   **E.** Choline acetyltransferase synthesizes ACh from choline and acetyl-coenzyme A. The ACh is transported into the vesicle by the ACh-H$^+$ exchanger, and after release it is hydrolyzed by AChE to acetate and choline.

[4.2]   **A.** GABA and glycine are the most important inhibitory neurotransmitters and produce their most common inhibitory effects by opening Cl$^-$ channels and producing a current that often causes a slight hyperpolarization and always tends to clamp the neuron close to its resting potential.

[4.3]   **D.** In contrast to other neuronal synapses, the individual EPSPs (or EPPs) at the neuromuscular junction are normally much larger than is required to evoke an action potential, and so temporal summation does not increase the probability of firing (although high-frequency firing of the motor neuron does lead to summation of twitches and to tetanization). All other features listed are shared by the neuromuscular junction and excitatory chemical synapses in the brain.

PHYSIOLOGY PEARLS

❖ Chemical synaptic transmission begins when an action potential depolarizes a presynaptic terminal sufficiently to open voltage-gated Ca^{2+} channels and thus trigger Ca^{2+}-dependent exocytosis of neurotransmitter.

❖ ACh at the neuromuscular junction and glutamate at central excitatory synapses bind to receptors on ligand-gated channels that are equally permeable to Na^+ and K^+.

❖ The duration of brief postsynaptic potentials mediated by ionotropic receptors is limited by **enzymatic degradation** of neurotransmitter, its **diffusion** away from the active zones and its **active transport** into the terminal and nearby cells.

❖ An individual EPP at the neuromuscular junction is very large (>40 mV) and reliably reaches the action potential threshold. Temporal and spatial summation is unnecessary and does not occur at the neuromuscular junction.

❖ In myasthenia gravis, the EPP is reduced by an autoimmune response to the ACh receptor and often fails to reach threshold during repetitive firing.

❖ Individual EPSPs in the CNS are very small (<1 mV) and require the summation of many separate EPSPs (temporal and/or spatial summation) to reach the action potential threshold.

❖ Inhibitory synapses utilize GABA or glycine and often open ligand-gated channels that are selective for Cl^-, which usually has an equilibrium potential that is slightly more hyperpolarized than is the resting potential. Opening these channels opposes the depolarizing effects of excitatory synapses that are active at the same time.

❖ In many modulatory synapses, neurotransmitter binds to metabotropic receptors that are coupled via G proteins to cell-signaling cascades, which can produce neuronal alterations ranging in duration from tens of seconds to weeks or longer.

REFERENCES

Byrne JH. Neuromuscular and synaptic transmission. In: Johnson LR, ed. *Essential Medical Physiology*. 3rd ed. San Diego, CA: Elsevier Academic Press; 2003: 97-122.

Moczydlowski, EG. Synaptic transmission and the neuromuscular junction. In: Boron WF, Boulpaep EL, eds. *Medical Physiology*. Philadelphia, PA: Elsevier Science; 2003: 204-229.

Moczydlowski, EG. Synaptic transmission in the nervous system. Ibid pp. 295-324.

❖ CASE 5

A 12-year-old girl is brought to the emergency room with difficulty in breathing. On examination she is found to have dyspnea with audible wheezes and is diagnosed with asthma. The patient is given an inhaled medication (albuterol), which provides immediate relief of the bronchial constrictive symptoms.

 What autonomic nervous system (ANS) receptor does this medication target?

 What is the mechanism of action when these receptors are stimulated?

◆ **What neurotransmitter normally activates these receptors?**

ANSWERS TO CASE 5: AUTONOMIC NERVOUS SYSTEM

Summary: A 12-year-old girl with an acute asthma exacerbation is given albuterol, a β-agonist sympathomimetic agent.

◆ **ANS receptor target:** β_2 receptors.

◆ **Mechanism of action:** Activation of adenylyl cyclase, increase in cyclic adenosine monophosphate (cAMP), and relaxation of bronchial smooth muscle, leading to bronchodilation.

◆ **Neurotransmitter:** Norepinephrine (NE).

CLINICAL CORRELATION

A good understanding of the autonomic nervous system is imperative in treating many medical conditions, such as asthma. Different cells throughout the body have different ANS receptors with differing agonist and antagonist properties, and medications targeting specific receptors can selectively relieve symptoms in particular organs while minimizing side effects that would be mediated by other receptors. The sympathetic β_2 receptor agonist albuterol selectively produces bronchial dilation and thus provides relief from bronchial constrictive disorders such as asthma. However, with some receptors it is not possible to achieve selective targeting because the same receptor is found in diverse organs, and many commonly used drugs act on more than one receptor. For example, propranolol, which is used to treat various cardiac and cardiovascular problems, blocks both β_1 and β_2 receptors. It would be contraindicated in patients with asthma because by blocking β_2 receptors, it would cause bronchial constriction and worsening of a patient's asthma. Many medications have side effects involving the ANS, but these effects can be predicted if one knows the distributions of different autonomic receptors in the body.

APPROACH TO AUTONOMIC NERVOUS SYSTEM

Objectives

1. Know the organization of the autonomic nervous system (ANS).
2. List the major neurotransmitters of the ANS.
3. Know the receptor types in the ANS.

Definitions

Parasympathetic nervous system: Division of the autonomic nervous system associated with resting visceral functions (e.g., digestion), defined anatomically by efferent preganglionic axons exiting the CNS via cranial nerves and sacral spinal nerves S_2 to S_4.

Sympathetic nervous system: Division of the autonomic nervous system associated with physiological responses to stress, defined anatomically by efferent preganglionic axons exiting the CNS via thoracic and lumbar spinal nerves T_1 to L_3.

Enteric nervous system: Division of the autonomic nervous system associated with direct control of gastrointestinal functions, defined anatomically by embedment within the gastrointestinal tract.

DISCUSSION

Bronchial smooth muscle, like most smooth muscle, cardiac muscle, and glands, is innervated by the ANS. The ANS mediates important homeostatic and emergency functions in a largely involuntary manner. It has **three major divisions:** the **sympathetic, parasympathetic,** and **enteric** nervous systems. The sympathetic and parasympathetic divisions have efferent (output) systems that evoke or modulate contractile, secretory, and metabolic responses throughout the body. The enteric division is a relatively independent nervous system embedded in the gastrointestinal (GI) tract and contains sensory neurons, interneurons, and motor neurons. Although the enteric system can function autonomously, its activity usually is modulated by the sympathetic and parasympathetic systems. The ANS also has central integrative components in the hypothalamus and brainstem autonomic nuclei that receive input from visceral and somatic afferents as well as from more rostral brain regions.

In the **sympathetic and parasympathetic systems,** the **final efferent pathway** consists of **central preganglionic neurons,** which synapse onto peripheral postganglionic neurons, which then synapse onto effector cells in target organs. In the **sympathetic** system, the preganglionic cell bodies are in the intermediolateral column of the spinal cord between levels T_1 and L_3 **(thoracolumbar).** The postganglionic cell bodies are in either the nearby paravertebral ganglia or the more distant prevertebral ganglia. Each preganglionic sympathetic fiber synapses with many postganglionic neurons across several ganglia, often producing widespread effects. Sympathetic postganglionic neurons usually send very long axons to effector targets. In the **parasympathetic** system, the preganglionic cell bodies reside in **nuclei of the medulla, pons, midbrain, and spinal segments S_2 through S_4 (craniosacral)** and send long axons to synapse with relatively few postganglionic neurons in terminal ganglia, which are close to or embedded in the walls of their target organs. **Sympathetic and parasympathetic systems usually have opposite effects** on visceral targets. Massive activation of the sympathetic system enhances the capacity for immediate physical activity (eg, exercise and **fight or flight** responses) and enables adaptive responses to physiologic emergencies such as hemorrhage, whereas more localized activation mediates discrete homeostatic reflexes. Parasympathetic activity enhances the functions of organs active during quiescent states (**rest and digest** functions) and often mediates actions opposite to those of the sympathetic system in homeostatic reflexes (eg, baroreceptor reflex, pupillary reflex).

All **preganglionic** fibers (sympathetic and parasympathetic) release **acetylcholine** (ACh) at synapses in autonomic ganglia; the ACh binds to nicotinic receptors and excites postganglionic neurons. Nearly all sympathetic postganglionic neurons release NE onto effector targets. The major exceptions are the

Table 5-1
ACTIONS MEDIATED BY AUTONOMIC RECEPTORS IN SELECTED EFFECTOR SYSTEMS*

| EFFECTOR | SYMPATHETIC ACTIVITY | | PARASYMPATHETIC ACTIVITY | |
	ACTION	RECEPTOR	ACTION	RECEPTOR

Heart
  Sinoatrial node
  Contractility
	Tachycardia
	Increase
		β_1, β_2
		β_1, β_2
			Bradycardia
			Decrease
			(atria)
				M
				M

Blood vessels
  Skin, viscera
  Skeletal muscle
	Constriction
	Dilation
		α_1, α_2
		β_2		

Sweat glands	Secretion, general Secretion, palms	M α_1		
Bronchial muscle	Relaxation	β_2	Contraction	M

Eye
  Radial muscle, iris
  Sphincter, iris
	Contraction	α_1	Contraction	M

Gastrointestinal tract
  Motility
  Secretion
	Decrease
	Decrease
		α_2, β_2
		β_2
			Increase
			Increase
				M
				M

Urinary bladder
  Detrusor
  Trigone, sphincter
	Relaxation
	Contraction
		β_2
		α_1
			Contraction
			Relaxation
				M
				M

Male sex organs	Ejaculation	α_1	Erection	M

*For a more complete list see Katzung (2004).

sympathetic fibers innervating most sweat glands, which release ACh (binding to muscarinic receptors), and the cells in the adrenal medulla, which are homologous with sympathetic postganglionic neurons but release epinephrine and some NE into the bloodstream. The major classes of receptors for NE and epinephrine are α_1 (important in blood vessels), α_2 (often on presynaptic terminals of sympathetic postganglionic axons), β_1 (important in the heart), and β_2 (concentrated in bronchial smooth muscle). All parasympathetic postganglionic neurons release ACh, which binds to muscarinic receptors on effector cells. Autonomic effects are often modulatory and are mediated by second messengers. Both muscarinic receptors and adrenergic receptors are metabotropic receptors that often are linked positively or negatively by **G proteins** to **adenylyl cyclase or phospholipase C,** which alter cAMP or Ca^{2+} levels in target cells. Table 5-1 lists some of the important autonomic effectors and the physiologic actions of each type of autonomic receptor found in them.

COMPREHENSION QUESTIONS

[5.1]   Which of the following is promoted by parasympathetic activity?

    A. Airway constriction
    B. Ejaculation
    C. Pupillary dilation
    D. Vasoconstrictor response to hemorrhage
    E. Secretion of sweat

[5.2]   Which type of receptor located on sinoatrial (SA) nodal cells mediate an increase in heart rate?

    A. α
    B. β
    C. Muscarinic
    D. Nicotinic

[5.3]   Which of following fibers release NE?

    A. Preganglionic fibers innervating the adrenal medulla
    B. Postganglionic fibers causing bradycardia
    C. Postganglionic fibers causing constriction of the iris
    D. Postganglionic fibers causing arteriolar constriction
    E. Sympathetic fibers innervating eccrine sweat glands

Answers

[5.1]   **A.** Parasympathetic fibers release ACh onto muscarinic receptors that cause contraction of bronchiolar smooth muscle. All the other listed effects are produced by sympathetic activation.

[5.2]   **B.** Sympathetic fibers release NE onto β_1 and β_2 receptors, which activate adenylyl cyclase, increasing the currents that generate the pacemaker potential. The other listed receptors are not present in the SA node or decrease heart rate (muscarinic receptors).

[5.3]　**D.** Sympathetic fibers release NE onto α_1 receptors in arterioles, which constrict these resistance vessels. The other listed fibers all release ACh, including sympathetic fibers that innervate eccrine sweat glands.

PHYSIOLOGY PEARLS

❖　The sympathetic and parasympathetic nervous systems are neural systems controlled by integrative regions in the brain, whereas the enteric nervous system has afferent, integrative, and efferent components that allow it to function autonomously (the term *autonomic* comes from Greek words meaning "self-governing").

❖　Massive activation of the sympathetic nervous system is vital for preparing for and responding to physiologic emergencies such as fight or flight situations and hemorrhage.

❖　Activation of more restricted parts of the sympathetic nervous system mediates discrete autonomic reflexes such as the baroreceptor reflex and ejaculation.

❖　The parasympathetic nervous system exerts more localized control over visceral functions such as digestion, micturition, and many sexual responses.

❖　ACh is released by all preganglionic fibers (sympathetic or parasympathetic) and binds to ganglionic nicotinic receptors that rapidly depolarize postganglionic cells.

❖　ACh is released by parasympathetic postganglionic fibers and binds to muscarinic receptors on effector cells, which often are coupled through G proteins to phospholipase C (positively) or adenylyl cyclase (negatively).

❖　NE usually is released by sympathetic postganglionic fibers and can bind to β_1 or β_2 receptors which are positively coupled to adenylyl cyclase. NE also can bind to α_1 receptors, which are coupled to phospholipase C, or to α_2 receptors, which are negatively coupled to adenylyl cyclase.

REFERENCES

Katzung BG. Introduction to autonomic pharmacology. In: Katzung BG. *Basic and Clinical Pharmacology*. New York: McGraw-Hill; 2004: 75-92.

Richerson GB. The autonomic nervous system. In: Boron WF, Boulpaep EL. *Medical Physiology*. Philadelphia, PA: Elsevier Science; 2003: 378-398.

Weisbrodt NW. Autonomic nervous system. In: Johnson LR. *Essential Medical Physiology*. San Diego, CA: Elsevier Academic Press; 2003: 145-154.

❖ CASE 6

A 21-year-old man presents to a rural emergency center with a 1-day history of progressive stiffness of the neck and jaw, difficulty swallowing, stiff shoulders and back, and a rigid abdomen. Upon further questioning, the patient reports that the stiff jaw was the first symptom, followed by the stiff neck and dysphagia. On examination he is noted to have stiffness in the neck, shoulder, and arm muscles. He has a grimace on his face that he cannot stop voluntarily and an arched back from contracted back muscles. The physician concludes that the patient has "tetanic" skeletal muscle contractions. A 3-cm laceration is noted on his left foot. The patient reports sustaining the laceration about 7 days ago while he was plowing the fields on his farm. He has not had a tetanus booster. He is diagnosed with a tetanus infection, and an injection of the tetanus antitoxin is given.

◆ **On which skeletal muscle filament is troponin located?**

◆ **What is the function of the sarcoplasmic reticulum (SR)?**

◆ **What is the molecular basis for initiation of contraction in skeletal muscle?**

ANSWERS TO CASE 6: SKELETAL MUSCLE

Summary: A 21-year-old man with acute tetanus presents with muscle rigidity in the face, jaw, shoulders, back, and upper extremities 7 days after sustaining a puncture wound while working on his farm. He is diagnosed with tetanus.

◆ **Troponin location:** Thin filaments

◆ **Sarcoplasmic reticulum function:** Storage and release of calcium

◆ **Molecular basis of contraction:** Calcium-troponin-C binding

CLINICAL CORRELATION

Tetanus is a neurologic disorder caused by the toxin produced in the bacterium *Clostridium tetani. Clostridium tetani* is an anaerobic gram-positive motile rod that is found worldwide in soil, inanimate environments, animal feces, and occasionally human feces. Contamination in wounds with spores of *C. tetani* is seen commonly, but germination and toxin production occur only in devitalized tissue, areas with foreign bodies, and active infection. The toxin that is released blocks the release of several inhibitory neurotransmitters, including γ-aminobutyric acid (GABA), altering the synaptic vesicle release apparatus. With diminished inhibition, the resting firing rate of motor neurons increases. Because of the increased repetitive stimulation of the motor neuron, the calcium released from the SR remains bound to troponin and extends the time for cross-bridge cycling, resulting in muscles that do not relax. Symptoms of tetanus often begin in facial muscles such as those in the jaw ("lockjaw") and then progress down the neck, shoulder, back, and upper and lower extremities. Generalized spasms may jeopardize breathing. Antitoxin is administered to bind and neutralize circulating and unbound toxin. Wounds should be explored, cleaned, and debrided. Muscle spasm can be controlled with medications such as diazepam (GABA agonist). Protection of the airway is essential.

APPROACH TO MUSCLE PHYSIOLOGY

Objectives

1. Describe striated muscle structure and arrangement.
2. List the steps in excitation–contraction.
3. Understand force–velocity relationships.
4. Describe summation and tetanus.
5. Describe motor unit recruitment.

Definitions

Sarcomere: The basic contractile unit comprising striated muscle.
Excitation–contraction (E–C) coupling: The events that describe the calcium movements within the muscle fiber.

DISCUSSION

All muscle cells can be divided into two groups—**striated and smooth**—on the basis of their microscopic structure. **Striated muscle** can be subclassified on the basis of location into three subgroups: **skeletal, cardiac, and visceral.** In addition, **skeletal muscle** can be classified on the basis of contractile behavior as **fast-twitch or slow-twitch** and on the basis of biochemical activities as oxidative or glycolytic.

Actin and myosin are proteins that form the basic structural characteristic of striated muscle and are arranged in **filaments: actin in thin filaments** and **myosin in thick filaments** (see Figure 6-1). In the **thin** filaments, the **monomers of actin** are **polymerized** together like **two strands of pearls** that are twisted in an α helix to form **F-actin (filamentous).** In the thick filaments, **complex myosin molecules** are arranged so that most of their filamentous tails intertwine to form the backbone of the thick filaments and parts of

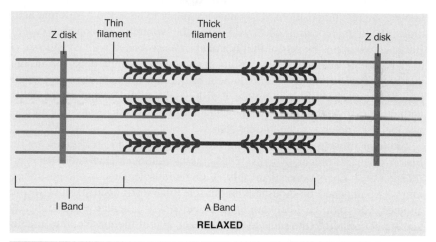

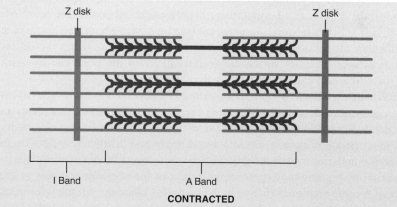

Figure 6-1. Relationships of thick and thin filaments and adjacent Z disks of a sarcomere in a relaxed and a contracted state.

their tails and their globular heads protrude from the backbone to form structures called **cross-bridges.**

These thick and thin filaments are very ordered in their anatomic arrangement within the striated muscle cell. Thin filaments extend in opposite directions from protein structures called **Z disks.** In relaxed muscle, the thin filaments from two opposing Z disks extend toward each other but do not touch or overlap. Bridging the gap between the thin filaments, and overlapping with them, are the thick filaments. This arrangement—Z disk, thin filament, thick filament, thin filament, Z disk—defines the functional unit called a sarcomere. In striated muscle, sarcomeres are arranged in transverse registry, accounting for the characteristic banding pattern or striations.

Arrangement of the contractile proteins in **sarcomeres** gives striated muscle cells the ability to shorten. When striated muscles contract, cross-bridges from the thick filaments attach to specific regions on the actin molecules. The cross-bridge heads then change angles, causing the thick and the thin filaments to slide over one another. The **cross-bridges** then release, and their angles assume the resting positions. They now are ready to attach to a different actin molecule, thus repeating the cycle until the stimulus to contract ceases. Because two opposing sets of thin filaments are associated with a single set of thick filaments, filament sliding results in movement of the Z disks toward one another without either the thick filament or the thin filament changing length (see Figure 6-1). Also, because the Z disks and the thin filaments are linked with other cytoskeletal elements, movement of the Z disks toward one another results in shortening of the muscle cell.

Skeletal muscle cells are among the largest cells and are formed by the fusion of many precursor cells. Thus, these multinucleated cells often are referred to as fibers rather than cells. A single muscle, such as the gastrocnemius, is composed of thousands of muscle fibers arranged parallel to one another. Although the fibers are bound together by connective tissue sheaths and are connected to the same tendons at each end of the muscle, they are not coupled electrically to one another. Thus, any muscle fiber can contract independently of its neighboring fibers. The tendons of a skeletal muscle are attached to bones in such a way that contractions bring about movement or stabilization of the skeleton. Attachment to the bone that is being moved most often is near the joint so that large movements of the bone can be accomplished by small changes in the length of the muscle.

Whether a muscle is contracting or relaxed depends on the level of **cytosolic calcium** available to interact with a regulatory protein complex, **troponin,** which is located on the **thin filament with actin.** In relaxed muscle, the level of free cytosolic calcium (calcium that is not bound to other structures) is low. Upon stimulation of the muscle, free calcium levels increase to initiate contraction by binding directly to a component of the troponin complex to bring about a conformational change in the complex. Once the stimulus for muscle contraction ceases, free calcium levels decrease and calcium dissociates from the regulatory proteins. The muscle then relaxes. Because calcium is the mediator between the events in the cell membrane that indicate excitation and the protein interactions that result in contraction, the events that describe calcium movements in muscle cells often are referred to as **excitation–contraction (E–C) coupling.**

The calcium that normally takes part in E–C coupling in skeletal muscle is stored inside the cell in the **SR.** The SR is highly developed and extensive in skeletal muscle and functionally serves as a storage place for calcium during muscle relaxation. Upon muscle excitation, calcium moves out of the SR and into the cytoplasm down a large concentration gradient. Once in the cytoplasm, calcium interacts with the tropomyosin-troponin complex to allow full activation of the contractile proteins. Calcium then is taken up by the SR by an active process that involves a calcium (adenosine triphosphatase) ATPase. This "pump" has a high affinity for calcium and can lower cytosolic calcium quickly to levels that do not support contraction.

Calcium is released by the SR in response to excitation of the cell membrane (sarcolemma). Each skeletal muscle fiber is innervated by a motor nerve. These nerves release **acetylcholine (ACh) at their junctions** with the muscle cell (neuromuscular junction). The ACh induces an **increase in permeability of that portion of the cell membrane to Na$^+$ and K$^+$.** This results in **depolarization** of adjacent areas of the membrane to threshold, at which point an action potential ensues.

When a muscle contracts, it develops force and usually shortens. A contraction that generates **only force, with no muscle shortening,** is called an **isometric** contraction. One that results in shortening against a constant force is called an **isotonic** contraction. Contractions of skeletal muscles are graded in force and in duration through activity of the central nervous system. Each skeletal muscle is innervated by a somatic nerve that is comprised of many axons of α-**motor neurons.** Each of these axons branches to innervate a number of fibers in the muscle. An α-**motor neuron and the muscle fibers** it innervates are called a **motor unit.** The force generated by a whole muscle depends on the number of its motor units that are active at any one time because the muscle fibers are arranged in parallel and parallel forces are additive. Thus, the central nervous system can regulate contraction force by regulating the **number of motor units activated** at any one time; this is called **recruitment. Muscle force** also can be regulated by the **frequency** at which the motor units are activated. A **single activation** to produce a single action potential of a muscle fiber will elicit a **small contraction** called a **twitch.** If the frequency of activation is increased, contraction duration and force increase up to a maximum. This process is called **summation and tetanus.** Force increases because, before the muscle relaxes from the previous excitation, the contractile proteins are activated again and again to add to the force. During summation and tetanus, each excitation releases calcium. The maximum calcium level is no higher than it is with a single isolated action potential, but it is maintained for a longer time. The continued elevation of calcium allows for continual activation of the contractile proteins, and the full force of cross-bridge cycling can be realized at the ends of the muscle.

If a muscle contracts isotonically, it will shorten, and the velocity of shortening will depend on the load being moved (often called the **afterload**).

By using different afterloads, which really are equal to the forces that the muscle must develop in order to shorten, a force–velocity relationship can be determined for a specific muscle. If the muscle is lifting **no afterload, the maximal velocity (V_{max}) is obtained.** With increasing afterload, velocity decreases until an afterload is reached against which the muscle cannot shorten. Now the muscle is contracting isometrically. Skeletal muscles differ from one another in their force–velocity relationships. Some, such as the extensor digitorum longus, contract more quickly than do others, such as the soleus. This difference is because of variations in the number and types of muscle fibers that make up the various muscles in the body. Although there is a spectrum of velocities among various muscle fibers, they have been divided into two main groups: **fast-twitch and slow-twitch. Fast-twitch** muscle fibers generally are found in muscles associated with **rapid movement; slow-twitch fibers** are found in muscles associated more with **endurance and posture.** Many muscles are composed of a mixture of fast- and slow-twitch fibers. Fast- and slow-twitch muscle fibers differ in the contractile protein isoforms that are present and in the ATPase activities of the myosin isoforms.

COMPREHENSION QUESTIONS

[6.1]   A researcher was examining some arrows sent from South America. He accidentally pierced his hand with one of the arrows. After a while he started to notice muscle weakness. He went to the hospital immediately. Electrical recordings from nerves innervating muscles in his arm indicated normal frequencies and amplitudes of impulses when stimulated; however, nerve-induced contractions of the muscles were weak. When the muscles were stimulated directly, normal contractions occurred. Which of the following is the most likely reason for the muscle weakness?

A. Decreased ability of ACh to stimulate the muscle fibers
B. Decreased ability of calcium to bind to troponin in the muscle fibers
C. Decreased ability of the muscle to produce adenosine triphosphatase (ATP)
D. Decreased ability of the muscle to undergo summation and tetanus
E. Depletion of intracellular calcium

[6.2]   If a person lifts weights routinely, the muscles involved in the lifting undergo hypertrophy and become capable of generating greater force. Which of the following is the best explanation for the basis for these adaptations?

A. Increased length of the muscle fibers
B. Increased maximal velocity (V_{max}) of contraction
C. Increased number of fast-twitch fibers in the muscle
D. Increased number of sarcomeres arranged in parallel
E. Greater specific activity of the myosin ATPase

[6.3]   While you are standing, holding a tray piled with dishes, an additional
        5 lb of dishes is placed on your tray. Your muscles that are holding the
        dishes increase their force of contraction through an increase in which
        of the following?

   A. Length of the muscle
   B. Number of motor units activated and the frequency of their activation
   C. Peak intracellular calcium concentration in the muscle
   D. Strength of each individual cross-bridge interaction with actin
   E. V_{max} of the muscles

Answers

[6.1]   **A.** Because the muscle responded normally to direct stimulation, the
        defect was not in the muscle itself. Therefore, the weakness was not
        because of decreased ability of calcium to bind to troponin in the mus-
        cle fibers, depletion of intracellular calcium, decreased ability of the
        muscle to undergo summation and tetanus, or decreased ability of the
        muscle to produce ATP. The lack of response also could not be because
        of a failure of action potentials in the motor nerves. Thus, the most
        likely explanation is a defect at the neuromuscular junction caused by
        a decreased ability of ACh to stimulate the muscle fibers. Curare,
        which is used by the inhabitants of South America as an arrow poison,
        is a drug that binds to ACh receptors, blocking access by ACh, and thus
        decreases the activation of skeletal muscles by motor nerves.

[6.2]   **D.** When a skeletal muscle undergoes hypertrophy, this is due mainly to
        an increase in the number of sarcomeres in existing muscle fibers and
        perhaps also to an increase in muscle fibers. Either way, the increased
        contractile units are added in parallel to existing units. This increases
        the force with which the muscle can contract. The length of the muscle,
        which is limited by its origin and insertion, will not change. The sar-
        comeres being added will be similar to the ones already present or more
        likely will have lower ATPase activity. Thus, there will not be increases
        in the maximal myosin ATPase activity, the maximal velocity of con-
        traction, or the number of fast-twitch fibers in the muscle.

[6.3]   **B.** The increase in the force of contraction of skeletal muscle is regu-
        lated by the number of motor units recruited by the central nervous sys-
        tem (CNS) and by their frequency of activation (summation and
        tetanus). V_{max} does not come into play because the muscle is contract-
        ing isometrically and V_{max} is determined by the maximal ATPase activ-
        ity of the myosin, which is not changing. The length of the muscle is
        not changing because this is an isometric contraction and because even
        during an isotonic contraction, the length of a skeletal muscle does not
        change appreciably. With each contraction, the amount of calcium
        released from internal stores is about the same, and so peak intracellular

calcium concentrations will not rise to higher levels. Finally, during an isometric contraction each individual cross-bridge interaction with actin will generate the same amount of force. The increase in total force is because of an increase in the number of actin–myosin interactions taking place at the same time.

PHYSIOLOGY PEARLS

❖ Contraction of skeletal muscle is due to interaction of the proteins actin and myosin, which constitute thin and thick filaments, respectively. ATP is consumed in the process.

❖ Upon stimulation, calcium released from the SR binds to troponin to initiate contraction.

❖ The force of muscle contraction is regulated by the number of motor units activated (recruitment) and by the frequency with which they are being activated (summation and tetanus).

❖ Contractions can be isometric (force generation but no change in length) or isotonic (force generation and changes in length).

REFERENCES

Watras J. Muscle. In: Levy MN, Koeppen BM, Stanton BA, eds. *Berne & Levy, Principles of Physiology.* 4th ed. Philadelphia, PA: Mosby; 2006:165-193.
Weisbrodt NW. Striated muscle. In: Johnson LR, ed. *Essential Medical Physiology.* 3rd ed. San Diego, CA: Elsevier Academic Press; 2003:123-136.

An 8-year-old boy is brought to the emergency room after being stung by a bee. His mother noticed that he was playing in the backyard when he suffered the sting, and within minutes he began having trouble in breathing. She also noticed that he had a "hive" rash over most of his body, along with increased difficulty breathing. When the emergency medical service (EMS) arrived, they administered epinephrine subcutaneously, which seemed to relieve most of the symptoms. In the emergency center, the boy was diagnosed with an anaphylactic reaction from the bee sting.

◆ **What type of smooth muscle (unitary versus multiunit) is present in the bronchi of the lungs?**

◆ **Why does smooth muscle not appear striated?**

◆ **What is the molecular basis for contraction in a smooth muscle?**

ANSWERS TO CASE 7: SMOOTH MUSCLE

Summary: An 8-year-old boy with bronchial constriction and an anaphylactic reaction from a bee sting is treated with epinephrine.

 Type of muscle unit: Multiunit smooth muscle.

 Appearance of smooth muscle: Thick and thin filaments are present but are not arranged in sarcomeres.

◆ **Molecular basis for contraction:** Calcium binds to calmodulin, which activates myosin light-chain kinase.

CLINICAL CORRELATION

Anaphylaxis is a life-threatening response of a sensitized human being to a specific antigen. Symptoms occur within minutes of the exposure. Some examples of common antigens are medications (penicillin), food (peanuts), pollen (ragweed), insect bites (honeybee, wasp), chemicals (ethylene oxide), and occupational exposure (latex). Symptoms of respiratory distress, angioedema, urticaria, vascular collapse, and possibly shock may ensue. The clinical symptoms are all a result of immune-mediated responses in different organs that lead to altered smooth muscle function. The offending antigen causes the release of various cytokines that affect various smooth muscles throughout the body. The patient may develop respiratory distress from bronchial constriction; cardiovascular changes from arteriolar dilation and increased capillary permeability; cutaneous manifestations of urticaria, pruritis, and angioedema; and gastrointestinal symptoms of nausea, vomiting, diarrhea, and crampy abdominal pain. Treatment with epinephrine provides both β- and α-adrenergic effects, causing bronchial dilation and vasoconstriction and thus relieving the symptoms of anaphylaxis. If the patient develops acute airway edema, control of the airway is paramount.

APPROACH TO SMOOTH MUSCLE PHYSIOLOGY

Objectives

1. Know the types of smooth muscles and their locations in the body.
2. Understand the arrangement of smooth muscle filaments.
3. List the steps in the excitation-contraction of muscle.

Definitions

Unitary smooth muscle: Muscle that contracts and relaxes as a unit.
Multiunit smooth muscle: Muscle that, like skeletal muscle, acts independently in contraction and relaxation.

DISCUSSION

Smooth muscle can be subclassified on the basis of location and contractile behavior. Smooth muscle is found in most organ systems and can be classified as, for example, airway, arterial, venous, intestinal, uterine among others. Although the muscle in each of these tissues is classified histologically as smooth muscle, there are many differences in the contractile activities and the regulation of contraction among the various smooth muscles. Some smooth muscles maintain a level of contraction most of the time and are called **tonic smooth muscles;** others contract and relax periodically and are called **phasic smooth muscles.** Part of this difference in behavior is because of the fact that in some smooth muscles the membranes of adjacent smooth muscle cells are coupled to one another through low-resistance electrical pathways (gap junctions) in their membranes. Thus, excitation of one cell will spread quickly, and a group of cells will contract in unison. This type of muscle also is called **unitary smooth muscle.** Other smooth muscles are arranged more like skeletal muscle, in which each muscle cell can act independently when stimulated. This type of muscle is called **multiunit smooth muscle.**

As in striated muscle, **actin and myosin** are the major contractile proteins in all smooth muscles. As in striated muscle, these proteins are arranged in two sets of filaments: **actin in thin filaments** and **myosin in thick filaments.** Myosin molecules are thought to be arranged in the thick filaments in the same way as are those in skeletal muscle, with cross-bridges extending to make contact with the actin filaments. Although there are thick and thin filaments in smooth muscle, they are **not organized into sarcomeres** and thus give a homogeneous smooth appearance under the light microscope. There are **many more thin filaments** than there are thick filaments, with the ratio being closer to 10:1 than to the 2:1 seen in skeletal muscle. Also, not every thin filament is in close proximity to a thick filament. In fact, there may be two or more populations of thin filaments: those associated with thick filaments and those associated with other actin-binding proteins and the cytoskeleton. Thin filaments are attached to elements of the cytoskeleton, but these attachments bear little anatomic resemblance to the Z disks found in striated muscle. Most common are thin filaments anchored to protein structures, which are called **dense bodies.**

Even though thick and thin filaments are not arranged in sarcomeres, the basic contractile model given for striated muscle—the sliding of one filament over the other as a result of cross-bridge cycling (see Case 6)—is thought to hold true for smooth muscle. The lack of a rigid structure may account for some of the quantitative differences seen in contractions of smooth muscle compared with those of striated muscle.

Smooth muscle myosin is an **adenosine triphosphatase (ATPase),** and its splitting of adenosine triphosphate (ATP) provides the energy required for muscle contraction. Although it is an ATPase, pure smooth muscle myosin exhibits low ATPase activity. Furthermore, myosin ATPase activity is not increased upon the addition of actin alone, unless myosin is phosphorylated. This indicates that the **regulation of smooth muscle contraction** is **mediated via the**

thick filaments rather than via the thin filaments as in striated muscle. The main mechanism for the initiation of contraction appears to involve **phosphorylation** of the **20,000-d light chains of myosin.** In resting smooth muscle, phosphorylation is low. **Myosin light chain kinase** is the enzyme that, on stimulation, is activated and quickly catalyzes the phosphorylation of the myosin light chains. This results in actin-activated ATPase activity and contraction. When the stimulus to contract ceases, kinase activity decreases, myosin light chains are dephosphorylated by phosphatases, and the muscle relaxes.

Although the regulatory proteins are different in smooth muscle, the sequence of events leading to contraction is caused by the actions of **calcium.** In relaxed muscle, the levels of "free" cytosolic calcium—calcium that is not bound to other structures, such as sarcoplasmic reticulum (SR), mitochondria, and nuclei—is low ($<10^{-7}$ M). Upon **stimulation of the muscle,** the **calcium level increases** into the micromolar, or higher, range to initiate contraction. **Calcium binds with calmodulin** (one of the calcium-binding proteins found in many tissues), and then the **calcium–calmodulin complex binds to and activates the myosin light chain kinase.** Once the stimulus for muscle contraction ceases, free calcium levels decrease, and calcium dissociates from the regulatory proteins. The muscle then relaxes. In addition to calcium levels regulating contraction, changes in the activities of myosin light chain kinase and phosphatases also influence contractions by altering levels of light chain phosphorylation in response to calcium.

The sources and sinks for calcium and, therefore, excitation–contraction coupling vary markedly from one smooth muscle to another. Some have an abundant SR. When these cells are excited, events initiated at the cell membrane cause the release of calcium from the SR. In some cells, the event is a depolarization, either sustained or phasic, of the cell membrane. Additionally, receptor activation by ligands may stimulate the intracellular production of second messengers, such as inositol triphosphate, that in turn cause the release of SR calcium. Other smooth muscle cells have almost no SR. These cells must rely on the entry of enough calcium through membrane calcium channels to activate their contractile proteins.

As in striated muscle, **cytoplasmic free calcium must be decreased** to allow for **relaxation.** In cells with abundant SR, most of this calcium is pumped back into the SR via a calcium ATPase. However, in these cells, and especially in cells with little SR, calcium also must be expelled from the cell across the cell membrane. Presumably, this is accomplished by a sodium–calcium exchange mechanism and perhaps by a membrane-bound calcium ATPase.

Smooth muscle cells vary in the manner in which they are excited. Many have membrane potentials that fluctuate rhythmically to reach threshold levels periodically. Others have stable resting potentials. In addition to this inherent activity, most smooth muscles are multiply innervated. Many have membrane receptors for circulating hormones and locally released paracrines and autocoids. In addition, many smooth muscles respond directly to stretching of their membranes. Also, in contradistinction to what occurs in striated muscle, certain ligand–receptor interactions in smooth muscle lead to inhibition of contraction rather than excitation. Thus, at any one time, a specific smooth muscle cell will be receiving multiple inputs, some excitatory and some inhibitory. In this particular clinical case, the **airway smooth muscle** is **contracting** in response to the **cytokine and paracrine mediators released by the allergic response.** This increases the resistance to airflow, making breathing difficult. Smooth muscle of the gastrointestinal tract also is stimulated by mediators released by the allergic response, resulting in the gastrointestinal symptoms. However, smooth muscle in some blood vessels is relaxed, and capillary permeability is increased by some of the same mediators. This can result in **hypotension and edema. Epinephrine** is able to counteract these actions because it can interact with **β-adrenergic receptors** on airway smooth muscle and gastrointestinal smooth muscle to elicit relaxation; it also can interact with **α-adrenergic receptors** on vascular smooth muscle to cause contraction, thus maintaining blood pressure.

All smooth muscles exhibit **length–force (tension) relationships** similar to those seen in striated muscle, even though sarcomeres are absent in smooth muscle. However, there are some quantitative differences compared with striated muscle. Smooth muscle cells can develop active force over greater variations in muscle length, and many can generate greater force than skeletal muscle can. All smooth muscles also exhibit force–velocity relationships that are similar to those seen in striated muscle. A major quantitative difference is that V_{max} is much lower. Finally, many smooth muscles resemble cardiac muscle in that changes in contractility occur. This probably is because of the varying amounts of calcium that enter and/or are released with a single action potential or another excitation event.

COMPREHENSION QUESTIONS

[7.1]   A patient is given a drug that causes inhibition of myosin light-chain kinase. Which of the following is the most likely clinical effect?

A. Arterial hypertension
B. Decreased airway resistance
C. Decreased force of contraction of the heart
D. Decreased tone of postural muscles
E. Diarrhea

[7.2]   A 55-year-old man has been taking a β-adrenergic receptor antagonist for treatment of a cardiac arrhythmia. Lately, he has noticed that he is experiencing some difficulty breathing, especially shortly after taking his medication. Which of the following is the most likely mechanism of the patient's respiratory difficulty?

A. Decreased levels of ATP in airways smooth muscle
B. Decreased levels of cytoplasmic "free" calcium in airways smooth muscle
C. Less phosphorylation of myosin in airway smooth muscle
D. Less production of inositol triphosphate in airway smooth muscle
E. The effect of endogenous relaxants on airway smooth muscle

[7.3]   A bundle of muscle cells is found to contract rhythmically and in uni-
         son even when its nerve supply is disrupted. Although muscle contrac-
         tions are dependent on the presence of extracellular calcium, the cells
         have poorly developed T tubules. Which of the following most likely
         describes the muscle type?
         A. Cardiac muscle
         B. Fast-twitch skeletal muscle
         C. Multiunit smooth muscle
         D. Slow-twitch skeletal muscle
         E. Unitary smooth muscle

Answers

[7.1]   **B.** Inhibition of myosin light chain kinase mainly affects smooth mus-
         cle, and so there would be minimal to no effect on cardiac or skeletal
         muscle. Because smooth muscle contraction would be inhibited, not
         stimulated, by the drug, arterial and intestinal smooth muscle would
         relax to produce hypotension and constipation. However, relaxation of
         airway smooth muscle would decrease resistance to airflow.

[7.2]   **E.** Airway smooth muscle has β-adrenergic receptors that when stimu-
         lated by endogenous catecholamines (mainly epinephrine) causes mus-
         cle relaxation. Blocking these receptors will prevent relaxation and
         allow endogenous contractile agents to predominate. Decreasing levels
         of ATP (smooth muscle does not undergo rigor), cytoplasmic "free" cal-
         cium, phosphorylation of myosin, and production of inositol triphos-
         phate all would result in relaxation, not contraction, of smooth muscle.

[7.3]   **E.** Although all muscles can contract rhythmically and in unison under the
         right conditions, skeletal muscle can do so only by being activated by its
         motor nerves. Skeletal muscle also does not require extracellular calcium.
         Cardiac muscle does not need innervation to contract rhythmically in uni-
         son and does require extracellular calcium; however, it has highly devel-
         oped T tubules. Among the smooth muscles, only unitary smooth muscle
         can contract rhythmically and in unison without extrinsic innervation.

PHYSIOLOGY PEARLS

❖ Smooth muscle is present in most organ systems, where it constitutes in part the walls of many structures.

❖ The pattern of contraction of smooth muscle varies from organ to organ and can be tonic and/or phasic.

❖ As in striated muscle, contraction is initiated by an increase in intracellular "free" calcium.

❖ Calcium initiates contraction by binding with calmodulin, which in turn activates a kinase that phosphorylates smooth muscle myosin, which then can interact with actin.

❖ Many endogenous chemicals and administered drugs act on receptors on smooth muscle membranes to cause contraction or relaxation. The state of contraction of a specific smooth muscle results from the interaction of these stimulatory and inhibitory mediators.

❖ Not all smooth muscles react the same way to any particular mediator.

REFERENCES

Watras J. Muscle. In: Levy MN, Koeppen BM, Stanton BA, eds. *Berne & Levy, Principles of Physiology*. 4th ed. Philadelphia, PA: Mosby; 2006:165-193.
Weisbrodt NW. Smooth muscle. In: Johnson LR, ed. *Essential Medical Physiology*. 3rd ed. San Diego, CA: Elsevier Academic Press; 2003:137-144.

❖ CASE 8

A 65-year-old man with a history of hypertension and coronary artery disease presents to the emergency center with complaints of left-sided facial numbness and weakness. His blood pressure is normal, as is his heart rate and other vital signs. On examination, the patient has clear lungs and a normal cardiac examination. Auscultation of the carotid arteries reveals a "whooshing sound" (bruits) bilaterally. There is evidence of slurred speech and left-sided facial droop. The patient is diagnosed with a stroke. A computed tomography (CT) scan of the brain is performed. The patient is taken immediately to the intensive care unit for stabilization.

◆ **What is the mechanism of the audible carotid bruit?**

◆ **How does one calculate the velocity of blood flow?**

◆ **Why is velocity of blood flow higher in arterioles than in capillaries? Why is this physiologically necessary?**

◆ **What is Reynolds number, and how would it apply to this case?**

ANSWERS TO CASE 8: CARDIOVASCULAR HEMODYNAMICS

Summary: A 65-year-old man has new-onset facial droop and weakness along with slurred speech, consistent with a left-sided cerebral stroke. He has findings suggestive of bilateral carotid insufficiency.

◆ **Carotid bruit:** Clinical evidence of turbulence in blood flow through a narrowed carotid artery.

◆ **Velocity of blood flow:** Velocity = Q (flow) ÷ A (cross-sectional area).

◆ **Difference in velocity of blood flow in arteries and capillaries:** Capillaries have a larger combined cross-sectional area, which decreases the velocity of flow. This allows capillaries to exchange substances across the capillary wall.

◆ **Reynolds number:** Predicts whether blood flow will be laminar or turbulent (the more elevated Reynolds number, the more turbulent the flow). This number is increased with increased blood velocity, which in this case is because of narrowed vessels.

CLINICAL CORRELATION

This patient has a classic presentation of a stroke probably resulting from atherosclerotic disease affecting the carotid arteries. The first step, as in addressing any patient, is to examine the ABCs (airway, breathing, circulation). Reversing any ischemia, correction of severe hypertension but not overcorrection, and oxygenation are the important principles. Strokes may be caused by ischemia (decreased oxygen delivery) resulting from arterial thrombosis (clot) or embolization (clot breaks off and lodges distally) or by hemorrhage (blood collection in the brain putting pressure on the normal brain cells). The CT scan helps in assessing for hemorrhagic stroke. Some patients are candidates for thrombolytic therapy when hemorrhagic stroke is ruled out. After stabilization, carotid ultrasound studies probably will be performed, perhaps followed, if carotid insufficiency is confirmed, by carotid endarterectomy.

Calculating and understanding cardiovascular hemodynamics are of utmost importance in clinically assessing patients. Pressure in the large conducting arteries such as the carotid normally is high compared with other vessels. These vessels normally offer little resistance to blood flow. When there is narrowing of a vessel, as in this case of peripheral vascular disease, resistance increases because of the narrowing and the change in flow from laminar to turbulent. Because of the increased resistance, blood flow to the tissues that the vessel supplies decreases. Blood flow to peripheral tissues also can be compromised by a decrease in pressure in the large conducting arteries. Rapid assessment of mean arterial pressure (MAP) can determine whether a patient is in shock and if vital organs such as the brain are perfused. As patients age, various hemodynamic changes occur, such as decreased arterial capacitance, which in turn can increase systolic blood pressure (systolic hypertension) and increase pulse pressure. Veins offer little resistance to blood flow but have the highest proportion of blood in the system. When a patient becomes hypovolemic, the adrenergic receptors are stimulated, causing constriction of the veins and thus limiting the decrease in venous return to the heart and the decrease in cardiac output.

APPROACH TO HEMODYNAMIC PHYSIOLOGY

Objectives

1. Know the components of the vascular system.
2. Know and be able to use the relationship among pressure, flow, and resistance.
3. Compare the different hemodynamic measurements between arteries and veins.
4. Be able to define systolic, diastolic, and pulse pressure.

Definitions

Cardiac output: The volume of blood the heart pumps per minute.
Mean arterial pressure: The average arterial pressure during a cardiac cycle.

DISCUSSION

Blood ejected by the heart (**cardiac output**) circulates through two vascular systems that are arranged in series: the **pulmonary and the systemic** systems. In this case, only the systemic system will be considered. This system is composed of a number of large conducting arteries such as the **aorta** and the **carotids** that subdivide multiple times until they give rise to the **arterioles.** With each subdivision, the radius of each individual vessel decreases, but the number of vessels in each subdivision increases dramatically, going from one aorta to tens of millions of arterioles. Each arteriole then feeds many **capillaries.** Physiologically, the focal point of this system is the billions of capillaries that function to bring each cell of the body to within a few microns of flowing blood so that exchange of substrates between the cells and the blood can take place. On the other end of the capillaries are the **venules,** which are about equal in number to the arterioles but are larger in diameter. The venules coalesce multiple times until they give rise to the **vena cava.**

The number and size of the vessels in each division markedly affect both the resistance to flow and the velocity of flow of blood in each division. The **resistance to blood flow** in any single vessel is **inversely proportional to its radius taken to the power of 4.** Thus, a **halving of the radius increases**

resistance 16 times. Conversely, the resistance offered by any division of vessels is inversely proportional to the number of vessels in that division because these vessels are arranged parallel to one another. Thus, the greater the number of vessels, the lower is the resistance. In the systemic circulation, this balance between vessel radius and vessel number is such that the small arteries, the capillaries, and, most important, the arterioles offer the greatest resistance to blood flow.

The velocity of blood flow through the vessels of any division depends on the volume of blood flow per unit of time (milliliters per second) and the combined cross-sectional area of all the vessels that constitute that division. Thus

$$\text{Velocity} = Q \text{ (flow)} \div A \text{ (cross-sectional area)}$$

Because all the divisions of the systemic circulation are in series with one another, the volume of blood flow per unit time (Q) will be the same through all divisions. However, velocity of flow will differ because the combined cross-sectional area of the vessels in each division will vary. The situation in the systemic circulation is such that the **peak flow velocity is highest in the large conducting arteries** and lowest in the capillaries. The low flow velocity in the capillaries allows time for exchange to take place between the cells of the body and the blood. The high velocity of flow in the large arteries is normally of little consequence. However, velocity can be increased in vessels that are partially occluded (thus decreasing cross-sectional area), as in this case, to the point where flow changes from laminar to turbulent. The conditions that produce clinically audible turbulent flow are expressed in the **Reynolds equation:**

$$R_e = \frac{D.v.\rho}{\eta}$$

which solves for the **Reynolds number (Re) when D is the diameter of the vessel, v is the velocity of flow, ρ is fluid density, and η is fluid viscosity.** The **larger the Reynolds number,** the more likely there is to be **turbulent flow;** and so the greater the velocity, the more likely there is to be turbulence. Turbulent flow is significant because it offers more resistance and produces clinically audible sounds termed bruits. The flow of blood through a vascular bed such as the central nervous system (CNS) depends not only on the resistance to flow but also on the pressure that is driving the flow. In a normal person who is lying down (to mitigate the influence of gravity), MAP (~100 mm Hg) is much higher than the pressure in the capillaries (~20 mm Hg) and in the veins (~5 mm Hg). Although it is the MAP that is useful in considering the force that drives blood across the capillaries and into the veins, pressure in the arteries fluctuates during the cardiac cycle. Pressure rises during systole, when blood is being ejected from the heart. The peak arterial pressure during this phase of the cycle is called systolic pressure. Pressure then falls to reach a minimum diastolic pressure as blood flows across the vascular beds during the phase of the cardiac cycle when no blood is being ejected from the heart. The arterial pressures that are estimated during the taking of blood pressure by auscultation are the systolic and diastolic pressures. The **MAP** can be estimated from these pressures by using the equation

$$MAP = DP + 1/3 \ (SP - DP)$$

where MAP is mean arterial pressure, DP is diastolic pressure, and SP is systolic pressure.

The difference between systolic pressure and diastolic pressure is also known as the **pulse pressure.** Pulse pressure provides some information about stroke volume and vascular capacitance. Stroke volume can vary from moment to moment and depends on cardiac output and heart rate. Vascular capacitance, in contrast, changes over a longer time, and that change appears to be a consequence of aging. With the decrease in capacitance with aging, systolic pressure tends to increase and diastolic pressure tends to decrease.

There is a relationship among **flow, pressure, and resistance** that can be expressed mathematically as

$$Q = \Delta P \div R$$

where Q is flow, ΔP is MAP minus venous pressure (VP), and R is resistance to flow across the bed.

Unless regulatory mechanisms are impaired, mean pressure in the large conducting arteries normally is held within fairly narrow limits. Thus, blood flow to any particular vascular bed normally is regulated by changes in resistance to flow provided mainly by the arterioles. However, in pathologic states such as the one described in this case, large conducting arteries can be obstructed to the point where they offer significant resistance as a result of decreased radius and turbulent flow. This can lead to decreased blood flow to the organs they perfuse, in this case the brain.

Because there are more veins than arteries and the diameters of the veins are greater, veins contain the greatest proportion of blood. Although veins offer little resistance to blood flow, they do contain smooth muscle that by contracting and relaxing can change their diameters and/or VP. This in turn can influence cardiac output by influencing preload.

COMPREHENSION QUESTIONS

[8.1] If one considers a single vessel within each division of the systemic circulation in a person who is lying down, one can arrange the vessels according to the end pressure, greatest to least, within each vessel. (If the vessel exhibits a pulse pressure, one can consider the mean end pressure.) Which of the following sequences of mean end pressure is correct in this case?

A. Large artery → large vein → arteriole → venule → capillary
B. Capillary → arteriole → venule → large artery → large vein
C. Large artery → arteriole → capillary → venule → large vein
D. Large vein → venule → capillary → arteriole → large artery
E. Capillary → venule → arteriole → large vein → large artery

[8.2] A patient is suspected of having reduced flow of blood to the brain. Her blood pressure taken from the brachial artery is normal. Bruits are detected in the right carotid artery but not in the left carotid artery. A comparison of hemodynamic events in the two carotid arteries would reveal which of the following?

A. A mean pressure in the right carotid artery proximal to the site of the bruit that is lower than the mean pressure in the left carotid artery
B. Equal blood flow in both carotid arteries
C. Lower resistance to flow in the right carotid artery
D. Increased velocity of flow in the right carotid artery
E. Turbulent blood flow in both carotid arteries

[8.3] A patient suspected of suffering a myocardial infarction is being monitored in the Coronary Care Unit. The following data are obtained on this individual.:

Arterial systolic blood pressure	121 mm Hg
Arterial diastolic blood pressure	82 mm Hg
Venous blood pressure	2 mm Hg
Cardiac output	4185 mL/min
Radius of the aorta	1.2 cm

Which of the following can be concluded from the monitored data?

A. The patient's MAP is 95 mm Hg
B. The pulse pressure is 80 mm Hg
C. Total resistance to flow is approximately 45 resistance units
D. The patient's blood flow in the carotid artery must be turbulent
E. The velocity of blood flow through the aorta is 3487 cm/s

Answers

[8.1] **C.** In a supine person, the effect of gravity is essentially nil and intravascular pressures are caused by contractions of the heart. Because fluid flows from regions of higher pressure to regions of lower pressure, pressures must be higher in the large arteries than in the arterioles, than in the capillaries, than in the venules, than in the large veins.

[8.2] **D.** The velocity of blood flow must be increased in the right carotid artery to produce the turbulence that is detected as bruits. Flow in the left carotid artery must be laminar because of the absence of bruits. The turbulent flow in the right carotid artery increases the resistance to flow in that artery, thus reducing blood flow, making it less than it is through the left carotid artery. Pressure in the right carotid artery distal to the site of the bruits will be decreased, but pressure proximal to the site of the bruits will be the same as the pressure in the left carotid artery.

[8.3] **A.** The MAP can be estimated by using the equation MAP = DP + 1/3 (SP − DP). The pulse pressure (SP − DP) is 39 mm Hg. (93 = 82 + 13). The resistance to flow can be calculated by using the equation $Q = \Delta P \div R$ rearranged to solve for R. Thus, R = (93 − 2) [MAP − VP] ÷ 4185, or approximately 0.022 resistance unit. From the data given, there is no reason to suspect turbulent flow anywhere in the vasculature. In the aorta, the velocity of flow can be calculated by using the equation $v = Q \div A$. Thus, v = 4185 cm³/60 s ÷ 4.52 cm², or approximately 15.4 cm/s.

PHYSIOLOGY PEARLS

❖ Transfer of material in and out of the blood, mainly by diffusion, takes place across capillary walls.

❖ In a healthy person, variations in blood flow through an organ come about through dilation and constriction of an organ's arterioles, thus changing resistance, rather than through changes in systemic arterial pressure.

❖ Arterial pressure and blood flow can be measured by using one of several techniques. Resistance, however, is calculated by using the equation

$$Q = \Delta P/R$$

where Q is flow, ΔP is MAP minus VP, and R is resistance to flow across the bed.

❖ The velocity of blood flow is highest in the large arteries, slowest in the capillaries, and intermediate in the veins because of variations in the total cross-sectional areas of these vascular beds.

❖ Blood flow in all regions of the vasculature normally is nonturbulent (laminar); however, it can become turbulent in diseased arteries as a result of the high velocity of flow.

❖ The pressure that causes flow is highest in the large arteries and lowest in the large veins. Pressure falls dramatically as blood flows through the small arteries and arterioles because of the high resistance to flow provided by these vessels.

❖ The difference between systolic and diastolic pressures is the pulse pressure. The amplitude of the pulse pressure is influenced mainly by stroke volume and the capacitance (stiffness) of the large arteries.

REFERENCES

Downey JM. Hemodynamics. In: Johnson LR, ed. *Essential Medical Physiology.* 3rd ed. San Diego, CA: Elsevier Academic Press; 2003:157-174.

Levy MN, Pappano A. Hemodynamics. In: Levy MN, Koeppen BM, Stanton BA, eds. *Berne & Levy, Principles of Physiology.* 4th ed. Philadelphia, PA: Mosby; 2006:276-287.

A 68-year-old woman presents to the emergency center with shortness of breath, light-headedness, and chest pain described as being like "an elephant sitting on her chest." She is diagnosed with a myocardial infarction. She is given oxygen and an aspirin to chew and is not felt to be a candidate for thrombolytic therapy. Her heart rate is 40 beats per minute (bpm). Although there are P waves, they seem to be dissociated from the QRS complexes on the electrocardiograph (ECG). The patient is diagnosed with complete heart block, probably as a result of her myocardial infarction. The patient is taken to the intensive care unit for stabilization, and plans are made for pacemaker insertion.

◆ **Where are the normal pacemaker and the backup pacemakers of the heart located?**

◆ **Why does this patient have a bradycardia?**

◆ **What parts of the heart have the fastest and slowest conduction velocities?**

ANSWERS TO CASE 9: ELECTRICAL ACTIVITY OF THE HEART

Summary: A 68-year-old woman with new-onset myocardial infarction presents with complete heart block that is symptomatic.

- ◆ **Location of pacemakers:** Normal, sinoatrial (SA) node; other pacemakers (in order of recruitment), atrioventricular (AV) node, bundle of His-Purkinje system.

- ◆ **Cause of bradycardia:** If the AV node is injured by the infarction, both its ability to conduct and its ability to serve as a backup pacemaker may be lost, allowing a slow intrinsic pacemaker in the bundle of His or the Purkinje system to generate the ventricular heartbeat.

- ◆ **Extreme conduction velocities:** Fastest in the Purkinje system and slowest at the AV node.

CLINICAL CORRELATION

Cardiac arrhythmias and heart block are common findings after a myocardial infarction. Depending on the location of the cardiac tissue injury, varying heart rate abnormalities can be seen. If the injury occurs in the AV node area, excitation from the SA node is not conducted to the ventricles, and healthy cardiac cells with the next fastest intrinsic rhythm take over. With complete heart block, the new pacemaker may be from cells in the bundle of His or the Purkinje system. There are varying degrees of heart block. First-degree heart block is defined as a prolongation of the PR interval in the ECG. This can result from slowed conduction through either the AV node or the His-Purkinje fibers. Second-degree heart block occurs when a fraction of the atrial impulses fail to conduct to the ventricles. In third-degree, or complete, heart block none of the atrial impulses reach the ventricle. This patient probably experienced right coronary artery occlusion that led to AV nodal disruption. Her bradycardia is symptomatic, leading to feelings of light-headedness. A pacemaker, first temporary (transvenous) and then permanent, is indicated.

APPROACH TO CARDIAC CONDUCTION SYSTEM

Objectives

1. Know the normal conduction through the heart.
2. Understand the mechanisms of cardiac action potentials.
3. Understand the mechanisms of pacemaking.
4. Describe regulation by the autonomic nervous system.

DISCUSSION

Excitation of the heart begins with **action potential** initiation in the cardiac tissue with the fastest intrinsic pacemakers, the **SA node.** Action potentials then are conducted through **gap junctions** in **intercalated discs** from fiber to fiber, proceeding sequentially through the **atria, AV node, bundle of His, Purkinje fibers, and contractile cells of the ventricles.** The small AV node is the sole conductive path to the ventricles, and its thin fibers and slowly rising action potentials greatly slow conduction, providing time for the ventricles to fill during atrial contraction. The **bundle of His and Purkinje fibers,** by virtue of their wide diameters and rapidly rising action potentials, **conduct extremely rapidly,** bringing excitation to all ventricular muscle cells simultaneously and ensuring that they contract in unison.

Cardiac action potentials are generated by the flow of currents through specific ion channels. Working muscle cells of the atria and ventricles, as well as the rapidly conducting fibers of the bundle of His and the Purkinje system, have **fast action potentials** that **depend on Na^+ influx** through depolarization-activated channels. The positive feedback between the opening of Na^+ channels and the consequent depolarization causes the **fast, regenerative upstroke (phase 0)** of the action potential (see Figure 9-1). **Early, partial repolarization (phase 1)** occurs because of slightly delayed, depolarization-induced closing (inactivation) of the Na^+ channels and because of the activation of a minor K^+ current. A **prolonged plateau (phase 2) follows,** which is produced by Ca^{2+} **influx** through depolarization-activated, L-type Ca^{2+} channels and is aided by the depolarization-induced closing of inward rectifier K^+ channels. Ca^{2+} influx during phase 2 is important for excitation–contraction coupling, mediating Ca^{2+}-induced Ca^{2+} release from the sarcoplasmic reticulum. **Complete repolarization (phase 3)** occurs because (1) the L-type Ca^{2+} channels spontaneously close (inactivate), (2) very slow, depolarization-activated K^+ channels open, and (3) the inward rectifier K^+ channels that had been closed by depolarization begin to open in response to the repolarization. During **rest (phase 4),** the hyperpolarized potential is maintained by K^+ current flowing out of the cell through both the leakage channels that are insensitive to voltage and the open inward rectifier K^+ channels.

Cells in the SA and AV nodes have "slow" action potentials because they lack fast, depolarization-activated Na^+ channels. Phase 0 is produced by a regenerative (positive feedback) interaction between depolarization and the opening of depolarization-activated, L-type Ca^{2+} channels. Phase 1 is absent, and the plateau and complete repolarization phases involve conductance changes similar to those in phases 2 and 3 in other cardiac cells. Most important for generating the heart beat, SA nodal cells have **no true resting potential;** instead a slowly depolarizing **pacemaker potential** begins immediately after complete repolarization from the action potential and continues until action potential threshold is again reached. The pacemaker potential has three

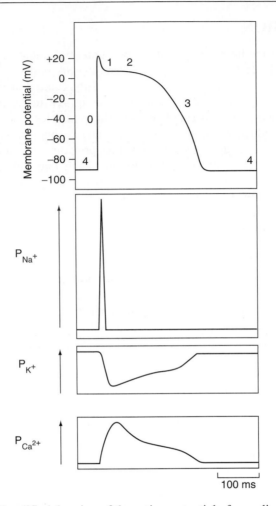

Figure 9-1. Simplified drawing of the action potential of a cardiac muscle cell. For simplicity, changes in permeability, P, rather than current, I, for different ions are plotted. Plots of I would show both magnitude and direction of ionic flow across the membrane.

major components. One is the slow closing of depolarization-activated K$^+$ channels that had been opened by the preceding action potential and served to repolarize the nodal cell's membrane. The second component is the opening of a **hyperpolarization-activated channel** permeable to Na$^+$ and K$^+$. This current is traditionally called the "**funny current**" (I$_f$, sometimes also called the hyperpolarization-activated current, I$_h$) because, before its role in pacemaking was appreciated, it seemed odd that a depolarizing current would be activated by hyperpolarization. As the pacemaker potential depolarizes the SA cell membrane, a level is reached where L-type Ca^{2+} channels begin to open. This third component of the pacemaker potential accelerates the depolarization, causing increasing numbers of Ca²⁺ channels to open, soon resulting in a regenerative, **Ca²⁺-mediated action potential.** Depolarization during the action potential closes the I_f channels, which then reopen after repolarization occurs, restarting the cycle. This spontaneously repeating cycle is responsible for generating the heart beat, and can occur even in completely isolated SA nodal cells. (See Figure 9-2 for action potentials for various parts of the heart.)

The AV node has two important functions. First, its extremely slow conduction properties (because of narrow fiber diameter, lack of fast Na⁺ channels, and low density of gap junctions) delay ventricular contraction until

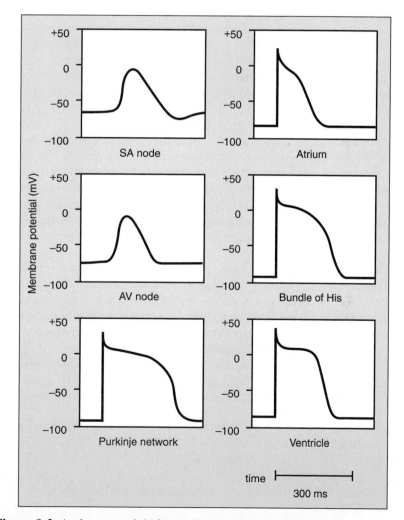

Figure 9-2. Action potentials for various parts of the heart.

after atrial contraction can fill the ventricles. Second, action potential conduction in the AV node is blocked easily because of the long refractory periods and other features of the action potential. This protects the ventricles from excessive frequencies of contraction, which can prevent effective filling, during **atrial tachycardia or atrial fibrillation.** Atrial tachycardia may be produced by elevated firing rates in the SA node (eg, from sympathetic stimulation) or by ectopic pacemakers, for example, generated by circulating impulses in reentry loops in the atrium and sometimes either the **AV node** or **abnormal accessory pathways** between the atria and ventricles. **Reentry** or other problems during chronic heart disease (as well as electrocution and certain drugs) also can lead to **fibrillation,** in which the atria or ventricles undergo continuous, completely uncoordinated excitation and contraction that precludes effective pumping. Ventricular fibrillation is lethal unless a strong shock (electric defibrillation) is used to force the entire myocardium simultaneously into a refractory state that allows the heart to relax and the SA node to regain control of the heartbeat.

The autonomic nervous system modulates electrophysiologic and contractile properties of the heart. Norepinephrine (NE) released by sympathetic postganglionic terminals acts through β receptors coupled to adenylyl cyclase to increase I_f, increase I_{Ca}, and increase depolarization-activated I_K. These effects increase heart rate by accelerating the pacemaker potential and shortening the action potential. Narrowing of the action potential, as well as NE-induced enhancement of the activity of the Ca^{2+} pump in the sarcoplasmic reticulum (which speeds relaxation), allows more beats to be accommodated per unit time. The increase in I_{Ca} also increases the amplitude of the action potential in the AV node, which makes conduction block in this node less likely. Finally, the increase in I_{Ca} in working cardiac cells increases Ca^{2+} influx and thus enhances contractility.

Parasympathetic input to the heart opposes the sympathetic actions. Acetylcholine **(ACh) inhibits adenylyl cyclase** and **increases the hydrolysis of cyclic adenosine monophosphate (cAMP),** directly antagonizing all the effects of NE mediated by the cAMP-protein kinase A (PKA) pathway. In addition, **ACh opens inward rectifier K⁺ channels, thus hyperpolarizing nodal cells.** Together these effects decrease heart rate and increase the chances of AV block. In the atria, parasympathetic stimulation decreases contractility by reducing background PKA activity, thus reducing I_{Ca} and Ca^{2+} influx. Few parasympathetic fibers innervate the ventricles.

COMPREHENSION QUESTIONS

[9.1] A 32-year-old woman is seen in the emergency center with supraventricular tachycardia. She is hypotensive. The cardiologist explains to the patient that the rapid heart rate does not allow for sufficient ventricular filling, thus reducing cardiac output. Which of the following best explains how ventricular filling is enabled during atrial contraction?

A. By the elevated contractility of ventricular muscle

B. As a functional consequence of narrow fiber diameter, slow depolarization, and low density of gap junctions in AV nodal cells

C. By the high density of depolarization-activated Na^+ channels in AV nodal cells

D. By the low basal activity of sarcoplasmic reticulum Ca^+ pumps in ventricular muscle

E. By the prolonged time it takes for action potentials to be conducted from the bundle of His to ventricular muscle

[9.2] A 59-year-old man is admitted to the intensive care unit for a myocardial infarction. He is given a β-adrenergic antagonist and instructed to avoid emotional turmoil to decrease sympathetic stimulation of the heart. From a cellular perspective, sympathetic stimulation of the heart does which of the following?

A. Decreases adenylyl cyclase activity in ventricular muscle

B. Decreases Ca^{2+} pump activity in the sarcoplasmic reticulum of atrial muscle

C. Decreases I_{Ca} in the AV node

D. Increases depolarization-activated I_K in the SA node

E. Increases hyperpolarization-activated I_K (inward rectifier) in the SA node

[9.3] A 28-year-old athlete is noted to have a baseline heart rate of 55 bpm, which his trainer attributes to excellent parasympathetic (vagal) tone. This parasympathetic effect, among other things, increases the ACh released in the SA and AV nodes. ACh released into the AV node increases which of the following in AV fibers?

A. Action potential amplitude

B. Conduction velocity

C. K^+ equilibrium potential

D. Probability of conduction failure (AV block)

E. Rate of depolarization of the pacemaker potential

Answers

[9.1]   **B.** Ventricular filling during atrial contraction depends on a sufficient delay in the propagation of action potentials from the atria to the ventricles. This delay is accomplished by requiring that all atrial-to-ventricular electrical communication be funneled through the AV node and by giving the AV nodal cells narrow diameters and slowly activating Ca^{2+} channels (rather than rapidly activating Na^+ channels), as well as a low density of gap junctions between AV cells; all these factors slow action potential conduction through the node. The bundle of His (answer E), in contrast, has the opposite features because it is specialized for rapid conduction. Elevated contractility of ventricular muscle (answer A) would not affect ventricular filling directly. The other properties listed (answers C and D) would impede rather than enhance ventricular filling.

[9.2]   **D.** By increasing the depolarization-activated I_K in the SA node, sympathetic stimulation decreases the duration of each action potential in the node; this allows more impulses to be generated per unit time, permitting higher heart rates to be produced. Most of the other effects listed (answers A, B, and C) are opposite to what sympathetic stimulation produces. The hyperpolarization-activated inward rectifier current found in working muscle cells, which is insensitive to ACh, is less important in SA nodal cells and is not increased by sympathetic stimulation.

[9.3]   **D.** ACh released by postganglionic fibers innervating the AV node hyperpolarizes the AV fibers, thus increasing the probability of blocking impulse conduction through the node. This also will decrease rather than increase action potential amplitude, conduction velocity, and the rate of rise of the pacemaker potential (answers A, B, and E). The K^+ equilibrium potential is not changed by vagal stimulation.

PHYSIOLOGY PEARLS

❖ Normal excitation of the heart proceeds from the SA node, through atrial muscle fibers, through the AV node (slowly, permitting the ventricles to fill), and rapidly through the bundle of His and Purkinje fibers, ending in the synchronous activation of all the working fibers of the ventricles.

❖ Working and conductile fibers in the atria and ventricles exhibit fast action potentials that depend on a high density of Na^+ channels that are activated rapidly by depolarization.

❖ During the long plateau of the action potential (phase 2), significant amounts of Ca^{2+} enter cardiac muscle cells through depolarization-activated Ca^{2+} channels, and this Ca^{2+} influx triggers contraction via Ca^{2+}-induced Ca^{2+} release from the sarcoplasmic reticulum.

❖ Nodal cells lack fast, depolarization-activated Na^+ channels and depend on slower depolarization-activated Ca^{2+} channels to produce the action potential.

❖ The heartbeat is initiated in the SA node by a spontaneously depolarizing pacemaker potential that is initiated by the hyperpolarization-activated, "funny" current, I_f (carried by Na^+ and K^+ ions). Slow waning of the depolarization-activated I_K and eventual activation of I_{Ca} also contribute to the pacemaker potential.

❖ The AV node is particularly vulnerable to conduction block because the same factors that decrease conduction velocity (narrow fiber diameter, low-amplitude action potentials) increase the probability that the action potential threshold will not be reached during propagation into nodal fibers. This protects the ventricles from excessive contraction frequencies during atrial tachycardia or atrial fibrillation.

❖ The probability of conduction block in the AV node is decreased by sympathetic stimulation, which increases action potential amplitude. Parasympathetic stimulation increases AV block by hyperpolarizing nodal cells and reducing action potential amplitude.

REFERENCES

Downey JM. Electrical activity of the heart. In: Johnson LR, ed. *Essential Medical Physiology*. San Diego, CA: Elsevier Academic Press; 2003: 175-186.

Lederer WJ. Cardiac electrophysiology and the electrocardiogram. In: Boron WF, Boulpaep EL, eds. *Medical Physiology*. Philadelphia, PA: Elsevier Science; 2003: 483-507.

❖ CASE 10

A 57-year-old man presents to the emergency center with complaints of chest pain with radiation to the left arm and jaw. He reports feeling anxious, diaphoretic, and short of breath. His past history is significant for type II diabetes mellitus and hyperlipidemia. On examination, the patient appears to be in moderate distress and anxious. His electrocardiograph (ECG) shows evidence of acute myocardial injury in the inferior leads. The emergency room physician suspects that the left anterior descending artery is involved.

◆ **What would the ST segment of this ECG look like?**

◆ **On which leads would you see this ST segment change?**

◆ **What does the T wave represent?**

ANSWERS TO CASE 10: ELECTROCARDIOGRAPHY

Summary: A 57-year-old man has chest pain and ECG evidence of acute myocardial injury (ST-segment elevation) in the inferior leads (leads II, III, and aV_F).

◆ **ST-segment appearance:** Elevation of the ST segments.

◆ **Inferior leads:** II, III, and aV_F.

◆ **T wave:** Represents ventricular polarization.

CLINICAL CORRELATION

This 57-year-old man has risk factors for coronary heart disease: diabetes mellitus and hyperlipidemia. His history is very suspicious for an acute coronary event. Oxygen should be administered quickly, followed by an aspirin to chew. Nitroglycerin can be given if the patient continues to have chest pain. The ECG often is helpful; however, a subset of patients with a myocardial infarction (MI) will not have ECG findings. Thus, a normal ECG does not rule out an MI. Cardiac enzymes should be drawn. These markers are sensitive indicators of myocardial injury.

Interpretation of an ECG is essential in managing patients with chest pain because a patient's clinical problem often can be determined from the ECG. Various abnormalities can be recognized, including cardiac arrhythmias, infarction, ischemia, and hypertrophy. This patient has typical symptoms of an MI. An ECG of a patient with an MI often will show elevated ST segments acutely and the presence of Q waves after several days. The location of ECG changes in certain leads helps localize where the injury may be occurring. In this case, leads II, III, and aV_F were affected and represent the inferior portion of the heart. When a patient with stable angina undergoes an exercise stress test, an ECG is performed, and the appearance of ST-segment depression or elevation will indicate cardiac ischemia and therefore be a positive stress test. Cardiac hypertrophy often leads to changes in the mean electrical axis, which can be determined by comparing the relative magnitude of the QRS complex on different leads.

APPROACH TO ELECTROCARDIOGRAPHY PHYSIOLOGY

Objectives

1. Know the ECG leads and electrical vectors.
2. Be able to understand the correspondence of parts of the ECG to the cardiac cycle.
3. Know the effects of heart block, hypertrophy, and acute MI on the ECG.

Definitions

ECG segment: Part of the ECG record measured in terms of voltage, usually relatively flat (e.g., the ST segment).

ECG interval: Part of the ECG record measured in terms of time (e.g., the QT interval).

First-degree heart block: Prolongation of the time taken for action potentials to propagate through the AV node (abnormally long PR interval).

Second-degree heart block: Failure of some but not all action potentials to propagate through the AV node (greater number of P waves than QRS complexes).

Third-degree heart block: Failure of all action potentials to propagate through the AV node (no correlation between P waves and QRS complexes).

DISCUSSION

The **electrocardiogram** records **small extracellular signals** on the **surface of the body** that are produced by **action potentials** generated synchronously by large regions of the heart. To obtain the standard 12-lead ECG, an electrode is attached to each forearm and ankle, and six electrodes are placed on standard locations across the chest (see Figure 10-1). The electrodes on the extremities are used to define six limb leads [three standard (I, II, and III) and three augmented (aV_R, aV_L, and aV_F)], and the chest electrodes define six precordial leads (V_1 to V_6). Individual leads refer to the potential difference measured between one electrode and one or more of the others. Each lead provides information from a unique angle. The six **limb leads** monitor electrical vectors (having magnitude and direction) in the **frontal plane,** and the six **precordial leads** monitor vectors in the **transverse plane.** Together, the leads provide a dynamic representation of the three-dimensional electrical vector resulting from the net flow of current from action potentials across the heart.

During the cardiac cycle, characteristic events are exhibited on most leads. The electrical signal depends on the mass of cardiac tissue in which current is flowing, and so electrical signals corresponding to events in small nodal regions are not detected by the leads. It also should be remembered that the ECG displays *changes* in potential (produced by changes in current) and not steady-state absolute values. When little net current is flowing (when most cells are at resting potential or in the plateau phase of the action potential), the ECG will be at its baseline value. The cycle begins with the **P wave,** generated by roughly **synchronous depolarization of atrial muscle cells** (see Figure 10-2). This is followed by a return to the isoelectric baseline during the period when action potentials are conducted through the **atrioventricular (AV) node, bundle of His, and Purkinje fibers,** which have relatively little mass. The **sharp QRS complex** then occurs when the large mass of **ventricular muscle cells** initiate, nearly synchronously, their **fast action potentials:** very large currents

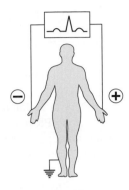
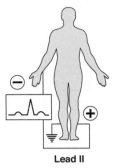
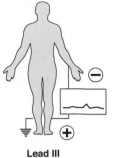

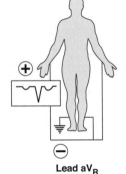

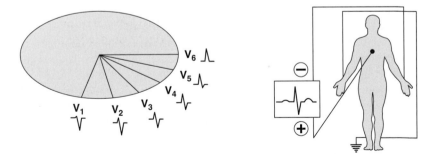

Figure 10-1. A diagram of the 12-lead placement for the ECG. The frontal plane is represented on leads I, II, and III as well as augmented leads aV_R, aV_L, and aV_F. The cross-sectional plane is depicted on the precordial leads of the chest.

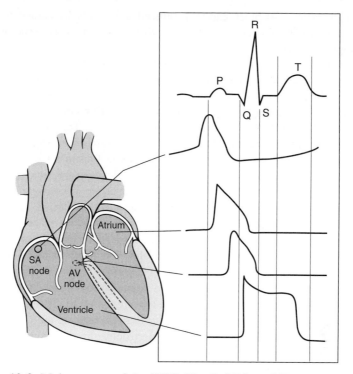

Figure 10-2. Major waves of the ECG. The P, QRS, and T waves are shown corresponding to characteristic action potentials in the key cardiac structures.

are produced by the coordinated opening of numerous Na^+ channels across the ventricles. Another isoelectric period follows during the **prolonged plateau (phase 2) of the ventricular action potentials,** when little net current flows. The **T wave** then occurs, produced by the **less synchronous repolarization (phase 3)** of the ventricular muscle cells.

First-degree heart block, which is produced by **slowing of conduction** through the **AV node,** is demonstrated on the ECG by a **prolongation of the PR interval. Second-degree heart block** occurs when a **fraction of the action potentials fail to propagate through the AV node.** This is demonstrated by a larger number of P waves than QRS complexes. Every QRS complex is associated with a preceding P wave, with the PR interval either remaining fixed or progressively increasing during successive cycles until a QRS complex is dropped. **Third-degree, or complete, heart block** occurs when no action potentials propagate through the AV node. In this case, the **P waves and QRS complexes are independent of each other,** and the QRS complexes occur less frequently than do the P waves because the **latent ventricular pacemaker that takes over** has a longer intrinsic cycle period. All three degrees of heart block can be produced transiently by parasympathetic stimulation of the AV node as well as by other causes, such as tissue injury.

Ectopic pacemakers can lead to atrial or ventricular tachycardia and to occasional premature contractions. **Premature atrial contractions** display an early P wave, often with an abnormal shape because the atrial discharge is initiated in a different part of the atrium than is normally the case. The following RR interval is usually normal. **Premature ventricular contractions** display an early QRS complex without any preceding P wave. The QRS complex is abnormal (broadened and sometimes inverted) because of the abnormal site of initiation and the lack of normal activation of the Purkinje fiber system. If reentry in the atria leads to **atrial fibrillation,** all P waves are lost and replaced by irregular voltage fluctuations and the RR interval becomes irregularly irregular. In **ventricular fibrillation,** all regular electrical signals in the ECG are lost while the ventricles quiver ineffectively.

Hypertrophy increases the mass of tissue that generates action potentials. If the hypertrophy is localized to one part of the heart, it alters the heart's mean electrical axis. This axis is determined by estimating the area under the QRS complex in different leads and plotting the vectors or by simply noting which lead is at right angles to the lead that is recording the minimal deflection. The normal mean electrical axis is down and to the left because the left ventricle has the greatest mass. In left ventricular hypertrophy, the axis would be shifted farther to the left. In right ventricular hypertrophy, it would be shifted to the right.

Acute MI can cause a **sustained, partial depolarization** of surviving myocardial cells in the **region of injury,** and this depolarization generates an **injury current** between those cells and normal cells in the heart. Because the ECG measures only changes in potential produced by changes in current, not absolute potentials, this steady injury current has no effect on the baseline of the ECG. However, during the plateau of the ventricular action potentials (the ST segment), membrane potential during the plateau phase of cells in the depolarized region will be close to that of cells in the remainder of the ventricle that are also in the plateau phase, and the recorded potential will be close to true zero. Because the baseline is not at true zero (because of the injury current), the ST segment will be elevated or depressed from the baseline (depending on the location of the injury and the lead examined) during an acute MI.

COMPREHENSION QUESTIONS

Choose one of these answers (A–E) for questions 10.1 through 10.3:

    A. P wave
    B. PR interval
    C. QRS complex
    D. ST segment
    E. T wave

[10.1]   Period when ventricular action potentials are in their plateau phase.

[10.2]   Prolonged during first-degree heart block.

[10.3]   Produced by depolarization of atrial fibers.

[10.4]   An emergency room physician performs carotid massage in an attempt to slow the heart rate of a patient with supraventricular tachycardia. The physician explains to the patient that this maneuver is expected to increase vagal stimulation. A dramatic increase in activity of vagal preganglionic axons is most likely to result in which of the following?

   A. Decrease the RR interval
   B. Decrease the number of QRS complexes relative to the number of P waves
   C. Decrease the PR interval
   D. Decrease the duration of the ST segment
   E. Shift the mean electrical axis of the heart to the right

Answers

[10.1]   **D.** Ventricular cells are in the plateau phase of the action potential during the ST segment, which is isoelectric (remaining at baseline) because there is no change in current flow and the net amount of current is very small.

[10.2]   **B.** The PR interval is prolonged because conduction through the AV node is slowed significantly during first-degree heart block.

[10.3]   **A.** The P wave is produced by atrial depolarization. The P wave is slower and shorter than the QRS complex because the atria lack a fast conducting system corresponding to the bundle of His-Purkinje fiber system to synchronize the depolarization of the atrial working fibers.

[10.4]   **B.** Dramatically increased release of acetylcholine (ACh) from postganglionic neurons strongly excited by vagal preganglionic axons will hyperpolarize AV nodal fibers sufficiently to block a fraction of the impulses being conducted through the AV node. This leads to partial (second-degree) or total (third-degree) heart block. Vagal activity also will decrease rather than increase heart rate (answer A) and conduction velocity through the AV node (answer C) and will have little effect on action potentials in the ventricles (answer D) because there is relatively little parasympathetic innervation of the ventricles. Parasympathetic stimulation has no effect on the mass of cardiac tissue in different regions of the heart and thus has no effect on the mean electrical axis of the heart (answer E).

PHYSIOLOGY PEARLS

❖ The ECG, which often is monitored with 12 extracellular electrodes on the surface of the body, detects small potentials produced by the generation of large extracellular currents during synchronous discharge of action potentials by enormous populations of cardiac muscle cells.

❖ In a single cardiac cycle monitored on an ECG lead, the P wave represents action potential initiation in the atria, the QRS complex represents action potential initiation in the ventricles, and the T wave represents the repolarization of the ventricles.

❖ In first-degree heart block, the number of P waves equals the number of QRS complexes, but the PR interval is prolonged. In second-degree heart block, the number of P waves exceeds the number of QRS complexes, but each QRS complex is coordinated with a preceding P wave. In third-degree heart block, the P waves and QRS complexes are completely independent, and the frequency of P waves exceeds the frequency of QRS complexes.

❖ Hypertrophy of part of the heart shifts the mean electrical axis in the direction of the increased mass of cardiac tissue.

REFERENCES

Downey JM. The Electrocardiogram. In: Johnson LR, ed. *Essential Medical Physiology*. San Diego, CA: Elsevier Academic Press; 2003: 187-200.

Lederer JW. Cardiac electrophysiology and the electrocardiogram. In: Boron WF, Boulpaep EL, eds. *Medical Physiology*. Philadelphia, PA: Elsevier Science; 2003: 483-507.

A 62-year-old woman with a history of atrial fibrillation presents to her primary care physician with worsening shortness of breath when she lies down flat in the supine position. She often has to sleep with several pillows at night and has frequent urination at night (nocturia). She has noticed that her ankles are more swollen than usual. Of note, she has run out of digoxin, which she takes to control her heart rate. On examination, she is noted to be slightly hypotensive with a blood pressure (BP) of 90/65 mm Hg. Her heart rate is 120 beats per minute (bpm) and is irregularly irregular, consistent with atrial fibrillation. She has bilateral pulmonary rales and increased jugular venous distention. Her heartbeat is irregularly irregular without a murmur. No S_3 or S_4 is noted. She has 3(+) (out of 4)-dependent peripheral edema of the legs. She is diagnosed with congestive heart failure and admitted to the hospital for further management.

◆ **What is the cause of the fourth heart sound?**

◆ **Why does this patient not have an audible S_4?**

◆ **What factors affect stroke volume?**

◆ **How does stimulation of muscarinic receptors affect contractility?**

ANSWERS TO CASE 11: MECHANICAL HEART ACTIVITY

Summary: A 62-year-old woman has atrial fibrillation with a rapid ventricular response and congestive heart failure. She has run out of digoxin.

◆ **Fourth heart sound:** Filling of the ventricle by atrial systole.

◆ **Reason this patient does not have an S_4:** She is in atrial fibrillation and has no atrial contraction.

◆ **Factors that affect stroke volume:** Contractility, preload (ventricular end-diastolic pressure and ventricular diastolic compliance), and afterload (aortic pressure).

◆ **Stimulation of muscarinic receptors:** Decreases contractility in atria (parasympathetic system).

CLINICAL CORRELATION

This 62-year-old woman has symptoms of congestive heart failure: fatigue, pedal edema, dyspnea, and orthopnea (needing to sleep on pillows). There are many causes for congestive heart failure. In this patient, atrial fibrillation with irregular ventricular rhythm leads to inadequate ventricular filling and decreased stroke volume. The likely explanation in this case is running out of medication (digoxin). Other factors that can present as congestive heart failure include myocardial infarction and cardiomyopathy (decreased contractility) as well as valvular problems (aortic valve stenosis). Clinically, these patients present with symptoms of fluid "backing up" in the cardiovascular system. They often have pulmonary edema, peripheral edema, and increased jugular distention. A chest x-ray will reveal bilateral pulmonary edema with cardiomegaly. An echocardiograph can be used to calculate the ejection fraction, a measure of contractility. The ejection fraction is the fraction of the end-diastolic volume ejected in each stroke volume (normal = 55%). Treatment of congestive heart failure depends on the etiology, but usually diuretics are given to relieve some of the excess fluid and medications are given (digitalis) to increase the contractility of the heart and improve cardiac output. A patient with atrial fibrillation would benefit from medications to decrease conduction through the atrioventricular (AV) node or cardioversion to convert heart rate back to normal sinus rhythm.

APPROACH TO PHYSIOLOGY OF CARDIAC MECHANICS

Objectives

1. Describe excitation–contraction coupling in the heart.
2. Describe factors regulating the force of myocardial contractions.
3. Describe the cardiac cycle.

Definitions

Systole: The period of time during which the heart muscle is contracting.
Diastole: The period of time during which the heart muscle is relaxed.
Heart sounds: The sounds produced by turbulent flow within the heart and by vibrations induced in structures comprising the heart.
Contractility: The ability of a muscle to shorten and/or develop force that does not depend upon a change in initial fiber length or afterload.

DISCUSSION

Cardiac and skeletal muscles have many similarities; however, there are important differences. **Both are striated muscles**, are excitable, and are **regulated by calcium** (see case 6). However, cardiac muscle fibers are smaller than skeletal muscle fibers, and, unlike skeletal muscle fibers, cardiac muscle fibers branch and are electrically coupled to one another.

Excitation of myocardial cells results from the propagation of action potentials from nodal cells, conduction fibers, or adjacent myocardial cells through low-resistance membrane junctions. There are no neuromuscular junctions as is seen in skeletal muscle. As in skeletal muscle, the mediator between membrane action potentials (excitation) and contraction is calcium. However, in contrast to skeletal muscle, a significant amount of calcium enters the cell through sarcolemma calcium channels during the action potential. This **increase in calcium permeability accounts in large part for the plateau phase of the myocardial action potential,** and the calcium that enters triggers the release of additional calcium from the sarcoplasmic reticulum. The entering and released calcium then binds to troponin C to initiate events that lead to contraction. Between action potentials, much of the calcium is taken back up into the sarcoplasmic reticulum by primary active transport. However, to maintain calcium balance, some calcium exits the cell by a secondary active process located on the sarcolemma. Calcium exit is coupled to and driven by the entry of sodium down its electrochemical gradient. The entering sodium then is expelled by the sodium pump.

The force of contraction of cardiac muscle can vary from beat to beat as a result of two basic mechanisms inherent to cardiac muscle. The first is the **length–tension (or force) relationship,** also known as the **Starling law of the**

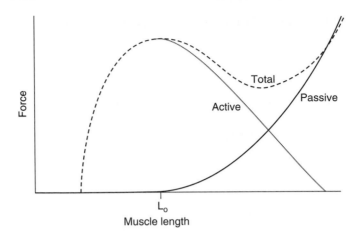

Figure 11-1. Relationship of muscle force and muscle length. The active and passive characteristics are added to supply a composite.

heart. A basic property of all muscles is that there is an optimal length for active force development. At lengths greater and less than this optimal length (L_o), less active force will be developed (see Figure 11-1). In vivo, this relationship is not important for skeletal muscles because their lengths are restricted close to L_o because of their attachment to tendons and bones. For the heart, however, the size of the chambers and hence the length of the cardiac muscle cells before systole will vary depending on the end-diastolic volume of blood. This volume in turn depends in large part on central venous pressure and the compliance of the ventricles. Under most conditions, myocardial cells operate at lengths at which an increase in end-diastolic muscle length leads to a more forceful contraction and a larger stroke volume. This helps balance venous return and cardiac output. The length–tension relationship may have both structural and biochemical bases. For active force to develop, myosin cross-bridges must interact with actin filaments. At L_o, the overlap of thick and thin filaments is such that every cross-bridge has easy access to actin (thin) filaments, allowing each one to develop force. At muscle lengths longer than L_o, some of the cross-bridges do not overlap thin filaments and thus cannot develop force. At muscle lengths less than L_o, the lateral distances over which the cross-bridges reach to attach to actin filaments is greater, and at very short lengths, thin filaments from one side can interfere with cross-bridge interactions on the other side. Biochemically, it appears that the calcium sensitivity of the actin–myosin interaction also is impaired at short muscle lengths. Thus, activation of the contractile machinery will be less.

The second mechanism responsible for regulating the force of myocardial contraction is referred to as **contractility.** Changes in contractility alter the force of contraction at any given muscle length, as shown in Figure 11-2. An increase in contractility will result in greater force and a greater stroke volume

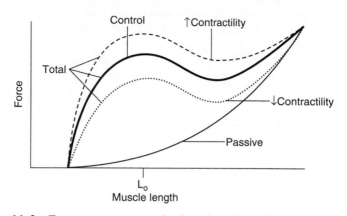

Figure 11-2. Force versus muscle length with different contractility characteristics.

at any muscle length (chamber volume), thus increasing the ejection fraction. A decrease in contractility will have the opposite effect. The **mechanisms** responsible for **changes in contractility** mostly involve **calcium metabolism** and include alterations in (1) calcium entry during the action potential, (2) calcium release from the sarcoplasmic reticulum, (3) calcium binding to troponin-C, (4) calcium uptake by the sarcoplasmic reticulum, and (5) calcium extrusion from the myocyte. Physiologically, changes in contractility result mainly from changes in sympathetic nerve activity. Activation of myocardial β-adrenergic receptors by norepinephrine and epinephrine results in stimulatory G protein activation of adenylyl cyclase and resultant increases in cyclic adenosine monophosphate (cAMP). Increased cAMP activates protein kinase A to phosphorylate key proteins involved in many of the steps of calcium metabolism listed above. The result is greater activation of the myosin–actin interactions and greater force. In contrast, stimulation of muscarinic cholinergic receptors by acetylcholine results in inhibitory G protein activation, inhibition of adenylyl cyclase activity, and less phosphorylation of the same proteins. This results in lesser activation of the myosin–actin interaction and less force.

The pumping of blood by the heart can be described best by considering events during a cardiac cycle, that is, during a **systole** and the following **diastole** (see Figure 11-3). During the time marked A, atrial depolarization, as indicated by the P wave of the electrocardiograph (ECG), leads to atrial contraction (**atrial systole**) and complete ventricular filling. In some cases, the turbulence caused by this filling results in an audible **fourth heart sound.** During the time marked B, **ventricular depolarization,** as indicated by the QRS complex of the ECG, leads to a period of ventricular contraction during which ventricular pressure rises, **closing the AV valves** (producing the **first heart sound**), but there is no ejection of blood into the aorta. This is the period

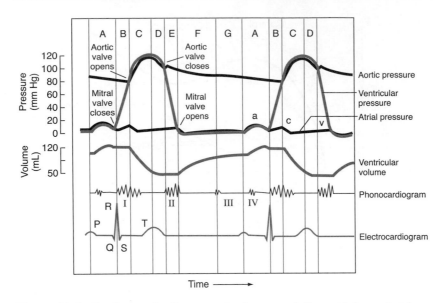

Figure 11-3. Cardiac cycle. Pressures in the aorta, left ventricle, and atrium. Key cardiac valvular events are superimposed on the auscultation of the heart and the electrocardiograph.

of **isovolumetric ventricular contraction.** During the time marked C, ventricular pressure surpasses aortic pressure and there is rapid emptying of blood, as indicated by the decrease in ventricular volume and the increase in aortic pressure. This constitutes the **rapid ventricular ejection** phase of the cycle. During the time indicated by D, the ventricles are repolarizing, as indicated by the T wave of the ECG; the force of ventricular contraction is decreasing; and the flow of blood into the aorta slows. This is the **reduced ventricular ejection** phase. During the time indicated by E, the ventricles continue to relax, and aortic pressure soon exceeds ventricular pressure. This results in closure of the aortic valve and the second heart sound. Ventricular pressure then falls with no change in volume. This is the **isovolumetric ventricular relaxation** phase. During the time indicated by F, ventricular pressure falls below venous pressure, the AV valve opens, and the ventricle begins to fill rapidly, as indicated by the increase in ventricular volume. This is the **rapid ventricular filling** phase that sometimes produces an audible third heart sound. The time indicated by G is the period of **reduced ventricular filling** that occurs before the next period of atrial systole.

COMPREHENSION QUESTIONS

[11.1]   A healthy 23-year-old medical student is participating in a cardiac echocardiography study. During the isovolumetric ventricular contraction phase of the cardiac cycle, which of the following findings take place?

A. Aortic blood pressure is falling
B. Aortic valve is open
C. AV valve is open
D. Second heart sound is produced
E. Ventricular muscle is undergoing repolarization

[11.2]   A 45-year-old man is seen by his cardiologist for increasing weakness and fatigue. He is diagnosed with an enlarged dilated poorly pumping heart (cardiomyopathy). The larger ventricular end-diastolic volumes ("enlarged hearts") can compensate somewhat for the reduced contractility that occurs in this condition because stretching of the ventricular muscle cells results in which of the following?

A. Decreases efflux of calcium during ventricular repolarization
B. Enhances reuptake of calcium by the sarcoplasmic reticulum
C. Enhances influx of calcium during the action potential
D. Enhances interaction of myosin cross-bridges with actin
E. Improves conduction among muscle cells

[11.3]   A 45-year-old male is prescribed an antihypertensive agent that affects calcium channel conductance. If this agent inhibits the influx of calcium into ventricular muscle cells during ventricular excitation, which of the following statements is true?

A. The amount of calcium bound to troponin C during ventricular contraction will be increased.
B. The amount of calcium released from the sarcoplasmic reticulum during ventricular contraction will be increased.
C. The force of ventricular contraction at any given ventricular volume will be decreased.
D. The overlap of thick and thin filaments during ventricular contraction will be increased.

Answers

[11.1]   **A.** During isovolumetric ventricular contraction, ventricular myocytes are depolarized and contract forcefully. Pressure within the ventricle is rising so that it is greater than atrial pressure but less than aortic pressure. Thus, both the AV and the aortic valves are closed. The first, not the second, heart sound is heard as the AV valve closes. Because blood is still flowing out of the aorta during this time, aortic pressure is falling.

[11.2] **D.** An increase in ventricular muscle cell length along its length-tension curve results in a more optimal interaction of cross-bridges with actin, thus producing more force than is produced at the shorter length. There is little if any effect on calcium fluxes or on conduction among muscle cells.

[11.3] **C.** Inhibition of calcium influx during the action potential also reduces the amount of calcium released from the sarcoplasmic reticulum, resulting in less calcium bound to troponin-C and a reduction in the force of contraction. These changes occur independently of ventricular end-diastolic lengths so that force developed at all lengths will be less than it was before drug administration. Because the change in force is length-independent (a change in contractility), the overlap of thick and thin filaments plays no role.

PHYSIOLOGY PEARLS

❖ Calcium influx during excitation is a major determinant of the force of contraction in cardiac muscle but not in skeletal muscle.

❖ During the rapid ventricular ejection phase, aortic pressure is rising, but during the reduced ventricular ejection phase, aortic pressure begins to fall.

❖ The majority of filling of the ventricle with blood occurs during ventricular diastole before atrial contraction.

❖ Ventricular muscle normally begins contracting when it is at lengths less than the optimal length for force development (on the ascending slope of the length–force relationship).

REFERENCES

Downey JM. The mechanical activity of the heart. In: Johnson LR, ed. Essential *Medical Physiology*. 3rd ed. San Diego, CA: Elsevier Academic Press; 2003:201-214.

Levy M, Pappano A. Cardiac pump. In: Levy MN, Koeppen BM, Stanton BA, eds. *Berne & Levy, Principles of Physiology*. 4th ed. Philadelphia, PA: Mosby; 2006:245-259.

Weisbrodt NW. Striated muscle. In: Johnson LR, ed. *Essential Medical Physiology*. 3rd ed. San Diego, CA: Elsevier Academic Press; 2003:123-136.

A 25-year-old pregnant woman is in labor at the hospital. She has no medical problems and has had no complications with this pregnancy. She is in the active phase of labor, feeling intense contractions, and wants pain relief. The anesthesiologist is called and administers an epidural nerve block (including sympathetic blockade) for anesthesia. Shortly after the administration of the epidural, the patient reports feeling light-headed and dizzy. She is noted to be tachycardic (rapid heart rate) and hypotensive (low blood pressure). The anesthesiologist notices the hypotension and gives an intravenous (IV) fluid bolus and a small amount of IV ephedrine. These measures resolve the patient's symptoms and hypotension.

◆ **Why would epidural analgesia cause these symptoms?**

◆ **How would increasing the blood volume change venous pressure (VP)?**

◆ **How would ephedrine counter the hypotension?**

ANSWERS TO CASE 12: REGULATION OF VENOUS RETURN

Summary: A 25-year-old pregnant woman in active labor develops hypotension and tachycardia after epidural analgesia is administered.

◆ **Effects of the epidural:** Sympathetic blockade resulting in decreased VP, and thus decreased cardiac output (CO), and decreased peripheral resistance resulting in hypotension.

◆ **Increase in blood volume:** Increases venous pressure.

◆ **Giving ephedrine:** Increases α_1 stimulation, leading to contraction of the venous musculature, increasing VP and thus CO and peripheral resistance.

CLINICAL CORRELATION

When using any medication, one must be able to anticipate potential adverse effects and be prepared to address them if they occur. This is evident with the epidural anesthesia often used in labor and delivery and in other types of surgeries for pain relief. The pain relief that results from blocking afferent nerves that innervate the uterus (T_{10} to L_3) is associated with a sympathetic blockade that in turn affects venous tone and peripheral resistance. When the sympathetic system is blocked, there is relaxation of venous and arteriolar smooth muscle, resulting in increased unstressed volume and decreased total peripheral resistance (TPR). These changes result in decreased VP, CO, and mean arterial pressure. Clinically, the drop in mean arterial pressure results in tachycardia if sympathetic innervation to the heart is not blocked. CO is calculated by multiplying the heart rate by the stroke volume, and so to try to maintain CO, the body compensates by increasing the heart rate. Anesthesiologists are aware of this complication and preload patients with isotonic IV fluids (500-1000 mL) before administering the epidural. This preload will increase VP (by shifting the vascular function curve to the right), resulting in increased CO. If this preload is not enough, ephedrine often is given to increase venous smooth muscle contraction (decreasing unstressed volume), further increasing VP and CO. The increased CO, plus ephedrine's actions to cause arteriolar constriction, thus increasing TPR, will combine to return mean arterial pressure toward control values.

APPROACH TO PHYSIOLOGY OF VENOUS RETURN

Objectives

1. Discuss the Frank–Starling relationship in terms of VP and CO.
2. Draw and label cardiac and vascular function curves.
3. Diagram the effects that changes in heart rate, contractility, blood volume, venous unstressed volume, and TPR have on the cardiac and vascular function curves and the resultant VPs and COs.

Definitions

Venous return: The volume of blood returning to the heart per minute.
Cardiac function curve: Depicts the dependence of CO on VP.
Vascular function curve: Depicts the dependence of VP on CO.

DISCUSSION

During a steady-state condition, CO and venous return are equal. The level of CO, and hence venous return, at any moment is determined by the interplay of factors that regulate cardiac function and factors that regulate vascular function. As can be seen in Figure 12-1, **CO is a function of VP.** The dependence of CO on VP is referred to as the **Frank–Starling relationship** and is displayed as a cardiac function curve. Blood that is flowing into the heart during diastole will stretch the muscle fibers. The volume of blood entering the heart depends on the VP driving the flow. The greater the VP (going from A to B), the more blood, the longer the muscle cell length, and the greater the force of contraction (see Case 10). Although CO is dependent on VP, the effect that a particular VP will have on CO is not constant. That is, there is not just one curve but a family of curves that adhere to the Frank–Starling relationship. The factors determining CO at any given VP are heart rate, myocardial contractility (see Case 11), TPR, and the pressure outside the heart (intrathoracic pressure).

The level of VP at any single moment is also determined by the interplay of factors that regulate cardiac function and factors that regulate vascular function.

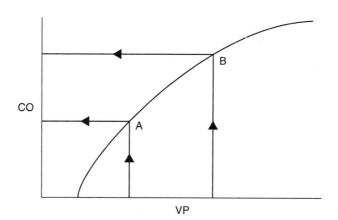

Figure 12-1. Cardiac output in relation to venous pressure. Going from A to B, an increased amount of blood enters the heart, stretching the cardiac muscle length and increasing the force of contraction. CO = cardiac output; VP = venous pressure.

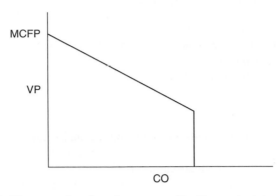

Figure 12-2. The vascular function curve. Cardiac output is a function of venous pressure. CO = cardiac output; VP = venous pressure; MCFP = mean circulatory filling pressure.

As can be seen in Figure 12-2, **VP is a function of CO.** If the heart is stopped, blood will continue to flow from the arteries into the veins until the pressure is the same throughout the cardiovascular system. Thus, arterial pressure will fall and VP will rise. The final pressure is called the mean circulatory filling pressure (MCFP). Once the heart starts pumping again, VP decreases, with the magnitude of the decrease being greater the greater the CO. There is a limit to how high CO can go because of the fact that the veins will collapse at low VPs. This **relationship between CO and VP** describes a **vascular function curve.** Just as the relationship between VP and CO depends on other factors, so does the relationship between CO and VP. The MCFP (VP at zero CO) depends on blood volume and the state of contraction of venous smooth muscle (unstressed volume). The **greater the blood volume** and the **greater the contraction of venous smooth muscle,** the **greater the MCFP.** The slope of the vascular function curve depends mainly on TPR. The greater the TPR, the greater the fall in VP for any given increase in CO.

The results of the interplay of the cardiac function curve and the vascular function curve, along with the effects of changing the factors that influence those curves, can be illustrated and understood by combining the two curves. Usually the vascular function curve is flipped so that VP is on the x-axis and CO is on the y–axis as in Figure 12-3. The point where the two lines cross— the **"equilibrium point" (A)**—defines the CO and the VP that exist under the current conditions. Changes in any of the factors that affect the cardiac function curve and/or the vascular function curve alter both CO and VP.

Increases in heart rate, increases in myocardial contractility, and decreases in TPR all increase CO at any VP. This can be viewed by **shifting the cardiac function curve upward** to yield a new equilibrium point (B in Figure 12-3). Of course, opposite changes in heart rate, contractility, and TPR will decrease

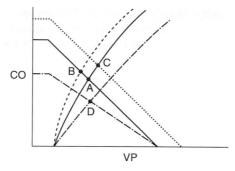

Figure 12-3. The equilibrium point. The equilibrium points indicate the CO and VP that exist under various conditions as described in the text. CO = cardiac output; VP = venous pressure.

CO at any VP and would shift the curve downward. Increases in blood volume and contraction of venous smooth muscle increase VP at any CO. This can be seen by shifting the vascular function curve to a higher MCFP but keeping the slope the same, producing a new equilibrium point (C in Figure 12-3). Note that CO also is increased if factors affecting the cardiac function curve do not change. Decreases in blood volume and relaxation of venous smooth muscle, as occurred in this case, would have the opposite effect, a decrease in VP (and a decrease in CO if factors affecting the cardiac function curve do not change). The effects of changes in TPR alone are a little more difficult to understand and visualize. Increases in TPR do not change MCFP, but they do decrease VP at all other COs. This can be visualized by shifting the vascular function curve counterclockwise. Viewing this shift in combination with the shift that an increase in TPR has on the cardiac function curve indicates that there will be a decrease in CO (point D in Figure 12-3). This decrease in CO will moderate the increase in mean arterial pressure (MAP) that results from the increase in TPR.

COMPREHENSION QUESTIONS

[12.1] A patient exhibits an elevated jugular venous pressure. This could be the direct result of which of the following?

    A. Decreased blood volume

    B. Decreased myocardial contractility

    C. Increased heart rate

    D. Increased total peripheral resistance (TPR)

    E. Relaxation of venous smooth muscle

[12.2]   A patient with a bleeding duodenal ulcer arrives at the hospital with a markedly low mean arterial pressure. In addition to the low MAP, this patient is likely to exhibit which of the following?

A. Decreased heart rate
B. Decreased myocardial contractility
C. Decreased TPR
D. Decreased VP
E. Increased CO

[12.3]   A 48-year-old male with malignant hypertension and a markedly elevated mean arterial pressure is given a drug that relaxes arterioles, thus reducing TPR. Which of the following is most likely to result from the reduction of TPR in this manner?

A. Decreased CO
B. Decreased heart rate
C. Decreased myocardial contractility
D. Increased blood volume
E. Increased VP

Answers

[12.1]   **B.** Elevations in central VP can result from contraction of venous smooth muscle and increases in blood volume, but most often they are caused by defects in cardiac function such as a reduction in myocardial contractility. The direct effects of a decrease in myocardial contractility can be viewed on a combined vascular and cardiac function curve by shifting the cardiac function curve downward.

[12.2]   **D.** Loss of blood will result in a decrease in MCFP and can be expressed as a decrease in VP and a decrease in CO. This will lead to a decrease in mean arterial pressure and a compensatory increase in heart rate, myocardial contractility, and TPR. The direct effects of a decrease in blood volume can be viewed on a combined vascular and cardiac function curve by shifting the MCFP to the left without changing the slope of the vascular function curve.

[12.3]   **E.** A decrease in TPR will result in a shift of blood from the arterial side to the venous side of the circulation, thus increasing VP and CO without changing blood volume. The decrease in TPR most likely also will result in a decrease in mean arterial pressure and a compensatory increase in heart rate and myocardial contractility. The direct effects of a decrease in TPR can be viewed on a combined vascular and cardiac function curve mainly by shifting the slope of the vascular function curve upward. (Note that a decrease in TPR also will shift the cardiac function curve upward, but the effect is not enough to bring VP back to its initial value.)

PHYSIOLOGY PEARLS

❖ CO at any given VP is a function of heart rate, contractility, TPR, and intrathoracic pressure and is represented by the cardiac function curve.

❖ VP at any given CO is a function of blood volume, unstressed volume, and TPR and is represented by the vascular function curve.

❖ The CO and VP at any one time is the result of the interplay of those factors determining the cardiac and vascular functions curves.

REFERENCES

Downey JM. Regulation of venous return and cardiac output. In: Johnson LR, ed. *Essential Medical Physiology*. 3rd ed. San Diego, CA: Elsevier Academic Press; 2003:215-224.

Levy M, Pappano A. Cardiac pump. In: Levy MN, Koeppen BM, Stanton BA, eds. *Berne & Levy, Principles of Physiology*. 4th ed. Philadelphia, PA: Mosby; 2006:320-331.

❖ CASE 13

A 57-year-old man with long-standing diabetes mellitus and newly diagnosed hypertension presents to his primary care physician for follow-up. The patient has been trying to alter his dietary habits and now exercises more frequently, but the hypertension has persisted. The patient is started on an angiotensin-converting enzyme inhibitor (ACE inhibitor) with good results. He is instructed to continue this medication and follow up in several months.

◆ **What neural and humoral pathways regulate arterial pressure?**

◆ **What are two effects of angiotensin II?**

◆ **How would inhibition of ACE decrease blood pressure?**

ANSWERS TO CASE 13: REGULATION OF ARTERIAL PRESSURE

Summary: A 57-year-old diabetic man is diagnosed with hypertension that is not controlled with lifestyle changes and requires medication (an ACE inhibitor).

◆ There are two pathways for the regulation of arterial blood pressure:

◆ **Neural:** Baroreceptor reflex (fast acting).

◆ **Humoral:** Renin-angiotensin-aldosterone system (slow acting).

◆ **Effects of angiotensin II:** Stimulates the adrenal cortex to synthesize and secrete aldosterone and causes vasoconstriction of the arterioles.

◆ **Inhibition of ACE:** Prevents conversion of angiotensin I to angiotensin II.

CLINICAL CORRELATION

The 57-year-old patient in this case has diabetes and hypertension. Tight control of the blood sugars helps slow down both the microvascular (small vessel) disease and macrovascular (atherosclerotic) disease. Aggressive control of the hypertension is also vital, particularly in helping to prevent heart disease and renal complications. In diabetic patients, ACE inhibitors are usually the best agents. ACE inhibitors stop the conversion of angiotensin I to angiotensin II. Decreased angiotensin II causes decreased secretion of aldosterone and decreased vasoconstriction of the arterioles, resulting in decreased blood pressure. Studies have shown that for diabetic patients with microalbuminuria, ACE inhibitors can slow progression to renal failure. Possible side effects for all ACE inhibitors include a cough, hyperkalemia, reversible decreased renal function, and, rarely, angioedema.

APPROACH TO ARTERIAL PRESSURE PHYSIOLOGY

Objectives

1. Discuss the determinants of mean arterial pressure (MAP).
2. Describe the baroreceptor reflex.
3. Describe the renin-angiotensin-aldosterone system.
4. Describe the effects of aldosterone on renal function and arterial blood pressure.

Definitions

MAP: The blood pressure in the large arteries averaged over time.
Total peripheral resistance (TPR): The resistance to blood flow in the systemic circulation.
Baroreceptor reflex: A neural reflex involved in the short-term regulation of arterial blood pressure.

DISCUSSION

MAP is determined by the interplay of **TPR** and **cardiac output (CO),** as is given by the equation

$$MAP = TPR \times CO$$

In reality, the equation should read (MAP – VP) = TPR × CO where VP is venous pressure. However, VP is so low (0-5 mm Hg) that it generally is ignored in the equation. Although VP can be ignored in this situation, it is of vital importance and cannot be ignored when the regulation of CO is considered (see Case 12).

TPR is **due mostly to the resistance** to flow offered by the **small arteries and arterioles** in the various vascular beds. These vessels are composed in large part by smooth muscle that contracts in response to the sympathetic nerve neurotransmitter norepinephrine and to the circulating hormones epinephrine, angiotensin II, and antidiuretic hormone (ADH, or vasopressin), among others. Contraction decreases vessel radius, thus increasing resistance to flow.

In young and middle-aged individuals, arterial blood pressure normally is maintained around 120/80 mm Hg. **Hypertension** currently is defined as systolic pressures of 140 mm Hg or more and/or diastolic pressures of 90 mm Hg or more. Regulation of blood pressure within rather narrow limits or set points is accomplished through a complex system of neural and humoral mechanisms that are not completely understood. Even less is known about the genetic and environmental factors that determine the set points.

Arterial pressure is determined by the interplay of **CO** and **TPR.** Thus, factors that influence either or both will influence blood pressure. One of the major factors is the **autonomic nervous system.** Afferent nerves that behave as stretch receptors (baroreceptors) are located mainly in the carotid sinus and the aortic arch and respond to intraluminal pressure. Nerve impulses from these receptors arrive and are processed in the brainstem. Regions within the brainstem then regulate the activities of sympathetic and parasympathetic efferent nerves, which in turn regulate both CO and TPR.

The sinoatrial (SA) and atrioventricular (AV) nodes of the heart are innervated by both sympathetic and parasympathetic efferent nerves. Norepinephrine released locally from sympathetic nerves and norepinephrine and epinephrine arriving from the adrenal gland increase the rate of depolarization of the SA node and increase conduction through the AV node, thus increasing heart rate. The same substances also stimulate receptors on myocardial cells to increase contractility. In contrast, acetylcholine (ACh) released locally from parasympathetic nerves decreases the rate of depolarization of the SA node and conduction through the AV node, thus decreasing heart rate. There appears to be minimal parasympathetic innervation of contractile myocardial cells; however, the decrease in heart rate itself will result in a decrease in myocardial contractility. As discussed in Case 12, changes in both heart rate and contractility can lead to changes in CO and thus MAP.

Arteries, especially arterioles, and veins are innervated by sympathetic nerves. Norepinephrine released from these nerves and norepinephrine and epinephrine released from the adrenal gland contract arteries to regulate TPR. As discussed in Case 12, changes in TPR directly affect MAP. Norepinephrine and epinephrine also contract veins to regulate mean circulatory filling pressure. As discussed in Case 12, changes in mean circulatory filling pressure affect venous pressure, which in turn affects CO and thus MAP.

The **neural reflex** described above, which is called the **baroreceptor reflex,** can respond rapidly to changes in MAP brought on by normal activity and by pathologic conditions such as those characterized by blood loss. For example, as a result of the forces of gravity, merely going from a supine to an upright position will cause a rapid increase in pressure in vessels of the lower extremities and a decrease in pressure in vessels of the upper extremities, including the carotid arteries. The increase in pressure in the veins below the heart leads to an increase in unstressed volume, a decrease in central venous pressure, and a decrease in CO (see Case 12). This decrease in CO decreases MAP to decrease the pressure in the carotid arteries further. The decreased pressure in the carotid sinus is sensed rapidly by the baroreceptors to initiate the reflex release of norepinephrine and epinephrine. These chemical mediators in turn rapidly contract the veins, thus increasing venous pressure, and rapidly increase heart rate and contractility; together, these changes increase CO. The mediators also contract the arterioles, rapidly increasing TPR. The increased CO and increased TPR quickly return MAP to the normal value, thus maintaining cerebral blood flow.

A second major factor regulating blood pressure is the hormonal **renin-angiotensin-aldosterone system. Renin** is an enzyme that is synthesized and stored in cells lining the renal afferent arteriole at the point where it contacts the thick ascending limb of the loop of Henle of the nephron in a region called the juxtaglomerular apparatus. Renin is secreted into the bloodstream in response to norepinephrine released from sympathetic nerves distributed to the afferent arteriole, to a decrease in afferent arteriolar pressure (the cells act as baroreceptors), and to unknown paracrine signals from cells that line the thick ascending limb of the loop of Henle. These paracrine signals are released in response to the rate of flow and the composition of the tubular fluid. Once released, renin cleaves the circulating α_2 globulin **angiotensinogen** to yield **angiotensin I.** Angiotensin I is relatively inactive itself, but it is cleaved rapidly by ACE to yield angiotensin II. ACE is found in many tissues but is present in relatively high amounts in the lung. Circulating angiotensin II has two major actions: It is a potent stimulator of arteriolar smooth muscle contraction, and thus it increases TPR. This is a relatively rapid response, but not as rapid as the baroreceptor reflex. Perhaps more important for the long-term regulation of blood pressure, angiotensin II stimulates the release of aldosterone from the adrenal cortex. As discussed in Case 22, aldosterone increases the reabsorption of sodium and water from the nephron. Thus, more of the salt and water that are ingested are retained, resulting in the expansion of blood and interstitial volume. The increase in extracellular volume, along with other actions that are understood less fully, results in a long-term increase in MAP.

COMPREHENSION QUESTIONS

[13.1] Patients with elevated MAP often are prescribed drugs that inhibit angiotensin-converting enzyme (ACE). Which of the following findings is most likely to be observed in patients on these drugs alone?

A. A further increase in TPR
B. Increased plasma renin levels
C. Decreased sympathetic nerve activity
D. Decreased plasma angiotensin I levels
E. Increased plasma aldosterone levels

[13.2] Licorice contains a chemical that enhances the aldosterone-like effects of cortisol. Thus, patients who ingest large amounts of licorice (which is an ingredient in some herbal medicines as well as a candy) will likely exhibit which of the following?

A. Increased blood pressure
B. Increased plasma renin levels
C. Increased plasma aldosterone levels
D. Increased TPR
E. Decreased central venous pressure

[13.3] In response to the loss of blood, compensatory mechanisms come into play at various times to blunt decreases in MAP and restore blood volume to normal. Which of the following most accurately depicts the temporal order of effectiveness of three of these mechanisms, from earliest to latest?

A. Aldosterone, sympathetic nerves, angiotensin II
B. Angiotensin II, aldosterone, sympathetic nerves
C. Angiotensin II, sympathetic nerves, aldosterone
D. Sympathetic nerves, aldosterone, angiotensin II
E. Sympathetic nerves, angiotensin II, aldosterone

Answers

[13.1]   **B.** Inhibition of ACE will reduce the formation of angiotensin II, a constrictor of arteriolar smooth muscle, thus reducing TPR. The decreased angiotensin II also will lead to a decrease in aldosterone secretion. However, the decrease in angiotensin II and in mean arterial blood pressure will result in an increase in plasma renin and angiotensin I concentrations and an increase in sympathetic nerve activity.

[13.2]   **A.** The aldosterone-like effects induced by licorice will result in NaCl
          and water retention and an expansion of blood volume. This will lead
          to an increase in venous pressure, CO, and MAP. Plasma levels of
          both renin and aldosterone will be decreased.

[13.3]   **E.** As part of the baroreceptor response, sympathetic nerve activity
          will increase almost immediately in response to the decrease in MAP
          induced by the loss of blood. The increased sympathetic nerve activ-
          ity and the reduced renal arterial pressure will result quickly in the
          secretion of renin, which initiates a cascade that results in the pro-
          duction of angiotensin II, a powerful constrictor of arterial smooth
          muscle. Although angiotensin II will induce the secretion of aldos-
          terone rather quickly, the onset of action of aldosterone is rather slow
          because expression of its actions requires the synthesis of proteins in
          renal epithelial cells.

PHYSIOLOGY PEARLS

❖   The level of MAP is determined by the interplay between TPR and
     CO, as given by the equation

$$MAP = TPR \times CO$$

❖   TPR is determined primarily by the state of contraction of the small
     arteries and arterioles.
❖   Rapid reflex changes in CO and TPR are accomplished through acti-
     vation of the sympathetic nervous system.
❖   Longer term regulation of CO and blood pressure results from regu-
     lation of extracellular (blood) volume by the renin-angiotensin-
     aldosterone pathway.

REFERENCES

Berne RM, Levy MN. Cardiovascular system. In: Berne RM, Levy MN, eds.
    Principles of Physiology. 3rd ed. St. Louis: Mosby; 2000:289-299.
Granger DN. Regulation of arterial pressure. In: Johnson LR, ed. *Essential Medical
    Physiology*. 3rd ed. San Diego: Elsevier Academic Press; 2003:225-234.

A 21-year-old woman presents to her primary care physician because she wants to begin an exercise program for weight loss. She is concerned because when she exercised in the past, she noticed that her heart seemed to beat rapidly. She has no known medical history and has no family members with medical problems. She denies chest pain. After a thorough physical examination, everything appears to be normal and the physician reassures the patient that her increased heart rate is probably a normal response to exercise.

◆ **In what two ways is blood flow to skeletal muscle controlled?**

◆ **What are some differences between cerebral circulation and skeletal circulation?**

◆ **What are some forms of extrinsic control of blood flow?**

ANSWERS TO CASE 14: REGIONAL BLOOD FLOW

Summary: A 21-year-old woman who is beginning an exercise program has a normal examination and normal physiologic increased heart rate with exercise.

◆ **Control of blood flow in skeletal muscle:** Sympathetic innervation and local metabolic control.

◆ **Differences between cerebral circulation and skeletal circulation:** Cerebral blood flow demonstrates autoregulation and is controlled almost entirely by local metabolic factors. Skeletal muscle relies on input from both sympathetic innervation and local metabolic factors.

◆ **Forms of extrinsic control of blood flow:** Sympathetic innervation and vasoactive hormones (bradykinin, serotonin, prostaglandins, angiotensin II, antidiuretic hormone [ADH], etc.).

CLINICAL CORRELATION

A more complete understanding of the cardiovascular changes that take place under varying physiologic conditions and under the influence of medications requires knowledge about the factors that regulate blood flow to specific vascular beds. Exercise is a common physiologic condition during which there are many changes. Increases in blood flow to contracting skeletal muscle are caused by both extrinsic and intrinsic factors. With increased muscle metabolism, there is an increase in vasodilator metabolites such as lactic acid, potassium, and adenosine. The increase in vasodilator metabolites represents intrinsic control over skeletal circulation. Extrinsic factors include sympathetic system activation, which results in increased heart rate and elevated venous pressure, thus increasing cardiac output. If the exercise is intense, sympathetic stimulation results in increased arteriolar resistance in the gastrointestinal tract, kidneys, and other organs, resulting in shunting of blood toward the exercising muscles. Adequate blood flow to a tissue allows for exchange of substrates and metabolites between cells of the tissue and the blood as blood flows through capillaries.

APPROACH TO REGIONAL BLOOD FLOW

Objectives

1. Describe the mechanisms of intrinsic control of regional blood flow.
2. Describe the mechanisms of extrinsic control of regional blood flow.
3. Compare and contrast the control of blood flow to the heart, brain, skeletal muscle, and skin.
4. Describe the transfer of substrates, metabolites, and volume between capillaries and interstitial fluid.

Definitions

Autoregulation: The process of maintaining blood flow constant in the face of varying mean arterial pressures.

Active hyperemia: The increase in blood flow in response to an increase in metabolic activity.

Reactive hyperemia: The temporary increase in blood flow seen following a period of ischemia.

Edema safety factor: Compensatory mechanisms (mostly increases in lymph flow) that can accommodate increases in capillary filtration and mitigate edema formation.

DISCUSSION

Blood flow to any organ of the body over any period of time normally is correlated closely with that **organ's metabolic activity.** If activity increases, blood flow increases to that organ, but not to others unless their levels of activity change as well. This local control of blood flow is accomplished by intrinsic and extrinsic factors that act to alter the resistance of small arteries and arterioles in the vascular beds of the organ.

Local changes in resistance can result in local changes in blood flow, as described by the following equation:

Local flow = mean arterial pressure/local resistance

As discussed in Cases 12 and 13, mean arterial pressure (MAP) is maintained at a fairly constant level and is determined by the interplay of cardiac output (CO) and total peripheral resistance (TPR). Because a change in resistance in any vascular bed will affect TPR, the only way MAP can remain constant is for CO to change or for there to be equal and opposite changes in resistance in other vascular beds to keep TPR constant. Normally, unless the local changes in resistance are great, CO will change so that the metabolic demands of all the organs of the body are met.

Many organs, especially the brain, exhibit **autoregulation** of their blood flow. As long as their metabolic activities do not change, they are able to maintain a **constant blood flow over a wide range of mean arterial pressures.** Thus, in circumstances in which MAP does deviate from normal levels, local arteriolar resistance will change so that blood flow still matches metabolic demand.

All organs, especially skeletal and cardiac muscles, exhibit active and reactive hyperemia. **Active hyperemia** is the increase in blood flow that occurs as the metabolic activity of an organ increases. The mechanism for the increased blood flow is a decrease in local resistance in the face of a stable MAP. The result is a matching of blood flow to metabolic demand. **Reactive hyperemia** is the increase in blood flow that occurs after restoration of blood flow to an organ that has been deprived temporarily of blood. The mechanism also is a decrease in local resistance, but one that develops during the period of ischemia.

The **changes in local arteriolar resistance** that occur during autoregulation, active hyperemia, and reactive hyperemia are due mostly, if not solely, to local intrinsic mechanisms. During autoregulation, a change in MAP initially causes a change in blood flow. If MAP is increased, flow initially increases and local concentrations of metabolites (CO_2, K^+, H^+, adenosine) decrease as a result of washout; local concentrations of substrates (O_2) increase because supply is greater than demand. Opposite changes in metabolite and substrate concentrations occur if MAP is decreased to decrease flow initially. Because metabolites relax and substrates support the contraction of arteriolar smooth muscle, changes in their local concentrations alter local resistance to blood flow to bring flow back to its previous state.

During active hyperemia, increased organ metabolic activity tends to increase metabolite concentrations and decrease substrate concentrations and thus bring about relaxation of arteriolar smooth muscle, decreased local resistance, and increased local blood flow. During reactive hyperemia, local metabolites accumulate and local substrates decrease during the period of ischemia, causing arteriolar dilation and a decrease in local resistance. Then, when the obstruction causing the ischemia is removed, blood flow is increased as a result of the arteriolar dilation. Most often, reactive hyperemia is thought of in relation to those times when flow is obstructed by resting on an arm or leg in such a way that flow is obstructed temporarily. However, reactive hyperemia also occurs along with active hyperemia during muscle contraction. For example, during contraction of ventricular muscle, vessels embedded in the myocardium are compressed to block flow. Metabolites continue to build further, relaxing resistance vessels, so that when flow can begin again during ventricular relaxation, it is increased.

In addition to the intrinsic control described above, regional blood flow may be regulated by **extrinsic factors,** mainly the sympathetic nervous system. The degree of sympathetic innervation of small arteries and arterioles varies from organ to organ. In some organs (eg, skin, intestine, kidney) it is quite dense, and sympathetic tone exists even under normal resting conditions. The norepinephrine released by these nerves contracts the smooth muscle of these vessels to varying degrees, thus regulating local resistance to blood flow. Under most conditions, this extrinsic mechanism works in concert with intrinsic mechanisms to provide blood flow that is adequate to meet the metabolic demands of the organs or, in the case of the kidney, to fulfill its role in maintaining homeostasis. However, under conditions in which the baroreceptor reflex or other reflexes are elicited, sympathetic tone will increase to override intrinsic mechanisms temporarily. This will result in an increase in both local and total peripheral resistance to restore MAP. The result of this is a decrease in blood flow to organs with a high degree of extrinsic regulation (eg, skin, intestine, kidney) and a maintenance or increase in blood flow to organs with a lower degree of extrinsic control (eg, brain and heart).

Capillary Physiology

Exchange of substrates and metabolites between the blood and tissues of the body takes place at the **level of the capillary.** Exchange is possible because every cell of the body is within a few microns of one of the billions of capillaries in the body and because the capillary wall is thin, being composed of a single layer of endothelial cells. In addition, endothelial cells abut one another in such a way that there are clefts between them, resulting in a **high permeability.** Thus, small molecules such as oxygen, carbon dioxide, ions, glucose, amino acids, urea, and lactate, as well as water, can move readily between the capillary lumen and the interstitial fluid. The majority of exchange between the capillary and the interstitium takes place by means of **diffusion.** However, the relatively high permeability results in bulk flow of volume either out of (filtration) or into (absorption) the capillary, depending on the balance of forces across the capillary wall.

There is a **hydrostatic pressure** in the capillary (P_c) that is owing to the forces responsible for blood flow. This pressure favors filtration. There also is a **hydrostatic pressure** exerted by the interstitial fluid (P_{IF}). This pressure, if above atmospheric pressure, will favor **absorption into the capillary.** The other forces across the wall are **osmotic forces** that are due mainly to the presence of proteins in the blood and the interstitium. **Proteins in the blood,** mainly albumin, cannot cross the capillary wall readily and thus exert an osmotic force (often called an oncotic force, π_c). This force favors absorption. **Proteins in the interstitial fluid** exert a force (π_{IF}) that favors filtration. The interaction of all these forces can be expressed in what is called the **Starling equation for the capillary:**

$$J_v = K_f \left[(P_c - P_{IF}) - (\pi_c - \pi_{IF}) \right]$$

where J_v represents the net flux of volume and K_f is the filtration coefficient (a measure of the permeability of the capillary wall that will vary from one capillary bed to another). If the algebraic sum of the forces favoring filtration exceeds the sum of those favoring absorption, fluid will leave the capillary at a rate determined by K_f and the net force.

Capillary hydrostatic force (P_c) changes along the **length of the capillary,** being higher at the arteriolar end than at the venule end. This can result in net filtration at the arteriolar end and absorption at the venule end. P_c also can change from moment to moment because of contraction and relaxation of arteriolar and precapillary sphincter smooth muscle. The presence of this muscle also means that pressure in the large arteries can increase and decrease with little change in P_c. In contrast, changes in venous pressure always result in changes in P_c. Elevations in venous pressure often lead to a marked increase in filtration and the development of **edema.**

Although capillary oncotic pressure (π_c) does not change acutely, decreases in plasma albumin do occur with many liver and kidney diseases. With **hypoalbuminemia,** the main force responsible for absorption, π_c **will decrease,** and this too can result in **edema.**

Interstitial fluid hydrostatic force (P_{IF}) is interesting in that it normally is subatmospheric and thus **favors filtration** rather than the expected absorption. P_{IF} is subatmospheric as a result of the action of lymphatic vessels. These blind-ended vessels are responsible for the return of the net filtered fluid and protein to the circulation via the thoracic duct. Because of their pumping action, small increases in capillary filtration can be accommodated without interstitial volume increasing to the point of edema. Thus, **lymphatics** are responsible for an **edema safety factor.** However, if lymphatic function is impaired, edema will form even if capillary forces are normal.

COMPREHENSION QUESTIONS

[14.1]   A 22-year-old subject who is sitting quietly begins to squeeze a rubber ball repetitively in her right hand, using moderate strength. During this time her mean arterial pressure does not increase. Using her cardiovascular state prior to the exercise as a baseline, which of the following would best describe her cardiovascular state during the exercise?

A. Increased blood flow through her right brachial artery
B. No change in cardiac output
C. Increased total peripheral resistance
D. Decreased blood flow through her left brachial artery
E. Decreased heart rate

[14.2]   A 25-year-old otherwise healthy patient is involved in a motor vehicle accident, and suffers appreciable blood loss. The cardiac output is falling because of a loss of blood. As a compensatory mechanism, the total peripheral resistance increases to attempt to maintain MAP. Which of the following vasculature corresponding to the listed organ is contributing the least to the elevated TPR?

A. Brain
B. Small intestine
C. Kidney
D. Skeletal muscle
E. Skin

[14.3]   If blood flow to an arm is obstructed for more than 30 seconds or so during the process of a blood pressure measurement, the release of the blood pressure cuff will be followed by a temporarily higher than resting level of blood flow through the arm. Which of the following best describes the temporarily higher blood flow?

A. Accompanied by an increase in total peripheral resistance
B. Called active hyperemia
C. Caused by a temporary increase in mean arterial pressure
D. Caused by local vasodilation resulting from the buildup of local metabolites
E. Caused by the shifting of blood flow from other organs

[14.4]   A patient has a renal condition that results in the loss of albumin in the urine that exceeds the body's albumin production. The resulting hypoalbuminemia will lead to edema of the hands, face, and feet. Which of the following is likely to be noted?

A. Decrease in interstitial fluid hydrostatic pressure (P_{IF})
B. Increase in capillary hydrostatic pressure (P_c)
C. Increase in lymph flow
D. Increase in plasma oncotic pressure (π_c)
E. Increase in the filtration coefficient (K_f) of capillaries in the skin

Answers

[14.1]   **A.** The increased metabolic activity of the muscles in the subject's right arm will induce relaxation of small arteries and arterioles, thus reducing local resistance as well as total peripheral resistance. This, along with no change in mean arterial pressure, will result in an increase in blood flow through her right brachial artery. The increased blood flow to the right arm will be accomplished by an increase in heart rate and cardiac output, not by a decrease in flow to other organs.

[14.2]   **A.** In cases in which cardiac output is inadequate, compensatory mechanisms come into play so that blood flow to vital organs such as the heart and brain is preserved as much as possible. One of these mechanisms is activation of sympathetic nerves to constrict small arteries and arterioles in organs whose vessels are heavily innervated. Vessels in the brain and heart undergo the least vasoconstriction.

[14.3]   **D.** During the occlusion, metabolites build up in the arm tissues. These metabolites cause relaxation of arteriolar smooth muscle and decreased local vascular resistance. When the dilated local vessels are exposed again to blood under normal mean arterial pressure, flow is greater than it was before occlusion. This reactive hyperemia is temporary because the increased flow will return metabolites to their normal resting value. Neither mean arterial pressure nor blood flow to other organs need be altered during this time.

[14.4]   **C.** Hypoalbuminemia results in a decreased π_c, the major force favoring absorption. This results in an increase in capillary filtration, an increase in lymph flow, and an increase in P_{IF} to levels above atmospheric. Once the edema safety factor is exceeded, edema results. Unless endothelial cells were damaged, there would be no change in K_f. Also, hypoalbuminemia has no direct effect on P_c (it most likely would decrease as a result of arteriolar constriction to maintain mean arterial pressure).

PHYSIOLOGY PEARLS

❖ Local resistance to blood flow in all tissues changes such that blood flow is adequate to meet the metabolic demands of the tissues.

❖ In certain tissues—skin, gastrointestinal, renal—but not in others—heart, brain—local regulation can be temporarily overridden by extrinsic factors in attempts to maintain mean arterial pressure.

❖ Changes in blood flow through any vascular bed normally are met by changes in cardiac output.

❖ The exchange of substrates and metabolites between blood and tissue occurs at the level of the capillaries, mostly by means of diffusion.

❖ Fluid filtration out of and absorption into capillaries depend on the balance between hydrostatic and osmotic forces across the capillary wall. Disruptions in this balance can lead to edema.

REFERENCES

Granger DN. Regulation of regional blood flow and capillary exchange. In: Johnson LR, ed. *Essential Medical Physiology*. 3rd ed. San Diego, CA: Elsevier Academic Press; 2003:235-258.

Levy M, Pappano A. Cardiovascular system. In: Levy MN, Koeppen BM, Stanton BA, eds. *Berne & Levy, Principles of Physiology*. 4th ed. Philadelphia, PA: Mosby; 2006:298-319.

A 34-year-old woman with diabetes presents to the emergency department with complaints of fever, chills, back pain, dizziness, and shortness of breath. She reports a new-onset nonproductive cough and denies having chest pain. She reports no sick contacts. On examination, she is ill-appearing, febrile, hypotensive, and tachycardic. She has marked right costovertebral (flank) tenderness. Her lung examination demonstrates course rales and rhonchi throughout both lung fields. Her heart rate is tachycardic, but with a regular rhythm. Her oxygen saturation on room air is very low at 80% (normal > 94%). Urinalysis reveals numerous bacteria and leukocytes, consistent with a urinary tract infection. She is diagnosed with pyelonephritis and septic shock and has evidence of adult respiratory distress syndrome (ARDS) with bilateral pulmonary infiltrates on chest x-ray. The emergency room physician explains to the patient that pulmonary injury has led to leaky pulmonary capillaries.

◆ **How does pulmonary capillary leakage cause hypoxia?**

◆ **After a patient takes a normal breath and exhales, what lung volume remains?**

◆ **How do obstructive lung diseases such as asthma affect forced expiratory volume?**

ANSWERS TO CASE 15: PULMONARY STRUCTURE AND LUNG CAPACITIES

Summary: A 34-year-old diabetic woman has pyelonephritis, septic shock, and ARDS.

◆ **Pulmonary capillary leakage and hypoxia:** Accumulation of excess fluid outside the capillaries leads to altered local ventilation and perfusion and makes gas exchange inefficient.

◆ **Lung volume remaining after normal breath:** Functional residual capacity (FRC; cannot be measured with spirometry alone).

◆ **Forced expiratory volume with obstructive airway disease:** Decreased.

CLINICAL CORRELATION

Knowledge of respiratory physiology is essential for understanding, diagnosing, and treating many medical conditions. When a patient presents with hypoxia, there may be many different etiologies, but there are two general categories: diseases that affect perfusion of the lungs (pulmonary embolus) and diseases of the bronchial tree (eg, pneumonia, pneumothorax, ARDS, pulmonary edema, asthma, bronchitis). A patient's history and physical examination will help determine the cause of most disorders. A chest x-ray and other radiologic studies may help as well. A patient with pulmonary difficulties may undergo pulmonary function tests to measure and test many of the lung volumes, capacities, and flows. For example, patients with a decrease in forced expiratory volume could have an obstructive lung disorder such as asthma. When the normal balance of reabsorption and lymphatic drainage is overwhelmed by the filtered fluid, fluid will accumulate in the interstitium. The edema can be hydrostatic, which may occur with fluid overload or congestive heart failure, or may be protein-rich, as with ARDS. ARDS is characterized by increased permeability of the capillary endothelium, resulting in a protein-rich fluid collection.

APPROACH TO PULMONARY PHYSIOLOGY

Objectives

1. Diagram lung volumes and capacities.
2. Describe the anatomy of the pulmonary tree.
3. Discuss pulmonary blood flow and regulation.

Definitions

Dead space: The volume of airways and of alveoli in which gas exchange does not take place.

FRC: The volume of air in the lungs when all the muscles of respiration are relaxed.

Vital capacity: The volume of air that can be expelled from the lungs during a forced expiration that starts at total lung capacity (TLC).

FEV$_1$: The volume of air expelled from the lungs during the first second of a forced expiration that starts at TLC.

DISCUSSION

The **exchange of oxygen and carbon dioxide** necessary for metabolism requires that **air and blood be brought into close contact** over a large surface area. This is accomplished by **matching ventilation** of the approximately **300 million alveoli** that constitute the lungs with blood flow to those alveoli. Neither the distribution of alveolar ventilation nor the distribution of blood flow is uniform within the lung; certain regions receive more of both, whereas other regions receive less of both. Normally, however, ventilation and flow are matched to provide optimal gas exchange.

Ventilation of alveoli is accomplished by the regulated movement of air into and out of the lung. During normal breathing while a person is at rest, a fairly constant volume of air moves in and out of the alveoli and airways with each breath. This is called the **tidal volume** and can be measured with a device called a **spirometer.** There are several kinds of spirometers, but all are able to monitor airflow without adding extra resistance or causing significant changes in air composition. In addition to tidal volume measurements, several other lung volumes and lung capacities can be measured with a spirometer (Figure 15-1).

If one makes a normal inspiration and then continues to inhale as much air as possible, the additional air inspired after the tidal volume is the **inspiratory reserve volume.** In a similar manner, the **expiratory reserve volume** is the volume of air exhaled if as much air as possible is exhaled after the exhalation of a normal tidal volume. The **vital capacity (VC),** which can be determined by inhaling as much as possible and then exhaling as much as possible, is composed of the **tidal volume** and the **inspiratory and expiratory reserve volumes.**

Although spirometry can provide much useful information, **residual volume (RV), functional residual capacity (FRC),** and **total lung capacity (TLC)** cannot be measured using spirometry alone. However, FRC can be determined by rebreathing air containing a known volume and concentration of an inert gas that is not readily absorbed and then determining its concentration in the expired gas at the end of the exhalation of a normal tidal volume. If one knows the initial volume and concentration of inert gas inhaled and the concentration of the inert gas at equilibrium, FRC can be calculated. With knowledge of this capacity, both RV and TLC also can be calculated.

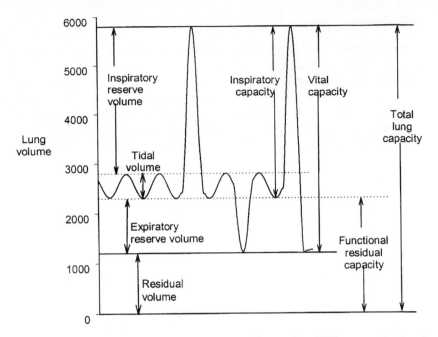

Figure 15-1. Pulmonary spirometry. Lung volumes in milliliters are depicted.

Measuring lung volumes can provide much information. For example, FRC, which is the **volume of air in the lungs when no air is moving and the muscles of respiration are relaxed,** is determined by the balance of lung elastic recoil and chest wall elastic recoil. Thus, changes in tissue composition of the lung (eg, fibrosis) or chest wall will affect FRC.

Combining lung volume measurements with airflow measurements can provide information about resistance to airflow. If a person inhales to TLC and then exhales as forcefully and completely as possible, the **forced expired volume during the first second of expiration (FEV_1)** and the **forced vital capacity (FVC)** can be determined. The ratio **FEV_1/FVC** provides information about **resistance to airflow.** Normally, about **80%** of the FVC will be exhaled during the first second. If resistance is increased, the percentage exhaled during the first second will be decreased. Resistance to airflow lies almost completely in the **airways** and is a function mainly of airway radius. A small decrease in radius will lead to a large increase in resistance because resistance to flow through a tube is inversely proportional to the fourth power of its radius. Airway radius can be affected in a number of ways. Many airways are enveloped in smooth muscle whose contraction can decrease radius. Many airways have **mucus**-secreting cells and glands; increased or abnormally thick mucus secretion can occlude airways partially. Inflammation and edema also can reduce airway radius.

As a result of the structure of the lung, not all the inspired air takes part in gas exchange even in a normal individual. Starting with the **trachea,** which branches into the **right and left bronchi,** each lung is composed of a set of **branching airways** that increase in number and decrease in radius with each branching. The airways that constitute the final seven or so branches have out-pouches or alveoli, and those forming the final branching end blindly, feeding millions of alveoli. There is just one set of airways leading to and from the alveoli; thus, not all the air inhaled reaches the alveoli and not all the gas leaving the alveoli during expiration is expelled into the air. Because exchange of gas between the air and the blood occurs only within alveoli, the volume of air remaining in the airways at the end of inspiration is called **dead space volume.** In a **normal individual with a tidal volume of 500 mL,** the **dead space volume is around 150 mL.**

The pulmonary circulation delivers blood to and from the lungs. The **main pulmonary artery divides to the right and left** to supply each lung. Each of these arteries branches to form smaller, more numerous arteries, which themselves branch. Successive branching continues and provides **capillaries** to each **alveolus** and to many of the airways. The capillaries then coalesce into **venules,** which coalesce into **larger veins** and finally into the **pulmonary vein,** which returns oxygenated blood back to the heart to be pumped through the systemic circulation. Although blood flows through the pulmonary and systemic circulations are equal, **pressures and resistances in the pulmonary circulation are about one-tenth of those in the systemic circulation.** In fact, in a person who is standing or sitting upright, pulmonary arterial pressure is not sufficient to perfuse the tops of the lungs as well as other regions. Also, resistance to flow in the pulmonary circulation, in contrast to resistance in the systemic circulation, depends as much if not more on the diameter and number of capillaries that are open as on the arteriolar radius.

Optimal gas exchange requires a **thin alveolar-capillary interface.** As in the systemic circulation, there is a net filtration of fluid out of the capillaries into the interstitial space. This fluid normally flows along the surface and is carried away in the lymphatic vessels in the walls of the small airways. However, during inflammatory conditions such as the one encountered in this case and in conditions in which pulmonary capillary hydrostatic pressure is increased, such as left-sided heart failure, capillary filtration exceeds lymphatic flow and pulmonary edema occurs. The **edema fluid fills alveoli, disrupting ventilation and gas exchange.**

COMPREHENSION QUESTIONS

[15.1]   In a 58-year-old woman with difficulty breathing, the TLC and FRC
         are lower than normal and FEV_1/FVC is slightly higher than normal.
         These findings are most consistent with which of the following?

         A. Decreased pulmonary blood flow
         B. Decreased strength of the chest wall muscles
         C. Increased airway resistance
         D. Increased chest wall elastic recoil
         E. Increased lung elastic recoil

[15.2]   A patient has reduced TLC and increased RV. FRC is normal. These
         findings are most consistent with which of the following?

         A. Decreased pulmonary blood flow
         B. Decreased strength of the muscles of respiration
         C. Increased airway resistance
         D. Increased chest wall elastic recoil
         E. Increased lung elastic recoil

[15.3]   A chest x-ray of a patient with left-sided heart failure indicates pul-
         monary edema. Additional examination probably would reveal which
         of the following?

         A. Decreased pulmonary artery pressure
         B. Decreased pulmonary lymph flow
         C. Increased pulmonary venous pressure
         D. Normal arterial oxygen partial pressure
         E. Normal vital capacity

Answers

[15.1]   **E.** A lung with increased elastic recoil (decreased compliance) will be
         harder to fill on inspiration and will tend to pull the chest wall inward
         on relaxation of the muscles of breathing. Thus, both TLC and FRC
         will be decreased. Because airway radius is normal or even increased,
         FEV_1 normalized to FVC will be normal or increased even though
         FVC will be reduced. Decreased muscle strength could cause a
         decrease in TLC, but it would not alter FRC.

[15.2]   **B.** If the muscles of inspiration are weak, lungs cannot be inflated as
         well, thus reducing the inspiratory reserve volume and TLC. If the
         muscles of expiration are weak, not as much air can be forced from
         the lungs and expiratory reserve volume will be decreased, thus
         increasing RV. Increases in elastic recoil of either the chest wall or the
         lungs and increases in airway resistance will alter TLC and/or FRC.

[15.3]   **C.** As a result of the decrease in myocardial contractility, end diastolic pressure in the left ventricle increases, leading to an increase in
the pulmonary venous and pulmonary capillary pressures. The
increased pulmonary capillary hydrostatic pressure leads to increased
pulmonary capillary filtration, and when filtration exceeds lymph
flow, pulmonary edema develops. Pulmonary artery pressure is likely
to be increased in this condition. The edema interferes with gas
exchange and with lung inflation; thus, arterial oxygen partial pressure and vital capacity will be decreased.

PHYSIOLOGY PEARLS

❖   Changes in FRC point toward changes in lung and chest wall struc-
    ture such as those caused by pulmonary fibrosis.
❖   Decreases in forced airflow, especially normalized to FVC, point
    toward increased airway resistance such as that seen in asthma,
    bronchitis, and emphysema.
❖   Pulmonary edema results in a ventilation-perfusion inequality and a
    decrease in diffusion of oxygen, leading to a decrease in oxygen
    transfer and arterial oxygen partial pressure.
❖   In a normal person who is standing or sitting upright, both blood
    flow and alveolar ventilation are lowest at the top of the lung and
    greatest near the bottom of the lung.

REFERENCES

Powell FL. Mechanics of breathing. In: Johnson LR, ed. *Essential Medical
    Physiology*. 3rd ed. San Diego, CA: Elsevier Academic Press; 2003:277-288.
Powell FL. Pulmonary gas exchange. In: Johnson LR, ed. *Essential Medical
    Physiology*. 3rd ed. San Diego, CA: Elsevier Academic Press; 2003:299-314.
Powell FL. Structure and function of the respiratory system. In: Johnson LR, ed.
    Essential Medical Physiology. 3rd ed. San Diego, CA: Elsevier Academic Press;
    2003:259-276.

A 24-year-old pregnant woman presented to the hospital in preterm labor and subsequently delivered a premature infant at only 27 weeks gestation (normal term pregnancy is 37-42 weeks). After the delivery, the infant cried, but it subsequently began to grunt and showed signs of hypoxia despite oxygen supplementation. The baby immediately was intubated by endotracheal tube and given surfactant down the endotracheal tube. The baby's hypoxia resolved, and he was transferred to the neonatal intensive care unit for further stabilization.

◆ **What is the role of surfactant in the lung?**

◆ **Where is the major site of airway resistance?**

◆ **How does stimulation of the parasympathetic system affect airway resistance?**

ANSWERS TO CASE 16: MECHANICS OF BREATHING

Summary: A premature infant at 27 weeks gestation develops respiratory distress syndrome (RDS) that requires intubation and surfactant.

◆ **Role of surfactant:** Reduces surface tension.

◆ **Major site of airway resistance:** Medium-sized bronchi.

◆ **Stimulation of parasympathetic system:** Increased airway resistance because of smooth muscle constriction in bronchi.

CLINICAL CORRELATION

The use of surfactant has decreased the mortality of infants with RDS dramatically. Infants who are born prematurely are at much greater risk of having this disorder than are term infants. Surfactant production begins in utero and increases throughout pregnancy. Infants beyond 36 completed weeks have a low incidence of RDS. Infants born with RDS present with grunting, hypoxia, atelectasis, retraction, and excess use of accessory muscles such as the intercostal muscles. During pregnancy, it is possible to perform an amniocentesis to assess for lung maturity. Patients with pregestational diabetes or a history of previous cesarean delivery who want a repeat cesarean often are delivered before labor begins, and if there is any question about the gestational age, an amniocentesis can be performed to assess lung maturity before delivery.

APPROACH TO MECHANICS OF BREATHING

Objectives

1. Discuss the relative roles of the muscles involved in breathing.
2. Discuss the roles of compliance of the lung and compliance of the chest wall in determining lung volumes and capacities.
3. Define surface tension and discuss its role in the mechanics of breathing.

Definitions

Surfactant: A lipoprotein produced by type II alveolar cells.
Compliance: The ability of a structure to yield elastically when a force is applied.
Interdependence: A condition in which the size and shape of a structure is dependent upon the size and shape of adjacent structures.

DISCUSSION

When all the muscles involved in respiration are relaxed, the volume of air in the lungs, called the **functional residual capacity (FRC),** is determined by the interplay between the elastic recoil of the lungs inward and the elastic recoil of the chest wall outward. This interplay results in an **intrapleural pressure** that is **subatmospheric. Inspiration** is accomplished by **expanding the volume of the chest,** making **intrapleural pressure even more subatmospheric.** This drop in pressure outside the alveoli results in the flow of air from the atmosphere into the alveoli, thus expanding them. During respiration at rest, chest expansion is accomplished largely by means of **contraction of the diaphragm. Expiration** is accomplished by simply **relaxing the diaphragm, allowing the elastic recoil of the lung** to return intrapleural pressure to its previous resting value, thus providing the force to move air out of the alveoli so that they return to their resting size. Contraction of the external intercostal muscles to stabilize and/or move the ribs upward and outward to expand the chest also occurs during inspiration. Deeper inspirations involve greater contraction of the diaphragm and external intercostals as well as the scalene and the sternomastoids. During increased breathing, expiration is aided by contraction of the abdominal muscles (rectus abdominis, internal and external obliques, and transversus abdominis) and the internal intercostals.

The lung volumes, capacities, and flows (eg, forced expired volume during the first second of expiration [FEV_1]) discussed in Case 15 depend not only on the **muscles of respiration** but also on the **compliance** of the lungs and the compliance of the chest wall. **Compliance** is defined by the equation

Compliance = Δvolume/Δpressure

Lung compliance basically is a **measure of the stiffness of the lung** and is **inversely related to lung elastic recoil:** The lower the compliance, the greater the elastic recoil and the greater the compliance, the lower the elastic recoil. In part, lung compliance depends on lung architecture. In a healthy lung, there is little connective tissue in the terminal airways and alveoli. Thus, the connective tissue contributes little to compliance. (However, fibrous tissue is increased in several disease states and can decrease compliance significantly.) **Compliance in the normal lung** comes primarily from two sources: **surface tension and alveolar interdependence.**

Alveolar membranes present a surface where air and fluid interface. The **fluid lining** this interface exerts a surface tension that **tends to collapse the alveoli,** thus decreasing compliance. If this fluid were just a saline solution, surface tension would be quite high; however, **type II alveolar cells** secrete a **phospholipid-protein solution** that acts as a **surfactant to lower surface tension.** If this solution is missing or is not of the proper composition, as in this case, surface tension and elastic recoil will be high. This decreased compliance will **make the work of breathing greater,** and accessory muscles of respiration will be used for normal breathing. **Surfactant** is unique and differs from a simple detergent in that the magnitude to which it **can lower surface tension is inversely related to surface area.** Alveoli communicate with one another and vary in size. If surface tension were the same in all alveoli, small alveoli would tend to collapse and larger ones would tend to expand. (This is the case because pressure is directly related to surface tension and indirectly related to radius, as stated in the **Laplace law.**) This does not happen because **surfactant is more compressed in the smaller alveoli,** thus lowering surface tension to a greater degree.

Although **alveoli** often are depicted as a bunch of grapes, they **actually are connected to one another** and to small airways to form a meshwork. In this arrangement, if one alveolus tended to collapse, it would tend to expand adjacent alveoli, and that expansion of adjacent alveoli would oppose its collapse. This is referred to as **interdependence.** In diseased areas of lung in which the alveolar structure is lost, as is seen in **emphysema, interdependence is reduced and lung compliance is increased.**

Changes in **compliance** alter the elastic recoil of the lung and are reflected in the **FRC.** With decreased compliance as is seen in fibrosis and in lack of surfactant, FRC is reduced. With increased compliance as is seen in emphysema, FRC is increased.

COMPREHENSION QUESTIONS

[16.1]   A 24-year-old medical student awakens to get ready for classes. When he arises from a lying down to a standing up position, changes occur to his lungs. Which of the following describes the alterations that occur in the alveoli at the top of his lungs compared with those at the bottom of his lungs?

   A. Exhibit greater compliance
   B. Have a lower ventilation-perfusion ratio
   C. Have larger radii
   D. Receive a greater percentage of the pulmonary blood flow
   E. Receive a greater percentage of the tidal volume

[16.2]   A premature newborn infant is noted to have a deficiency of pulmonary surfactant. Which of the following muscles will the infant likely require to use to accomplish adequate respiration?

   A. Diaphragm, internal intercostals, scalene, sternomastoids
   B. Diaphragm, internal intercostals, sternomastoids, rectus abdominis
   C. Diaphragm, external intercostals, internal intercostals, rectus abdominis
   D. Diaphragm, external intercostals, scalene, rectus abdominis
   E. Diaphragm, external intercostals, scalene, sternomastoids

[16.3] A pulmonary physiologist notes that the lung characteristics of individuals who lack surfactant and those with pulmonary fibrosis are similar. Which of the following occurs in patients who lack surfactant but not in patients with pulmonary fibrosis?

A. Collapse of small alveoli and expansion of large alveoli
B. Decreased lung compliance
C. Decreased total lung capacity
D. Increased work of breathing
E. Intrapleural pressures more subatmospheric than normal

Answers

[16.1] **C.** Under the influence of gravity, the weight of the lung stretches structures at the top of the lungs and compresses those at the bottom. Thus, alveoli are larger at the top of the lung. Because they are stretched, these alveoli are less compliant and have smaller changes in volume with changes in intrapleural pressure upon inspiration. Thus, they are less well ventilated. Because pulmonary artery pressures are relatively low, blood flow to these alveoli also is low. However, ventilation is not as low as blood flow; thus, ventilation/perfusion (V/Q) is high.

[16.2] **E.** As a result of the lack of normal surfactant, surface tension in the lung is higher than normal. This results in a tendency for alveoli to collapse and a decrease in lung compliance. Thus, greater than normal muscular effort is needed to expand the lung during inspiration. Contraction of the internal intercostals and the rectus abdominis occurs with a forced expiration.

[16.3] **A.** The lack of surfactant not only results in an overall decrease in compliance as does fibrosis, it also results in unstable alveoli. Without surfactant, surface tension will be nearly the same in alveoli of all sizes. Thus, pressures will be greater in smaller alveoli, as predicted by the Laplace law. This leads to the collapse of small alveoli into larger alveoli. The decreased compliance in both conditions leads to decreased total lung capacity, increased work of breathing, and intrapleural pressures that are more negative than normal.

PHYSIOLOGY PEARLS

❖ During quiet respiration, inhalation is accomplished mainly by contraction of the diaphragm. Exhalation is passive because of elastic recoil of the lungs.

❖ Compliance of the lung is due in large part to the surface tension of fluid lining the alveoli.

❖ Stability of alveolar size is maintained by the presence of surfactant in the fluid lining the alveoli and by the interdependence among adjacent alveoli and small airways.

❖ In the absence of surfactant, the work of breathing is markedly increased.

REFERENCES

Cloutier MM, Thrall RS. Respiratory system. In: Levy MN, Koeppen BM, Stanton BA, eds. *Berne & Levy, Principles of Physiology*. 4th ed. Philadelphia, PA: Mosby; 2006:361-426.

Powell FL. Mechanics of breathing. In: Johnson LR, ed. *Essential Medical Physiology*. 3rd ed. San Diego, PA: Elsevier Academic Press; 2003:277-288.

A 55-year-old man with a history of a chronic lung disease presents to his primary care physician with worsening shortness of breath. He was diagnosed about 1 year ago. He gives a history of smoking cigarettes (one pack a day for 30 years) but has no other medical problems. His general appearance is that of a thin male who appears to be in mild distress. His cardiac examination is normal, but he is noted to have an expanded anterior-posterior diameter of the chest with expiratory wheezes and breathing through pursed lips. A chest x-ray reveals hyperinflated lung fields bilaterally and no infiltrates. The patient's physician recommends spirometry to differentiate emphysema, which is an obstructive pulmonary disorder, from restrictive lung diseases.

◆ **What effect does emphysema have on the functional residual capacity and FEV_1?**

◆ **What effect does a restrictive lung disease process have on the functional residual capacity and FEV_1?**

◆ **What are some nonrespiratory functions of the lung?**

ANSWERS TO CASE 17: FUNCTION OF THE RESPIRATORY SYSTEM

Summary: A 55-year-old man with a long smoking history has emphysema and increasing shortness of breath.

◆ **Emphysema:** Increases the functional residual capacity, decreases FEV_1.

◆ **Restrictive lung disease:** Decreases the functional residual capacity and decreases FEV_1.

◆ **Nonrespiratory functions of the lung:** Airway and immune defense mechanisms and biosynthetic functions.

CLINICAL CORRELATION

Emphysema is a pulmonary disease that results in destruction of the elastic tissue in the lungs. α_1-Antitrypsin, which normally is produced by the liver and certain inflammatory cells, acts within the lung to inhibit neutrophil elastase and other serine proteases. Serine proteases destroy lung tissue when they are not inhibited. Smoking is a contributing factor to emphysema because it inhibits the action of α_1-antitrypsin, resulting in destruction of the elastic tissue in the lungs. A patient also may have a genetic deficiency for α_1-antitrypsin. Destruction of the elastic tissue of the lung results in increased lung compliance and a tendency for the airways to collapse during expiration, thus trapping air in the lungs. The decreased lung compliance allows for greater recoil of the chest wall, which results in an increase in functional residual volume. This is visualized during the physical examination as an increased anterior-posterior diameter (barrel-shaped chest) and on chest x-ray as hyperinflated lungs.

APPROACH TO RESPIRATORY PHYSIOLOGY

Objectives

1. Understand compliance of the chest wall.
2. Discuss dynamic compression of the airways and its importance in limiting airflow during expiration.
3. Understand the nonrespiratory functions of the lung.

Definitions

Dynamic compression: Narrowing of the airways because of increases in intrathoracic pressure.

Mucociliary transport: The trapping of inhaled particles in the mucus secreted by the airways and the subsequent transport of those particles orally by the directed beating of airways ciliated epithelial cells.

DISCUSSION

Compliance of the lung was discussed in Case 16 in relation to a premature infant with a deficit in pulmonary surfactant. In that patient there was a decrease in lung compliance as a result of abnormally high surface tension at the alveolar-capillary interface. The infant presented with atelectasis, retraction of the chest, and labored breathing. The increased elastic recoil of the lung (decreased compliance) was pulling the chest wall inward and made inspiration difficult. In **emphysema,** the **compliance of the lung is increased** because of **loss of lung elasticity** and **destruction of alveoli and small airways.** Emphysema has minimal to **no effects on the compliance** (elastic recoil) of the **chest wall.** Therefore, the increased lung compliance (decreased lung elastic recoil) allows the elastic recoil of the chest wall to expand the chest more than normal and induce **hyperinflation** of the lungs, with a resultant **increase in functional residual capacity.**

As discussed in Case 16, expiration is accomplished mostly by elastic recoil of the lungs. Although airflow during expiration can be increased through activity of the muscles of expiration, their effect is limited by what is called **dynamic compression of the airways.** Contraction of the muscles of expiration will increase intrathoracic pressure to values above atmospheric, and this increase will compress alveoli to aid in expelling air. However, because many divisions of the airways are within the thorax, the airways are being compressed by that same increase in intrathoracic pressure. As the airways are compressed, resistance to airflow increases dramatically. The increased resistance limits airflow such that a large part of a forced vital capacity (FVC) is **effort independent.** In emphysema, the decrease in elastic recoil and the destruction of alveoli and airways, which decreases interdependence, magnifies the effect of dynamic compression such that air is trapped resulting in a hyperinflated lungs.

The elastic and bony structures that constitute the chest wall are arranged so that at **functional residual capacity, the chest wall has a tendency to spring outward.** Not until lung volumes of approximately 75% of vital capacity are reached is the chest wall at an equilibrium position. This elastic recoil of the chest wall at any lung volume depends on the compliance of the chest wall. **Chest wall compliance** can be altered in states such as **scoliosis** and **ankylosing spondylitis,** in which the spine, ribs, and vertebral joints are altered so that compliance is decreased. This can result in a reduction in all lung volumes, including functional residual capacity. Although they do not affect chest wall compliance, **neuromuscular diseases** can affect respiration; functional residual capacity often will be normal, but **residual volume will be increased,** and other volumes, **capacities,** and **forced volumes will be reduced.**

In addition to gas exchange, the pulmonary system is involved in a number of other functions, many of which are related to defense. The air people breathe is far from pure, and there are both **mechanical and chemical defenses** to protect the lungs and prevent invasion of the body through the lungs. Before its arrival in the alveoli, the bulk of inspired air, especially particles larger than 1 mm, come into contact with the walls of the conducting airways. Those walls are lined with cells that secrete mucus and possess **cilia** that beat with a motion that moves particles toward the oropharynx, where they can be swallowed. Smaller particles that can reach terminal airways and alveoli are removed by **macrophages.** There also is an abundant **immune system** composed of **lymphocytes and dendritic cells.** Many of the phagocytic and immune cells produce **reactive oxygen molecules,** which can be detrimental to lung tissue, especially in the face of the relatively high oxygen levels existing within the alveoli. To deal with these molecules, lung surfactant contains high levels of the **antioxidant glutathione.**

The lung also is very metabolically active. Many **biogenic amines** are inactivated in the lung, including serotonin, bradykinin, and several arachidonic acid metabolites. In contrast, the relatively inactive **angiotensin I is converted to the very active angiotensin II as it passes through the lungs.**

COMPREHENSION QUESTIONS

[17.1] A 35-year-old man is noted to have generalized weakness of the skeletal muscles but is otherwise normal. Which of the following lung volumes or lung capacities most likely would be normal?

A. Inspiratory reserve volume
B. Functional residual capacity
C. Residual volume
D. Total lung capacity
E. Vital capacity

[17.2] A 15-year-old female has the autosomal recessive disease cystic fibrosis. The airway epithelial cells secrete mucus that is more viscous than normal. Which of the following happens as a consequence?

A. Bacteria are cleared more readily from the airways
B. Cilia on the epithelial cells beat more easily
C. Inhaled particles are not trapped
D. Mucus is propelled orally more slowly

[17.3] A 56-year-old female is brought into the office complaining of difficulty breathing for several weeks. Physical examination is performed, and office spirometry is utilized. The, total lung capacity (TLC) and functional residual capacity (FRC) are noted to be greater than normal, and forced vital capacity (FVC) and FEV_1/FVC are lower than normal. These findings are most consistent with which of the following?

A. Decreased lung compliance
B. Decreased strength of the chest wall muscles
C. Increased airway resistance
D. Increased chest wall compliance

Answers

[17.1]   **B.** Functional residual capacity is the volume of air in the lungs when no muscular effort is being expended. It depends only on the balance in elastic forces of the lung and the chest wall. All the other volumes and capacities in the lungs depend at least in part on muscular effort.

[17.2]   **D.** The thick mucus still can trap particles, including bacteria. However, the thick mucus impairs ciliary function, thus impeding oral transport of the mucus-trapped particles.

[17.3]   **C.** The finding of an increase in total lung capacity and functional residual capacity indicates that compliance of the lung is increased. This allows for an increase in dynamic compression of the airways upon a forced expiration. Dynamic compression increases airway resistance and decreases airflow, which is typical of an obstructive pulmonary process.

PHYSIOLOGY PEARLS

❖   Intrapleural pressure is subatmospheric because of the balance of the elastic recoil of the lungs inward and the elastic recoil of the chest wall outward.

❖   During a forced expiration, airflow is limited by dynamic compression of the airways, which is greater in lungs with increased compliance.

❖   Neuromuscular diseases affecting muscles of respiration do not alter functional residual capacity and may not affect tidal volume, but residual volume is increased and all other volumes and capacities are decreased.

❖   Angiotensin I, which is formed by the action of renin on angiotensinogen, is converted to angiotensin II in the lung through the action of angiotensin-converting enzyme.

❖   Particles larger than 1 mm that are inhaled with the air are trapped by the mucus that coats the airways. The ciliary action of airway epithelial cells transports the particles to the pharynx, where they are swallowed.

REFERENCES

Cloutier MM, Thrall RS. Respiratory system. In: Levy MN, Koeppen BM, Stanton BA, eds. *Berne & Levy, Principles of Physiology*. 4th ed. Philadelphia, PA: Mosby; 2006:361-426.

Powell FL. Respiratory physiology. In: Johnson LR, ed. *Essential Medical Physiology*. 3rd ed. San Diego, CA: Elsevier Academic Press; 2003:273-288.

A 36-year-old woman presents to her primary care physician with complaints of shortness of breath, arthritic pain, and multiple skin lesions. The patient is short of breath on examination with a slightly low pulse oximetry reading, consistent with mild hypoxemia. She has multiple skin lesions, and a biopsy reveals noncaseating granulomas consistent with sarcoidosis. Chest x-ray findings revealing hilar adenopathy are also suggestive of sarcoidosis. The physician explains to the patient that he likely has a restrictive disease process, and recommends formal pulmonary function testing.

◆ **What parameters are measured in a pulmonary function test?**

◆ **What changes in pulmonary function would be consistent with a restrictive disease?**

◆ **How would a restrictive lung process lead to hypoxemia?**

◆ **What changes in pulmonary function might be observed in this patient?**

ANSWERS TO CASE 18: GAS EXCHANGE

Summary: A 36-year-old woman with sarcoidosis has both skin and lung involvement. Her physician explains that sarcoidosis is a restrictive lung disease.

◆ **Parameters measured in a pulmonary function test:** Changes in the volume of inspired air versus time. Lung capacities and airflow rates can be measured. Figure 15-1 in Case 15 shows a spirometry measurement.

◆ **Pulmonary function consistent with restrictive disease:** Decreased vital capacity and decreased functional residual capacity (FRC) or resting lung volume. Conditions that restrict lung expansion are neuromuscular conditions, problems with the chest wall, pleural disease, and decreased lung compliance. Depending on the nature of the restrictive disease, there may be little or no change in rates of airflow.

◆ **How restrictive lung processes cause hypoxemia:** Thickening of alveolar membrane, which increases the diffusion distance.

◆ **Changes in pulmonary function with sarcoidosis:** Decreased lung compliance (Δvolume/Δpressure), increased lung elastic recoil, decreased resting lung volume (FRC), decreased vital capacity. Gas exchange will be affected:

N_2O gas exchange: perfusion-limited exchange
CO gas exchange: diffusion-limited exchange

CLINICAL CORRELATION

Both restrictive and obstructive lung diseases can **affect gas exchange** in the lung. Examples of **restrictive diseases** are **sarcoidosis, connective-tissue disorders, interstitial pneumonia, environmental exposure, and pulmonary vascular disease.** Restrictive diseases result in poor gas exchange because of a **thickening of the alveolar membrane** that results in **restriction of oxygen diffusion with increased diffusion distance.** Obstructive diseases include emphysema, chronic bronchitis, and asthma. Obstructive disorders result in poor gas exchange because of decreased surface area for diffusion of gases. These two pulmonary problems can often be distinguished from each other by pulmonary function tests, but the clinical presentation is the most important method of diagnosis.

APPROACH TO GAS EXCHANGE PHYSIOLOGY

Objectives

1. List lung volumes and lung capacities.
2. Define lung compliance and elastic recoil.
3. Explain how measurements of lung volumes and gas flow rates can be used to distinguish between obstructive and restrictive lung diseases.
4. Discuss alveolar gas exchange and factors that determine the rate of O_2 diffusion.

Definitions

Obstructive disease: Disorders that cause an increase in the airway resistance to flow such as narrowing of the passages due to inflammation or compression.

Restricive disease: Disorders that impair or increase the work necessary for lung expansion.

DISCUSSION

Pulmonary function tests are used to identify and distinguish obstructive from restrictive lung diseases. The mechanical factors that contribute to lung function fall into the following categories:

1. Resistance to airflow through the airways.
2. Elastic recoil of the lungs.
3. Elastic recoil of the chest wall.
4. Strength of respiratory muscles.

An easy way to remember the distinction is to realize that **obstructive diseases** manifest themselves as **increased resistance to airflow and restrictive diseases** manifest themselves as **restriction of lung expansion.** Pulmonary function tests measure the **velocity of airflow** and **lung volumes.** These parameters provide an accurate assessment of lung disease.

Sarcoidosis is a disease that causes **inflammation in the tissues.** It is characterized by **noncaseating granulomas,** and although it may occur in any tissue, the inflammation generally starts in the **lungs or lymph nodes.** In the present case, lung injury has occurred because of granule formation in the bronchioles and alveolar sacs and chronic inflammation resulting in scarring or formation of fibrotic tissue. **Fibrosis** in the lung tissue has a marked effect on the elasticity, or compliance, of the lung. **Compliance** is the **change in volume of the lung for a given change in pressure.** Physically, the lung volume is dependent on two factors: the elastic recoil of the lung to collapse on itself and the outward recoil of the chest wall. The **interpleural pressure** is the result of these two opposing forces.

Lung volumes are determined in a pulmonary function test by a spirometer (see Case 15). The patient breathes through a mouthpiece that is attached to an instrument which measures the volume of air that the patient is moving as a function of time. During normal quiet breathing, expansion of the chest wall reduces the interpleural pressure, causing an expansion of the lung volume. Relaxation of the inspiratory muscles allows a return of the chest wall and a decrease in lung volume. The volume is referred to as the **tidal volume (TV).** The amount of air that remains in the lungs at the end of normal, quiet expiration is referred to as the **FRC,** which for a **normal individual is around 2300 mL.** The FRC is an important and useful value in the evaluation of a lung disorder. Physiologically, the **FRC** is dependent on two factors: the **outward recoil of the chest wall** and the **elastic recoil of the lung.** Compliance is the inverse of the elasticity (compliance = Δvolume/Δpressure) of the lung tissue; therefore, the volume under these conditions will be dependent on and may be used as an estimate of lung compliance. A **fibrotic lung** compared with a normal lung is **less compliant (higher elastic recoil);** therefore, a given pressure change will cause a smaller change in volume and the **FRC will be lower than normal.** This can be contrasted to a high-compliance lung, which will undergo a larger volume change for a given pressure. Thus, a lower FRC would indicate a low-compliance (higher elastic recoil) lung consistent with a restrictive disease such as fibrosis. **Pulmonary fibrosis** is one of several causes of restrictive disease.

There are other mechanical factors that cause restrictive disease, such as **neuromuscular weakness of the respiratory muscles,** which can prevent full expansion of the chest. **Scoliosis** or malformations that interfere with chest movements or pneumothorax (air in the chest cavity) can prevent full expansion of the lungs. Rates of airflows may be affected in restrictive diseases, but usually can be identified on the basis of other factors. For example, with **muscle weakness, the forced expiratory volume in the first second (FEV_1)** is likely to be **reduced** simply as a result of the **inability to exhale forcefully.** In **pulmonary fibrosis, the FEV_1** also may be **reduced** because of the **reduced volume of air available;** however, looking at the **FEV_1/FVC** (forced vital capacity) ratio can show a normal or elevated value in **fibrosis.**

Obstructive diseases usually can be distinguished by increased resistance to airflow. **Resistance to airflow** will occur under conditions in which there is a diminished diameter of the airway. For example, mucus reduces the airway diameter and increases airway resistance. Asthma causes active smooth muscle contraction with constriction of the airways. Another cause of airway constriction is dynamic compression of airways during expiration. Dynamic compression of airways is more pronounced in high-compliance tissues and is one of the major factors limiting pulmonary function in chronic obstructive pulmonary disease.

The **diffusion of a gas** through a barrier is described by the **Fick law of diffusion,** which states that the **rate of diffusion of a gas** through a barrier is dependent on the **surface area** of the barrier, the **thickness** of the barrier, the

diffusion coefficient of the gas, and the concentration gradient of the gas across the barrier. **Pulmonary gas exchange** is dependent on the **surface area and thickness of the pulmonary capillary, the partial pressure difference of the gas between the alveolar and blood compartments**, and the **residence time of the blood in the alveolar capillary.** Thus, factors that affect the surface area or thickness of the pulmonary capillary can have a profound effect on the rate of diffusion of a gas between the two compartments.

Gases with different diffusion coefficients illustrate the limitations of gas transfer across the pulmonary capillary. **Nitrous oxide (N_2O) diffuses very rapidly** and **equilibrates** across the pulmonary capillary in about **0.1 second;** beyond that point, there is no further net gas transport across the barrier. Since the residence time of blood in the capillary is about 0.75 second, N_2O equilibrates fully by the time the perfusing blood leaves the capillary. This is referred to as **perfusion-limited gas exchange.** In contrast, a gas such as **carbon monoxide binds avidly to hemoglobin** with a reaction time that is faster than the rate of diffusion across the capillary barrier. This means that the partial pressure of CO in the blood will be less than that in the alveolar compartment until the hemoglobin is saturated. The **residence time of blood in the capillary required for this to occur is more than 0.75 second;** thus, the partial pressure of CO in the blood leaving the capillary is lower than its alveolar concentration. This is referred to as **diffusion-limited gas exchange.**

Pulmonary capillary **O_2 exchange** is **intermediate** between **N_2O** and **CO exchange.** The binding of O_2 to hemoglobin is slower than that of CO; however, its diffusion across the barrier allows it to reach equilibrium with the alveolar PO_2 in about 0.25 second. The higher arterial PO_2 increases the rate of O_2 binding to hemoglobin such that by the time the blood leaves the capillary, binding is complete. In other words, **O_2 transfer is normally perfusion limited.** As stated above, the rate of diffusion is dependent on the surface area of the barrier and the thickness of the barrier. Physiologically, conditions that alter either of these two properties can have serious impact on gas transfer from the lungs into the blood. These conditions can limit the rate sufficiently to the point that **O_2 transport becomes diffusion limited,** creating a significant alveolar–arterial O_2 gradient. In an individual with pulmonary fibrosis, as in the present case, there is a thickening of the alveolar-capillary barrier causing a reduction of O_2 exchange. Diffusion may also be reduced because of an accumulation of fluid in the alveolar-capillary membrane, increasing the barrier thickness. Alternatively, the effective surface area can be diminished because of tissue damage or destruction observed in emphysema. Any of these states will lead to decreased oxygenation of arterial blood.

COMPREHENSION QUESTIONS

[18.1] The lung function tests of a patient show a markedly reduced FEV_1 and an FRC of 4.2 L (normal 2.3 L). Which of the following is the most likely cause of the reduced FEV_1?

A. Weak expiratory muscles
B. Small-diameter airways
C. Pulmonary congestion
D. Dynamic compression of airways
E. Pulmonary fibrosis

[18.2] Mr Smith complains of shortness of breath and difficulty with moderate exercise. Pulmonary function tests indicate a reduced FRC, and his FEV_1 was 2.6 L (78%). His FVC was 3.1 L (70%). Which of the following is the most likely cause of Mr Smith's problems?

A. Weak expiratory muscles
B. Small-diameter airways
C. Pulmonary congestion
D. Dynamic compression of airways
E. Pulmonary fibrosis

[18.3] A 36-year-old woman undergoes chemotherapy with bleomycin for an ovarian germ cell cancer. She develops mild pulmonary fibrosis secondary to the chemotherapy. Which of the following agents is most likely affected in its diffusion across the alveoli-pulmonary capillary barrier?

A. CO
B. CO_2
C. N_2O
D. O_2

Answers

[18.1] **D.** The decrease in the FEV_1 indicates that there is a decrease in the rate of expiration. This is indicative of an obstructive disease; however, it also could result from weakened musculature, for example (restrictive). The FRC normally would be in the range of 2.3 L. In this individual the FRC is 4.2 L. The FRC can be used to estimate lung compliance ($\Delta V/\Delta P$), and a value this high suggests a high-compliance lung. High compliance is most consistent with dynamic compression of airways.

[18.2]   **E.** Mr Smith has pulmonary fibrosis. The first indication is the reduced FRC, suggesting a decrease in lung compliance that would be consistent with a restrictive disease. Generally, changes in rates of change obtained in lung function tests are associated with obstructive disease. With Mr Smith, however, there is a decrease in the FEV_1. However, analysis of the FVC also shows a reduction and comparison to the FVC yields an FEV_1/FVC of 85%, which is normal. In patients such as Mr Smith, the FEV_1 is reduced, but not as a consequence of obstruction; simply, there is a smaller starting volume as a result of the fibrosis. The ratio FEV_1/FVC calculates to a normal value because there is a proportionate decrease in both of these parameters.

[18.3]   **A.** Carbon monoxide binds avidly to hemoglobin and presents a remarkable "deep sink" for CO to enter the capillary network; therefore, it is considered diffusion limited. Thus, in pulmonary fibrosis, this gas is most likely to be affected. In contrast, nitrous oxide is perfusion dependent; carbon dioxide and oxygen are intermediate.

PHYSIOLOGY PEARLS

❖   Obstructive diseases manifest themselves as increased resistance to airflow. Restrictive diseases manifest themselves as restriction of lung expansion.

❖   Pulmonary gas exchange is dependent on the surface area and thickness of the pulmonary capillary wall, the concentration gradient of the gas between the alveolar and blood compartments, and the residence time of blood in the pulmonary capillary.

❖   Diffusion limitation for O_2 can be corrected by increasing the O_2 concentration in inspired air.

REFERENCES

Powell FL. Pulmonary gas exchange. In: Johnson LR, ed. *Essential Medical Physiology*. 3rd ed. San Diego, CA: Elsevier Academic Press; 2003:299-314.

Powell FL. Structure and function of the respiratory system. In: Johnson LR, ed. *Essential Medical Physiology*. 3rd ed. San Diego, CA: Elsevier Academic Press; 2003:259-276.

Staub NC, Sr. Mechanical properties of breathing. In: Berne RM, Levy MN, eds. *Physiology*. 4th ed. St. Louis, MO: Mosby; 1998:534-547.

Staub NC, Sr. Structure and function of the respiratory system. In: Berne RM, Levy MN, eds. *Physiology*. 4th ed. St. Louis, MO: Mosby; 1998:517-533.

A 23-year-old man with no medical problems is brought to the emergency center by family members who found him to be confused, nauseated, short of breath, and complaining of a headache. The patient was found in the basement of their home next to a furnace, where he was trying to stay warm on a cold winter day. On examination, the patient is lethargic and confused. His lips appear a bright pink. A urine drug screen is obtained and is negative. His serum carboxyhemoglobin level is elevated. The patient is diagnosed with carbon monoxide poisoning and is admitted to the hospital for further treatment.

◆ **What is the mechanism by which carbon monoxide causes hypoxia?**

 In which direction (right or left) would the hemoglobin–oxygen dissociation curve shift with fetal hemoglobin compared with adult hemoglobin?

◆ **What is the most common way in which carbon dioxide is transported in venous blood?**

ANSWERS TO CASE 19: OXYGEN-CARBON DIOXIDE TRANSPORT

Summary: A 23-year-old man has confusion, nausea, shortness of breath, and headache after being found near a furnace in the basement. The patient has clinical and laboratory findings consistent with carbon monoxide poisoning.

◆ **Hypoxia with carbon monoxide:** Decreased oxygen-binding capacity of hemoglobin.

◆ **Fetal hemoglobin–oxygen dissociation curve:** Shift to the left.

◆ **Most common way carbon dioxide is transported in the blood:** Bicarbonate (HCO_3^-).

CLINICAL CORRELATION

Carbon monoxide is a gas that is produced commonly by internal combustion engines, fossil-fuel home appliances (heaters, stoves, furnaces), and incomplete combustion of nearly all natural and synthetic products. Poisoning with carbon monoxide, if a person is exposed for a long period, can be fatal. Symptoms include headache, shortness of breath, confusion, impaired judgment, nausea, respiratory depression, coma, and even death. It is particularly a challenging problem because the gas is odorless and colorless; also, because the hemoglobin molecule is saturated, the patient is "pink" but hypoxemic. Carbon monoxide is inhaled through the lungs and binds to the oxygen-binding site of hemoglobin with a significantly higher affinity than does oxygen. The combination of carbon monoxide and hemoglobin makes carboxyhemoglobin, which can be measured in a patient's blood. The elevation of the carboxyhemoglobin level may give some indication of the severity of the disease. After a person's removal from the carbon monoxide exposure, the carbon monoxide slowly dissociates and is excreted through the lungs. Treatment of the poisoning includes removal from the carbon dioxide exposure and the administration of 100% oxygen (non-rebreather mask). At times patients need intubation (coma, seizures, or cardiovascular instability) or treatment with hyperbaric oxygen (extremely elevated carboxyhemoglobin levels).

APPROACH TO OXYGEN-CARBON DIOXIDE TRANSPORT

Objectives

1. Know about the structure and function of hemoglobin.
2. Understand the hemoglobin–oxygen dissociation curves and the factors which may change them.
3. Know about carbon dioxide transport in the blood.

Definitions

Oxygen carrying capacity of blood: The sum of the amount of dissolved O_2 plus the amount of O_2 bound to hemoglobin in the presence of 100% O_2.

Oxygen content of blood: The sum of the amount of dissolved O_2 plus the amount of O_2 bound to hemoglobin at any given PO_2.

Bohr effect: In the presence of CO_2 hemoglobin has a lower binding affinity for O_2. Because of the Bohr effect, increasing CO_2 or lowering the pH of the blood decreases the O_2 affinity of hemoglobin favoring O_2 release.

Haldane effect: Deoxygenation of hemoglobin increases its ability to bind CO_2.

DISCUSSION

Oxygen Transport

Metabolism consumes O_2 and produces CO_2. Gas exchange in the lungs occurs when blood passing through the **pulmonary capillaries releases CO_2 and takes up O_2.** The arterial concentrations of CO_2 and O_2 are in equilibrium with their concentrations in the alveolar compartment. The gas concentration in the blood is expressed as its **partial pressure,** and its **content** is determined by its partial pressure and its solubility in blood. The **solubility of oxygen in aqueous solution is low,** and the amount of O_2 that can be dissolved in normal plasma, or the **O_2 content, at 37°C is 0.3 mL/100 mL** at a normal arterial partial pressure of 100 mm Hg. The O_2 content of plasma is much too low to meet a person's metabolic demands; however, **hemoglobin** greatly increases the amount of O_2 the blood can carry. The **O_2-carrying capacity of blood** is **dependent on the hemoglobin concentration.** At saturating oxygen levels, **hemoglobin** binds about **1.34 mL of O_2 per gram of hemoglobin.** Normal blood has about **15 g of hemoglobin per 100 mL;** thus, at saturation, the amount of O_2 bound to hemoglobin is

15 g Hb × 1.34 mL O_2/g Hb × 100% saturation = 20.1 mL O_2/100 mL blood

The amount of O_2 bound at saturation is the O_2-**binding capacity** of hemoglobin. The normal arterial PO_2 is about 100 mm Hg. At this partial pressure, hemoglobin is 97.5% saturated and the amount of O_2 that is bound is

15 g Hb × 1.34 mL O_2/g Hb × 97.5% saturation = 19.6 mL O_2/100 mL blood

The total amount of O_2 in the blood is the sum of the dissolved O_2 and the bound O_2:

$$O_{2dis} = 0.3 \text{ mL/100 mL blood}$$
$$O_{2bound} = 19.6 \text{ mL/100 mL blood}$$
$$O_{2content} = 19.9 \text{ mL/100 mL blood}$$

The majority of O_2 is transported in the blood bound to hemoglobin. Any factors that influence the amount of functional hemoglobin will influence O_2 transport in the blood.

Hemoglobin is the major blood protein constituent; it is contained within the **red cells** of the blood and is central to gas transport and maintenance of hydrogen ion homeostasis and acid–base balance. It is a **tetrameric complex of two α subunits and two β subunits, each of which binds an O_2 molecule.** The binding of the first oxygen to hemoglobin causes a structural shift that favors the binding of additional oxygen molecules. This **cooperativity** yields a characteristic **sigmoidal affinity curve for O_2 binding.** Several important physiologic parameters contribute to the binding affinity of hemoglobin for O_2 and affect the shape of the curve. Variables such as **temperature, pH, and CO_2** alter the binding affinity for O_2. The structural shift induced by O_2 binding alters the ionization state of important amino acid residues, causing a shift in their H^+ dissociation constant (pK_a). O_2 binding results in a decreased affinity of hemoglobin for H^+ and a release of H^+ from the molecule. The reaction is readily reversible and is in equilibrium. Thus, not only does O_2 binding or release cause a change in $[H^+]$, the H^+ concentration influences O_2 binding by hemoglobin. Although seemingly minor, the **O_2 binding affinity of hemoglobin is pH-dependent** and is important to the overall physiologic function of hemoglobin. Also, **hemoglobin contributes to H^+ ion homeostasis** by becoming a weaker acid (higher affinity for H^+) upon O_2 dissociation. This shift in the pK_a is the basis of both the **Haldane effect and the Bohr effect.** Finally, hemoglobin also binds CO_2 with the formation of carbamino groups. The binding is weak and readily reversible but has two important consequences: The binding of CO_2 alters O_2 affinity, and hemoglobin contributes to CO_2 transport in the blood.

An **increase in H^+ or PCO_2 will shift the O_2 dissociation curve to the right** with a resultant **decrease in the affinity for O_2.** This phenomenon is known as the **Bohr effect.** Another important regulator of the O_2 binding affinity of hemoglobin is **2,3-diphosphoglycerate (DPG).** DPG is produced by red cells and is increased during hypoxia. An increase in **DPG shifts the affinity curve to the right,** decreasing the affinity for O_2 and favoring oxygen release in the tissues (See Figure 19-1).

The effect of pH, PCO_2, temperature, and 2,3-DPG on O_2 binding to hemoglobin is central to gas transport by the blood. Figure 19-1 is the oxygen-binding curve of hemoglobin. Because of the steeply sigmoidal nature of the curve through much of the physiologic range, even slight changes in the binding affinity for O_2 can cause large changes in the percent of O_2 saturation at a given PO_2. Thus increases in H^+, CO_2, temperature, or 2,3-DPG will cause O_2 dissociation from hemoglobin. Conversely, a decrease in any of these factors will increase the affinity for O_2 favoring its binding to hemoglobin.

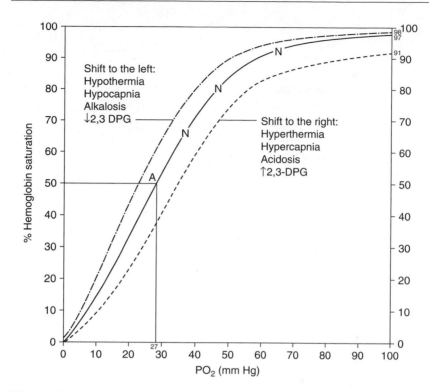

Figure 19-1. Oxygen dissociation curve with shifts based on various factors.

Carbon Dioxide Transport

The transport of CO_2 by the blood occurs through several different mechanisms. **CO_2 has a higher solubility than does O_2;** therefore, a larger fraction is carried as dissolved CO_2. More important, CO_2 spontaneously reacts with water to form carbonic acid:

$$CO_2 + H_2O \rightarrow H_2O\, CO_3 \rightarrow H^+ + HCO_3^-$$

Carbonic acid dissociates to H^+ and **HCO_3^-.** The enzyme **carbonic anhydrase** catalyzes this reaction and is **contained in red cells.** CO_2 freely diffuses into the red cell and reacts with water to form H^+ and HCO_3^-. The HCO_3^- is transported rapidly out of the red cell by the $Cl^-/\ HCO_3^-$ exchanger in the red cell membrane. The H^+ remains in the cell and is in part buffered by the hemoglobin. Physiologically, this arrangement works to advantage because the increase in H^+ favors the dissociation of bound O_2 (Bohr effect). At the same time, dissociation of O_2 causes hemoglobin to become a weaker acid (higher affinity for H^+), increasing the buffer capacity of hemoglobin. **About two-thirds of metabolically produced CO_2 undergoes this reaction and is carried to the lungs as HCO_3^-.**

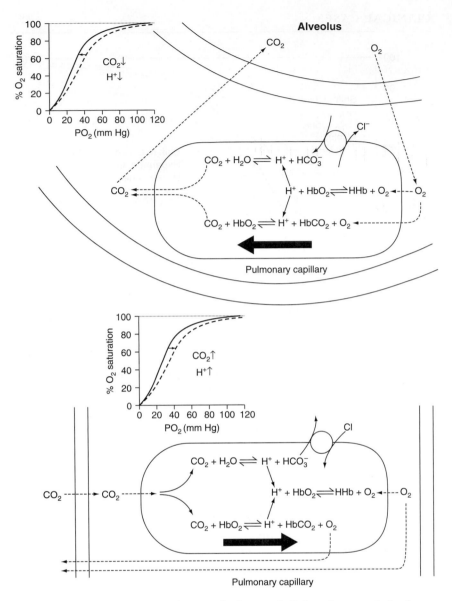

Figure 19-2. Gas transport from actively metabolizing tissue and the lungs. Tissue production of CO_2 in the peripheral capillary will cause CO_2 to diffuse into the red cell. In the red cell, CO_2 will react with H_2O via the action of carbonic anhydrase to form H^+ and HCO_3^-. The HCO_3^- is transported out of the cell in exchange for Cl^-. Both CO_2 and H^+ will facilitate O_2 release by causing a shift in the O_2 dissociation curve of hemoglobin, lowering its O_2 affinity. At the same time, O_2 dissociation will increase the affinity of Hb for H^+ and CO_2. As the blood enters the pulmonary capillary, the arterial O_2 will rise decreasing the affinity for CO_2. CO_2 will diffuse down its concentration gradient into the alveolus resulting in HCO_3^- reacting with H^+ to form CO_2. As H^+ and CO_2 fall, the O_2 affinity of hemoglobin increases facilitating oxygenation.

Hemoglobin also binds CO_2 directly through the formation of carbamino groups on terminal amines. There is **no cooperativity of CO_2 binding,** and the dissociation curve is much flatter over the normal physiologic range. The binding affinity for CO_2 is dependent on the O_2 concentration. **Increasing O_2 causes a shift to the right** with a decrease in affinity for CO_2. The effect is known as the **Haldane effect.**

Physiologic Relevance

Physiologically, the Bohr effect and the Haldane effect are important in the understanding of gas transport, O_2 delivery to tissues, and H^+ homeostasis (summarized in Figure 19-2). In metabolically active tissues, there is increased production of CO_2, which freely diffuses into the red cell. In the red cell, two-thirds of the CO_2 is converted by carbonic anhydrase to H_2CO_3 which dissociates to H^+ and HCO_3^-. The HCO_3^- is transported into the blood in exchange for Cl^-. The elevation in CO_2 and H^+ will favor release of O_2 from hemoglobin, facilitating O_2 delivery to the tissue. The blood leaving the tissue will have elevated H^+, CO_2 and HCO_3^-. In the lungs, O_2 diffuses into the pulmonary capillary and CO_2 diffuses into the alveolar compartment. In the red cell, the increase in O_2 drives the release of CO_2 from the hemoglobin. The fall in CO_2 reverses the reaction of HCO_3^- and H^+ to form H_2CO_3 which is converted to CO_2 and H_2O. The fall in both H^+ and CO_2 increase the affinity for O_2, favoring maximal saturation of the hemoglobin

COMPREHENSION QUESTIONS

[19.1]   A 32-year-old woman is theorizing that breathing 100% oxygen should increase the amount of oxygen in her blood about fivefold, because room air is composed of approximately 21% oxygen. Which of the following statements is the most accurate answer to her hypothesis?

   A. The amount of oxygen carried by her hemoglobin probably will increase markedly, but the amount soluble in her serum will remain the same.
   B. The amount of oxygen carried in her blood will not rise appreciably.
   C. The amount of oxygen in her blood will rise about fivefold.
   D. The partial pressure of oxygen in her blood probably will remain unchanged.

[19.2]   A 56-year-old man is admitted to the coronary care unit (CCU) for an acute inferior wall myocardial infarction. The cardiologist is trying to optimize the oxygen delivery to the myocardial tissue. Supplemental oxygen is provided by nasal cannula at 3 L/min. Which of the following best describes the oxygen-carrying capacity of whole blood?

A. Dependent on the alveolar PO_2
B. The amount of O_2 dissolved in the blood
C. The sum of the dissolved O_2 plus the amount bound to hemoglobin
D. The sum of the dissolved O_2 plus the amount of O_2 bound to hemoglobin under saturating conditions
E. Limited by O_2 diffusion

[19.3]   In the case above, the patient had been sleeping in a small room at his house heated with a space heater. He suffered from carbon monoxide poisoning.

The carbon monoxide has bound to hemoglobin and reduced its oxygen-binding capacity. Which of the following best describes the PO_2 level in the patient's arterial blood when the paramedics were called to evaluate him?

A. Dependent on the alveolar PO_2
B. Dependent on the amount of CO bound to hemoglobin
C. Increased from normal because of displaced oxygen from hemoglobin
D. Reduced from normal because of the CO bound to hemoglobin

[19.4] O_2 binding to hemoglobin in the pulmonary capillary is inhibited by which of the following?

A. CO_2 dissociation from hemoglobin
B. Diffusion of CO_2 from pulmonary capillary to alveolus
C. Reaction of bicarbonate with H^+
D. Shift to more acidic pH than is found in venous blood

Answers

[19.1]   **B.** Because the vast majority of oxygen content in blood is carried by hemoglobin, breathing 100% oxygen will increase the partial pressure of oxygen but will not affect the content or oxygen-carrying capacity.

[19.2]   **D.** The oxygen-carrying capacity is the total amount of oxygen that can be carried by blood. The capacity is measured under saturating conditions for O_2. Therefore, the maximum amount of dissolved oxygen and the maximal amount of bound oxygen are obtained. It is dependent on the amount of hemoglobin in the blood.

[19.3]   **A.** The O_2 concentration is dependent only on the partial pressure of O_2 in the gas phase in contact with the blood, or the alveolar PO_2. The binding capacity of the blood is compromised because CO binding to hemoglobin blocks O_2 binding; therefore, the total amount of oxygen will be reduced, but not its concentration.

[19.4]   **D.** In the pulmonary capillary, CO_2 diffusion down its concentration gradient into the alveolar compartment shifts the entire equilibrium to promote O_2 binding to hemoglobin. The fall in CO_2 in the capillary leads to the dissociation of CO_2 from hemoglobin. The fall in CO_2 also causes a shift in the equilibrium of the CO_2-HCO_3^- buffer driving the reaction of H^+ and HCO_3^- toward CO_2 production with an increase in the pH. Both the fall in CO_2 and the rise in pH increase the oxygen-binding affinity of hemoglobin.

PHYSIOLOGY PEARLS

❖   The O_2 content of arterial blood is the sum of the amount of dissolved O_2 plus the amount of O_2 bound to hemoglobin. The O_2 concentration is the partial pressure of O_2 in the blood and is determined by the partial pressure of O_2 in the alveolar compartment.

❖   About two-thirds of the CO_2 produced by metabolism is transported by the blood in the form of HCO_3^-. The HCO_3^- is produced from the reaction of CO_2 with water and catalyzed by carbonic anhydrase in the red cells. The remaining CO_2 is either dissolved or bound to hemoglobin.

❖   The affinity of O_2 binding to hemoglobin is dependent on the pH, $[CO_2]$, temperature, and 2,3-DPG. The combined effects of pH and $[CO_2]$ favor O_2 dissociation in the tissues and binding of O_2 in the pulmonary capillary.

❖   In conditions such as anemia and CO poisoning, the O_2 concentration of arterial blood can be normal. The O_2 content is lower than normal because the amount of hemoglobin or its oxygen-binding capacity is reduced.

REFERENCE

Powell FL. Oxygen and carbon dioxide transport in the blood. In: Johnson LR, ed. *Essential Medical Physiology*. 3rd ed. San Diego, CA: Elsevier Academic Press; 2003:289-298.

A 19-year-old woman with a history of depression is found by her college roommate lying on the floor, vomiting and having seizures, with an empty bottle of aspirin beside her. The roommate states that she has not been taking her depression medications and has been overwhelmed by the upcoming final examinations. The roommate bought the bottle of aspirin earlier that morning. In the emergency center, the patient is lethargic and confused with a low-grade fever and is hyperventilating. Her urine drug screen is negative, but the arterial blood gases reveal an anion gap metabolic acidosis, probably as a result of the aspirin overdose.

◆   **What is the anion gap and what is its significance?**

◆   **What effect does metabolic acidosis have on the respiratory system?**

◆   **What chemoreceptors are involved in the response to an acid–base disturbance?**

◆   **Are the lung stretch receptors fast- or slow-acting reflexes?**

ANSWERS TO CASE 20: CONTROL OF BREATHING

Summary: A 19-year-old college student with a history of depression presents to the emergency center with salicylate poisoning and an anion gap acidosis.

◆ **Significance of the anion gap:** Anion gap = $[Na^+] - ([Cl^-] + [HCO_3^-])$. An increase in the rate of production (eg, lactic acid or ketoacids) or ingestion of noncarbonic acids or substances that increase lactic acid or ketoacid production will cause a decrease in the plasma concentration of bicarbonate. The anion gap helps identify the type of acidosis and estimate the magnitude of the acid load to the system.

◆ **Effect of metabolic acidosis on the respiratory system:** Increases ventilation to lower the arterial $[CO_2]$ to compensate for the fall in plasma pH.

◆ **Chemoreceptors involved in response to an acid–base disturbance:** Two groups of chemoreceptors respond to a metabolic acidosis:

  1. Peripheral chemoreceptors located in the carotid bodies detect changes in arterial $[H^+]$, $[CO_2]$, and $[O_2]$.

  2. Central chemoreceptors located on the medulla (reticular segment). They are separated from the blood by the blood–brain barrier and detect changes in the arterial $[CO_2]$.

◆ **Lung stretch receptors:** Slow-acting reflexes.

CLINICAL CORRELATION

Overdosing on over-the-counter medications is a commonly seen problem in emergency centers. A thorough history and physical examination often will reveal clues necessary to make the diagnosis. In this case, the history of depression with stressful final examinations coming up and an empty bottle of recently purchased aspirin make one think of the possibility of salicylate poisoning. Salicylate poisoning may cause clinical symptoms of vomiting, sweating, tachycardia, fever, lethargy confusion, coma, seizures, cardiovascular collapse, and possibly pulmonary or cerebral edema. Salicylate ingestion can cause a multitude of effects, depending on the magnitude of the ingestion. A complication is that salicylates can alter metabolic processes, causing an increase in lactic acid production, and directly stimulate central respiratory centers, causing hyperventilation and a fall in arterial PCO_2. Symptoms usually occur 3 to 6 hours after an overdose. Abnormal laboratory findings may include anion gap metabolic acidosis, hypokalemia, hypoglycemia, and a positive urine ferric chloride test. Other agents are also possible, including acetaminophen, alcohol, and illicit drugs. Treatment of salicylate toxicity includes activated charcoal to decontaminate the stomach (possibly gastric lavage), correction of electrolyte abnormalities, supportive care with intravenous (IV) fluids, and alkalization of urine (promotes excretion of salicylates). Elevated levels of salicylates increase the sensitivity of the respiratory center in the brain. The metabolic acidosis results in hyperventilation and a compensatory respiratory alkalosis.

APPROACH TO CONTROL OF BREATHING

Objectives

1. Know the central and peripheral centers for control of breathing.
2. Describe the different types of chemoreceptors.
3. Know the different types of receptors (lung stretch, irritant, etc.).

Definitions

Respiratory center: Located in the reticular formation of the medulla it is responsible for maintaining a rhythmical cycle of breathing and integrating neural input from a variety of receptors (e.g. central and peripheral chemoreceptors) to adjust the rate and depth of breathing in response to perturbations in environmental or physical conditions.

Central chemoreceptors: Located in the ventrolateral surface of the medulla directly respond to a change in the pH of the CSF, however, since the blood brain barrier is impermeable to either H^+ or HCO_3^-, these receptors detect changes in the arterial PCO_2.

Peripheral chemoreceptors: Located on the carotid and aortic bodies these receptors respond directly to changes in the arterial pH, PCO_2, and PO_2.

CO_2 / HCO_3^- buffering system: The central buffering system in the body for maintaining H^+ homeostasis. The importance of this buffering system is the ability to control the arterial PCO_2 by pulmonary function and $[HCO_3^-]$ through renal function to compensate for acid-base disturbances.

DISCUSSION

The pH of the arterial blood is normally 7.4 and is dependent mainly on the CO_2 / HCO_3^- buffering system in the blood:

$$CO_2 + H_2O \rightarrow H_2CO_3 \rightarrow H^+ + HCO_3^-$$

The control of the pH, or **hydrogen ion homeostasis** is dependent on an interaction of the **respiratory control of arterial PCO_2** and **renal control of arterial HCO_3^- and H^+** excretion. Acid–base disturbances are generally identified as being of respiratory or metabolic origin. **Respiratory acid–base disorders** are a consequence of a respiratory disturbance that results in a **change** in the arterial PCO_2. Until the disturbance is corrected, renal function will compensate the disruption. **Metabolic disturbances** are the consequence of a **change in the arterial pH** caused by initial changes in $[H^+]$ or $[HCO_3^-]$. The **respiratory system** serves to **compensate for metabolic disturbances**. The respiratory system is finely tuned to and highly sensitive to changes in CO_2 and H^+. The O_2 concentration is an important regulator, but has a minimal role until the arterial PO_2 falls to less than 55 to 60 mm Hg. Acid–base disturbances have immediate effects on respiration caused by specific chemoreceptors that are sensitive to changes in CO_2, H^+, and O_2.

This case involves a **metabolic acidosis** caused by the ingestion of an acidic substance. The respiratory system can compensate for this disturbance only by controlling the CO_2 concentration and shifting the equilibrium of the CO_2/HCO_3^- buffering system and maintaining hydrogen ion homeostasis. Acid–base balance is markedly disturbed, as indicated by the anion gap. Acid–base balance can be restored only by renal excretion of the acid and reabsorption of HCO_3^- (see Case 27 for the renal response to an acid–base disturbance).

Respiration is **spontaneously and rhythmically initiated by the respiratory center** located in the **reticular formation of the medulla.** Neural signaling to the inspiratory and expiratory muscle groups maintains the cycle of breathing. Numerous mechanisms are capable of modifying the signal to alter the frequency and depth of breathing in response to voluntary stimuli, reflexes and other neural stimuli, and a variety of chemical or mechanical stimuli. **Acid–base disturbances** are characteristically identified by their effects on plasma pH, PCO_2, and $[HCO_3^-]$. **Chemoreceptors** located centrally and in the periphery respond to changes in arterial pH and PCO_2 with input to the respiratory center that causes compensatory changes in breathing. **Peripheral chemoreceptors** are located in the **carotid bodies and the aortic bodies** and detect changes in pH, O_2, and to a lesser extent PCO_2. Under normal conditions, O_2 has little role in the control of ventilation. However, under hypoxic conditions in which the PO_2 begins to approach 50 mm Hg or lower, O_2 stimulates ventilation directly and increases sensitivity to H^+ and CO_2. Impulses from the peripheral chemoreceptors are carried by the **glossopharyngeal nerve** to the respiratory center. Stimulation of the peripheral chemoreceptors causes an increase in ventilatory rate. **Central chemoreceptors** located on the **medulla** are separated from the blood by the blood–brain barrier. These receptors are bathed by the cerebrospinal fluid (CSF), which is essentially a pure bicarbonate buffer. Because the blood–brain barrier is impermeable to H^+ and HCO_3^- but freely permeable to CO_2, a **change in the arterial CO_2** will cause a change in the CSF CO_2 with a concomitant change in the CSF pH. Thus, although directly sensing a change in CSF pH, central chemoreceptors respond to changes in the arterial PCO_2. A **fall in the arterial PCO_2 (hypocapnia)** will **increase the CSF pH and slow respiration.** An increase in the arterial PCO_2 (hypercapnia) will decrease the CSF pH and stimulate respiration.

Physiologically, a **metabolic acidosis** or an **initial decrease in pH** (an increase in H^+) stimulates the **peripheral chemoreceptors, resulting in hyperventilation.** The hyperventilation leads to a compensatory fall in PCO_2. Normally, the magnitude of the hyperventilation is limited and controlled by a negative feedback from the central chemoreceptors, which detect only a decrease in PCO_2. This important control mechanism serves to dampen the respiratory response to an acid–base disturbance. In the present case of **salicylate intoxication**, there also may be a **direct stimulation of the respiratory center** that will cause a further **increase in the respiratory rate with a resultant respiratory alkalosis (hypocapnia) superimposed on the metabolic acidosis.** This example emphasizes the importance of the interactions between the central and peripheral chemoreceptors. A metabolic alkalosis will have exactly the opposite response. The peripheral chemoreceptors respond to an increased pH (a fall in H^+) by slowing ventilation with a compensatory rise in PCO_2. The rise in arterial PCO_2 is sensed by central chemoreceptors, which respond with an increase in the ventilatory rate to dampen the response. In disorders in which one or the other chemoreceptor is blocked or nonfunctional, severe aberrations in breathing patterns are observed.

In addition to the chemoreceptors outlined above, there are three receptor groups that are located in the lungs. **J-receptors** (juxtapulmonary capillary receptors) are located in the interstitium near alveoli and blood capillaries. Increasing pressure in the interstitium by edema or capillary engorgement stimulates J-receptors, causing bronchoconstriction and tachypnea. **Irritant receptors** are located in the airways between epithelial cells. They are located in such a way that they have immediate contact with inhaled air and are stimulated by cigarette smoke, dust, fumes, and cold air. Stimulation of irritant receptors leads to bronchoconstriction, hyperpnea, coughing, and sneezing. **Pulmonary stretch receptors** are located in airway smooth muscle and are stimulated by distention of the lung and serve to protect the lungs against being overinflated.

COMPREHENSION QUESTIONS

[20.1] A 17-year-old male develops pneumonia, diabetic ketoacidosis, and metabolic acidosis. Respiratory compensation to a metabolic acidosis consists of hyperventilation to lower the arterial PCO_2. The cause of the hyperventilation is described by which of the following statements?

A. CO_2 produced from the reaction of the acid with bicarbonate stimulates central chemoreceptors.

B. A decrease in the bicarbonate concentration stimulates ventilation.

C. H^+ stimulates central chemoreceptors.

D. H^+ stimulates peripheral chemoreceptors.

[20.2]   A 21-year-old woman is admitted to the intensive care unit for an opi-
         ate drug overdose that probably has suppressed her central chemore-
         ceptor response to CO_2, diminishing the drive for ventilation. Her
         respiratory rate is diminished at eight breaths per minute. Which of
         the following is the best course of action for this patient?

         A. Administration of oxygen by mask
         B. Administration of benzodiazepine for possible alcohol withdrawal
         C. Leaving the patient on room air
         D. Placing the patient on a low opiate infusion to prevent opiate
             withdrawal

[20.3]   A 29-year-old man who lives at sea level drives up a mountain to a
         high altitude (17,000 feet) for over 3 hours. Which of the following
         statements best describes his condition after the elevation climb?

         A. Increased arterial PO_2
         B. Decreased arterial PCO_2
         C. Decreased arterial pH
         D. Decreased respiratory rate

Answers

[20.1]   **D.** A common mistake is thinking that elevated CO_2 produced by the
         reaction of the acid with bicarbonate is the stimulus for ventilation. To
         the contrary, as soon as the peripheral chemoreceptors sense an
         increase in the H^+, there will be an immediate increase in the rate of
         ventilation. The hyperventilation lowers the alveolar PCO_2, which low-
         ers the arterial PCO_2. This is the appropriate compensatory response
         because the initial perturbation was a decrease in the bicarbonate con-
         centration from the acid insult. From the Henderson-Hasselbalch equa-
         tion, it is apparent that a fall in the bicarbonate concentration can be
         compensated most rapidly by a proportionate fall in CO_2.

[20.2]   **C.** Because of the narcotic effect, the central receptors are insensitive to
         CO_2; therefore, CO_2 exerts no ventilatory drive. The only drive for ven-
         tilation is the fall in O_2 resulting from the near cessation of breathing.
         Applying oxygen will remove the remaining drive for ventilation, and
         breathing will stop. Thus, room air with oxygen saturation monitoring
         is the best action. Medications that further suppress respirations, such as
         sedatives (benzodiazepines, opiates, hypnotics), are contraindicated.

[20.3]   **B.** The partial pressure of oxygen decreases with increasing altitude.
         Rapid ascent to high altitude can result in hypoxia. The hypoxia stim-
         ulates pulmonary ventilation to increase alveolar PO_2. A consequence
         of the hyperventilation is to decrease the PCO_2, or hypocapnia. The
         fall in CO_2 shifts the equilibrium of the CO_2/HCO_3^- buffer system to
         decrease the H^+, resulting in a respiratory alkalosis.

PHYSIOLOGY PEARLS

❖ The rate and depth of respiration are controlled by a neural feedback loop that involves central chemoreceptors in the medulla and peripheral chemoreceptors in the aortic and carotid bodies. Central chemoreceptors are separated from the blood by the blood–brain barrier and detect changes in arterial $[CO_2]$. Peripheral chemoreceptors respond directly to $[H^+]$, CO_2, and O_2.

❖ The concentration of CO_2 in the blood is controlled by the alveolar PCO_2. Hyperventilation decreases the PCO_2, and hypoventilation increases the PCO_2. Raising the arterial $[CO_2]$ causes a hyperventilation with a compensatory decrease, and lowering the $[CO_2]$ causes a hypoventilation.

❖ The main buffer system in the body is the CO_2/HCO_3^- buffering system. One of its components, CO_2, is controlled by the ventilatory rate; therefore, one of the most effective ways of compensating for an acid or base disturbance is to alter the $[CO_2]$ in the blood. Increasing H^+ stimulates ventilation, which lowers CO_2. Conversely, a fall in $[H^+]$ slows ventilation, resulting in a rise in $[CO_2]$.

REFERENCE

Powell FL. Structure and function of the respiratory system. In: Johnson LR, ed. *Essential Medical Physiology*. 3rd ed. San Diego, CA: Elsevier Academic Press; 2003:259-276.

A 23-year-old man has been admitted to the surgical floor after suffering multiple injuries in a motor vehicle accident. Plain film radiographs have not indicated any fractures. At the time of admission, his abdomen had some bruising but no distention or tenderness. After 8 hours of observation, the nurse calls the physician because the patient's urine output has been decreasing steadily. His blood pressure is normal but lower than it was when he presented to the hospital, and he has a slightly increased heart rate. His abdomen is now distended and tender. An intravenous (IV) fluid bolus of 500 mL of normal saline is administered, and his urine output increases to a normal range. The surgeon makes a diagnosis of hypovolemia that probably is caused by intraabdominal hemorrhage and prepares the patient for exploratory surgery.

◆ **What is the response of the juxtaglomerular cells to decreased extracellular fluid and arterial pressure?**

◆ **What are two effects of angiotensin II?**

◆ **What are two mechanism by which autoregulation of renal blood flow occurs?**

ANSWERS TO CASE 21: RENAL BLOOD FLOW AND GLOMERULAR FILTRATION RATE

Summary: A 23-year-old man has hypotension, tachycardia, and oliguria secondary to intraabdominal hemorrhage after a motor vehicle accident.

◆ **Juxtaglomerular cells and decreased renal arterial perfusion:** Release of renin.

◆ **Two effects of angiotension II:** Increases vascular smooth muscle tone and increases aldosterone production by the adrenal cortex.

◆ **Mechanisms of autoregulation:** Myogenic mechanism and tubuloglomerular feedback.

CLINICAL CORRELATION

Monitoring urine output is an easy way to assess a patient's fluid status. Often after surgery or trauma, a Foley catheter is placed in the bladder to measure urine output accurately. Decreasing urine output may be because of hypovolemia or injury to the urinary tract system. In this case, the decreased urine output probably was secondary to hypovolemia, because the patient also has hypotension and tachycardia. The blood pressure remained relatively normal initially because of the renin-angiotensin system, which sensed the decreased blood flow to the renal artery, and the sympathetic nervous system, which sensed the decreased blood volume and pressure. The decreased blood flow through the renal artery will stimulate renin to be released, with the subsequent generation of angiotensin II, leading to increased systemic blood pressure and total peripheral resistance. Decreased blood volume and pressure will be sensed by volume and pressure receptors, leading to modest vasoconstriction and increased systemic blood pressure. With excessive blood loss (hypovolemic shock), the action of the autonomic (sympathetic) nervous system causes pronounced vasoconstriction of the renal arteries with shunting of blood to vital organs (brain, heart, lungs) and is seen clinically with decreased urine output. Replacement with crystalloid fluids and blood is necessary to maintain kidney perfusion and prevent acute tubular necrosis. If a patient is in shock and urine output is not responding to IV fluids and blood, low-dose dopamine often is used to cause renal artery dilation and increased renal blood flow. In any case, the source of bleeding must be addressed and intravascular volume must be replaced.

APPROACH TO GLOMERULAR FILTRATION RATE

Objectives

1. Know the concepts underlying regulation of renal artery blood flow.
2. Understand the concept of autoregulation.
3. Know the basics of how to measure the glomerular filtration rate (GFR).

Definitions

Renin: A proteolytic enzyme released from the juxtaglomerular cells of the afferent arteriole that splits off angiotensin I from angiotensinogen.

Angiotensin II: A potent vasoactive peptide produced by the conversion of angiotensin I to angiotensin II by angiotensin-converting enzyme (ACE).

Antidiuretic hormone (ADH, vasopressin): A posterior pituitary peptide hormone that functions both as a regulator of osmotic balance and a vasoconstrictor.

Autoregulation: The maintenance of normal blood flow to an organ during periods of altered arterial pressure.

Tubuloglomerular feedback: The process by which alterations in renal tubular flow are sensed by specialized cells in the macula densa and signal the afferent arteriole to constrict or dilate to bring about alterations in GFR, thereby negating the alteration in tubular flow.

DISCUSSION

Urine output is regulated by numerous factors, including alterations in extracellular fluid volume and blood volume (volume expansion or depletion). Typically, under conditions of volume expansion (eg, drinking a liter of water), urine output is increased, whereas under conditions of **volume depletion** (eg, hemorrhage, profuse sweating) **urine output is decreased.** In this case, the patient probably has had an intraabdominal hemorrhage during trauma that has led to modest volume depletion. The renal system responds by reducing urine output in an attempt to maintain volume-water balance. As this case demonstrates, several mechanisms come into play to regulate urine output during volume depletion, including the sympathetic nervous system, volume-sensitive hormonal systems, and intrinsic autoregulator mechanisms.

Renal autoregulation is an intrinsic property of the renal vasculature that serves to maintain renal blood flow and the GFR at nearly normal levels in the presence of alterations in renal arterial pressure. Although the mechanism of this response is not fully understood, it appears to be predominantly related to myogenic stretch receptors in the wall of the afferent arteriole, similar to what is observed in precapillary sphincters in muscle capillaries during autoregulation of muscle blood flow. The efferent arteriole does not appear to be involved in the autoregulation mechanisms. Under conditions of **elevated mean arterial pressures,** such as observed during volume expansion, hydrostatic pressures along the renal vasculature will be elevated, leading to an **initial increase in renal blood flow and the GFR** (secondary to elevation of glomerular capillary hydrostatic pressure). The elevated pressure in the afferent arteriole stretches the arteriole, causing the **arteriole to respond, inducing constriction.** This constriction returns blood flow to near normal and glomerular hydrostatic pressure and, hence GFR, to near normal. Conversely, under conditions of **depressed mean arterial pressure,** such as observed during volume depletion, hydrostatic pressure along the renal vasculature is decreased, leading to an initial decrease in renal blood flow and GFR (secondary to reduction of glomerular capillary hydrostatic pressure). The reduced pressure decreases the stretch of the afferent arteriole, causing the arteriole to respond, inducing **dilation.** This returns blood flow and GFR to near normal. Maximum dilation is approached when renal perfusion pressures decrease to 70 to 80 mm Hg so that further decreases in renal arterial pressure will lead to parallel decreases in renal blood flow and GFR.

Tubuloglomerular feedback also serves to autoregulate renal blood flow and GFR through a mechanism induced by alterations in tubular flow rate (**chloride delivery**) that is sensed by specialized cells in the **macula densa segment** of the **cortical thick ascending limb.** These cells are juxtapositioned to their own afferent arteriole and control constriction of the arteriole. Under conditions of an elevated GFR, for example, volume expansion, the tubular flow rate (chloride delivery) will increase; this will be sensed by the macula densa cells, and this leads to constriction of the afferent arteriole, bringing about a reduction in GFR and tubular flow rate. Conversely, under conditions of a reduced GFR, for example, volume depletion, the reduced tubular flow rate will be sensed by the macula densa cells, leading to dilation of the afferent arteriole, bringing about an increase in GFR and tubular flow rate. Hence, the tubuloglomerular feedback mechanism works in parallel with the normal autoregulatory process in an attempt to maintain renal blood flow and GFR at nearly normal levels.

Extrinsic factors play a significant role in regulating renal function during both hypo- and hypervolemia and normally overpower the intrinsic autoregulatory mechanisms. The **renin-angiotensin-aldosterone system** can play a major role in this process. In hypovolemic states, the reduction in blood volume results in reduced renal blood flow and reduced hydrostatic pressure along the renal vasculature. The decrease in pressure in the afferent arteriole is sensed by baroreceptors in the afferent arteriole, leading to stimulation of renin release from the juxtaglomerular cells of the afferent arteriole (increased sympathetic activity also increases renin release).

Renin   ACE

Angiotensinogen $\rightarrow$ Angiotensin I $\rightarrow$ Angiotensin II

Renin is a proteolytic enzyme that works on a plasma α_2-globulin, angiotensinogen, to produce angiotensin I, which in turn is converted to angiotensin II by ACE, which is present predominantly at the luminal surface of endothelial cells in the lungs, although significant levels are present in the renal afferent and efferent arterioles.

Angiotensin II is a **potent vasoactive peptide** that leads to **vasoconstriction, elevating mean arterial pressure toward normal. Angiotensin II** also leads to **vasoconstriction of both the afferent and efferent arterioles,** increasing renal vascular resistance and reducing renal blood flow. This leads to a modest decrease in glomerular capillary hydrostatic pressure and, in turn, GFR. The reduced GFR will contribute to a reduction in urine output (see below).

In a similar manner, hypervolemic states lead to elevated mean arterial pressure, bringing about an increase in renal blood flow and pressure along the renal vasculature. The afferent arteriole baroreceptors sense this change and signal to reduce renin release from the afferent arteriole, resulting in a reduction in angiotensin II and causing vasodilation and a reduction in mean arteriole pressure. A dilation of both the afferent and efferent arterioles will accompany the reduced angiotensin II levels, causing an increase in renal blood flow and a modest increase in GFR. This in turn contributes to an increase in urine output.

Angiotensin II plays a secondary role in volume regulation by regulating the synthesis of aldosterone, a mineralocorticoid hormone, by the zona glomerulosa cells of the adrenal cortex. Aldosterone, in turn, acts on the renal distal tubule and cortical collecting ducts to enhance sodium (and chloride) reabsorption, leading to salt retention and an associated retention of water with a corresponding decrease in urine output. Hence, adaptive responses to elevation of angiotensin II during volume depletion lead to aldosterone synthesis and thus increased fluid retention. The opposite occurs in volume expansion.

The sympathetic nervous system also is intimately involved in regulating renal function during alterations in volume balance. Volume depletion will be accompanied by a decrease in blood volume and venous return to the heart that will be sensed by baroreceptors (volume receptors) in the atria and pulmonary veins and pressure receptors in the renal afferent arteriole, leading to increased sympathetic activity. This will result in sympathetically mediated vasoconstriction and partial return of mean arterial pressure toward normal. If blood volume depletion is modest—less than 10% of blood volume—the changes are modest, but will help maintain blood pressure near normal. With more severe cases of hypovolemia (15% to 25% blood loss), there is a more pronounced sympathetic-mediated vasoconstriction. Increased sympathetic activity also will lead to constriction of both the afferent and efferent arterioles, which, like angiotensin II, will reduce renal blood flow and modestly reduce GFR (subsequent to a modest reduction in glomerular capillary hydrostatic pressure) and contribute to reduced urine output. Conversely, during volume expansion, baroreceptors will sense an increase in blood volume and mean arterial pressure, leading to a decrease in sympathetic activity which, in turn, will lead to vasodilation and a return of blood pressure toward normal. Dilation of both the afferent and efferent arterioles will bring about an increase in renal blood flow and a modest increase in GFR and urine output. Again, the response is to return blood volume toward normal.

A final modulator of water and volume balance is ADH. Although alterations in plasma osmolarity are the main factor regulating ADH release from the posterior pituitary, alterations in blood volume also are part of the response (see Case 24). During volume depletion, volume receptors lead to increased release of ADH into plasma. The ADH binds to receptors on the renal collecting ducts, leading to the insertion of water channels (aquaporins) into the luminal cell membrane, increasing cell water permeability and, in turn, stimulating water reabsorption from the tubule lumen. Water is retained, and urine output is reduced. Conversely, during volume expansion, volume receptors sense the change, leading to a decrease in ADH secretion with a subsequent decrease in the water permeability and hence, water reabsorption by the collecting ducts. Water is lost, and urine output is elevated.

GFR is a major factor controlling the function of the kidney and is a major indicator of abnormal functions of the renal system. Hence, estimating GFR in the clinical setting is critical to understanding the status of the kidney. GFR typically is estimated in the clinic by measuring **creatinine clearance** or is estimated indirectly from the **plasma levels of creatinine and blood urea nitrogen (BUN).** Both of these components are filtered at the glomerulus and excreted in the urine. As a result, both are **inversely related to GFR.** A reduction in GFR leads to reduced filtration and, in turn, excretion of these substances, resulting in elevated plasma levels. Hence, the time course of kidney diseases that affect GFR often can be monitored over years by following the changes in plasma levels of BUN and creatinine. A more direct assessment of GFR can be obtained by measuring the clearance of creatinine (see the references at the end of this case).

COMPREHENSION QUESTIONS

[21.1] An individual is known to be suffering from diabetes mellitus. Recently, he has developed hypertension. His doctor suspects that the patient may be developing renal insufficiency that is leading to a reduced glomerular filtration and, as a result, hypervolemia and hypertension. The doctor wishes to evaluate kidney function by measuring the glomerular filtration rate (GFR). She can estimate GFR best by performing a urine clearance study of which of the following substances?

   A. Creatinine
   B. Para-aminohippuric acid (PAH)
   C. Urea
   D. Glucose
   E. Sodium

[21.2] A 21-year-old man has been vomiting to the point where he has become hypovolemic, as evidenced by an accompanying decrease in blood pressure and a feeling of light-headedness. The kidneys respond by reducing urinary volume flow, thus limiting the potential extent of hypovolemia. Increases in the plasma levels of which of the following hormones will bring about the most dramatic decrease in urinary volume flow rate?

   A. Angiotensin II
   B. Atrial natriuretic peptide
   C. Parathyroid hormone
   D. Aldosterone
   E. Arginine vasopressin (ADH)

[21.3] A 56-year-old woman is diagnosed with small-cell carcinoma of the lung. She has a paraneoplastic effect from the cancer, with release of an ADH-like agent. Which of the following is most likely to be seen?

A. Elevated serum sodium
B. Elevated serum osmolarity
C. Elevated urine sodium
D. Elevated urine catecholamines

Answers

[21.1] **A.** Creatinine is a normal end product of muscle metabolism. It is freely filtered at the glomerulus and excreted in the urine. Although creatinine is not reabsorbed by the kidney tubules, it is partially secreted so that the rate of urinary excretion of creatinine overestimates the rate of filtration by a small percentage in healthy individuals (it overestimates more in individuals with a compromised GFR). Nonetheless, in the clinic the clearance of creatinine can provide a reasonable estimate of GFR.

[21.2] **E.** Increases in plasma levels of arginine vasopressin, or ADH, lead to water reabsorption by the collecting ducts, decreasing urine output.

[21.3] **C.** ADH allows for increased reabsorption of water from the collecting system, and thus decreases serum sodium and serum osmolarity The urine is concentrated with high sodium and high osmolarity.

PHYSIOLOGY PEARLS

❖ Baroreceptors in the renal afferent arteriole sense low blood pressure in the arteriole and induce release of renin from the juxtaglomerular cells of the arteriole.

❖ Both the renal afferent and efferent arterioles are innervated with sympathetic nerves that regulate contraction and dilation of the arterioles.

❖ Autoregulation in the kidney maintains constancy of both renal blood flow and GFR during periods of altered renal arterial pressure.

❖ Aldosterone regulates the reabsorption of sodium (and chloride) from the distal tubule and the cortical collecting duct, bringing about retention of salt and water and an increase in extracellular fluid volume.

❖ ADH acts on the collecting ducts to increase their water permeability, leading to an increase in water reabsorption from the tubular fluid, bringing about retention of water and an increase in extracellular fluid volume.

REFERENCES

Giebisch G, Windhager E. Integration of salt and water balance. In: Boron WF, Boulpaep EL, eds. *Medical Physiology: A Cellular and Molecular Approach.* New York: Saunders; 2003:Chap 39.

Schafer JA. Regulation of sodium balance and extracellular fluid volume. In: Johnson LR, ed. *Essential Medical Physiology.* 3rd ed. San Diego, CA: Academic Press; 2003:Chap 29.

A 27-year-old patient presents at her obstetrician's office for her first prenatal visit at 26 weeks gestation. She has no medical history and has had an uncomplicated pregnancy. Her examination is normal other than glycosuria noted on the urine dipstick. A 1-hour glucose challenge test is performed along with her other prenatal laboratories, and they are all normal. The obstetrician diagnoses the glycosuria as a normal physiologic response to the increased glomerular filtration rate (GFR) of pregnancy.

◆ **Where in the renal glomerulus-tubule structure is glucose reabsorbed actively (secondary active transport)?**

◆ **What other solutes are reabsorbed by a secondary active process?**

◆ **With what is glucose cotransported in the proximal tubule?**

ANSWERS TO CASE 22: RENAL TUBULE ABSORPTION

Summary: A 27-year-old pregnant woman presents at 26 weeks gestation with glycosuria and a normal diabetic screen.

 Location of glucose reabsorption: Proximal tubule.

 Other actively reabsorbed solutes: Organic acids, amino acids, proteins and peptides, phosphate, and sulfate.

 Cotransporter with glucose: Sodium.

CLINICAL CORRELATION

Glycosuria is present when the filtered load of glucose in the kidney is too large to be reabsorbed. This can be seen in patients with diabetes. The glycosuria acts as an osmotic diuretic and leads to the common symptoms of uncontrolled diabetes: urinary frequency, nocturia, and frequent thirst. During pregnancy, several factors influence glucose reabsorption in the kidney. At that time there is an increased GFR that increases the filtered load of glucose. Lactose and galactose will also be present in the urine in addition to glucose. The increase in GFR and filtered glucose load are normal changes that result in glycosuria during pregnancy. The presence of glycosuria is not suggestive of gestational diabetes, and a 1-hour diabetic screen must be performed to rule out that disease.

APPROACH TO RENAL TUBULE TRANSPORT

Objectives

1. Understand the function of the proximal tubule.
2. Know the importance of sodium reabsorption.
3. Describe the role of sodium with reabsorption of organic acids, amino acids, and proteins.

Definitions

Glycosuria: A condition characterized by the appearance of glucose in the urine.
Tubular transport maximum (Tm): The maximum rate of transport for a substance (eg, TmG denotes the maximum reabsorptive rate of glucose).

DISCUSSION

Most of the fluid filtered at the glomerulus is reabsorbed along the length of the nephron and collecting ducts (see Figure 22-1 for the parts of the glomerulus,

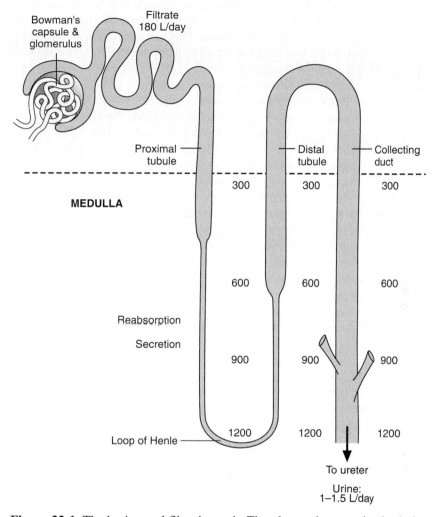

CORTEX

Bowman's capsule & glomerulus

Filtrate 180 L/day

Proximal tubule

Distal tubule

Collecting duct

MEDULLA

300   300   300

600   600   600

Reabsorption

Secretion

900   900   900

1200   1200   1200

Loop of Henle

To ureter

Urine: 1–1.5 L/day

Figure 22-1. The basic renal filtration unit. The glomerulus, proximal tubule, descending limb and ascending limb, distal tubule, and collecting duct.

nephron, and collecting duct). Approximately 60% to 70% of the filtered fluid is reabsorbed in the proximal tubule. The **primary transport process** underlying fluid reabsorption is **active sodium reabsorption.** Water and many other filtered solutes then are reabsorbed passively as an isosmotic reabsorbate.

Sodium ion is reabsorbed actively by the proximal tubule cells. The driving force for reabsorption is the **Na⁺ pump (also called the Na⁺-K⁺ exchange pump),** which is a Na⁺-K⁺-ATPase. The Na⁺ pump actively extrudes Na⁺

across the basolateral membrane in exchange for K^+, thereby keeping the $[Na^+]$ concentration inside the cell low and $[K^+]$ high. The high $[K^+]$ generates a diffusion potential across the basolateral membrane that is responsible for the cell's negative membrane potential (-70 mV) across the basolateral and luminal cell borders. The low intracellular $[Na^+]$ concentration and the cell's negative membrane potential create a favorable gradient for passive entry of Na^+ across the luminal membrane into the cell. The Na^+ then is extruded actively across the basolateral membrane, giving rise to Na^+ reabsorption. Chloride and bicarbonate ion are reabsorbed passively either through the cell or through the tight junctions between the cells (the proximal tubule has "leaky" tight junctions), providing a balance of charge. **The tissue is very leaky to water** so that as solute is reabsorbed through the cell into the interstitial space, **water follows passively** by osmotic coupling to the solute, moving through the cells or through the "leaky" tight junctions between the cells.

The entry step for Na^+ across the luminal cell membrane is normally a coupled process. The **two most dominant transport processes are Na^+-H^+ exchange,** which is important for Na^+ reabsorption and acid–base balance, and **Na^+-glucose cotransport,** which is important for both Na^+ and glucose reabsorption. Both processes are passive steps that are driven by the Na^+ gradient into the cell (set up by the Na^+ pump). For glucose, the downhill gradient for Na^+ entry across the luminal membrane can drive the cellular glucose concentration to higher levels than that apparent in the luminal fluid, thereby appearing to be active transport, but only secondary to Na^+ transport (see Figure 1-2). Hence, **glucose** entry often is referred to as **secondary active transport** even though the entry step is passive. Once inside the cell, glucose is transported passively across the basolateral membrane by a **facilitated diffusion process** (passive glucose transporter) into the interstitial space and taken up into the peritubular capillaries.

Under **normal conditions, all filtered glucose is reabsorbed,** except for trace quantities, from the tubular lumen of the proximal tubule, utilizing the Na^+-glucose cotransport process at the luminal border. However, both Na^+ and glucose must bind to specific, but saturable, sites on the **Na^+-glucose cotransport carrier protein,** making glucose reabsorption saturable. Hence, under conditions of **elevated plasma glucose levels,** such as in diabetes mellitus, or an **increased glomerular filtration rate,** such as in pregnancy, the filtered glucose load can exceed the capacity for glucose transport; that is, the **Na^+ glucose cotransporters become saturated,** leaving un-reabsorbed glucose behind in the tubular fluid which is swept away into the final urine (glycosuria). The **maximum rate of glucose reabsorption** (Figure 22-2) is defined as the **tubular transport maximum for glucose (Tm_G),** whereas the plasma concentration at which glucose first begins to appear in the urine is defined as the **renal plasma threshold.** In the presence of un-reabsorbed glucose, the "trapped" glucose will act as an osmotic solute, leading to an osmotic diuresis. The associated diuresis can be particularly problematic in patients with diabetes mellitus.

The reabsorption of other organic solutes in the proximal tubule also is coupled to Na^+ as a **Na^+-solute cotransporter at the luminal cell membrane,**

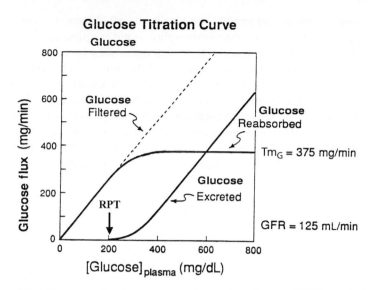

Figure 22-2. Tm_G: tubular transport maximum for glucose; RPT: renal plasma threshold for glucose.

similar to what has been described for glucose. Both sugars, such as galactose, and most amino acids, such as glutamate and glycine, are cotransported with Na^+ and display both a tubular transport maximum and a renal plasma threshold (the transport of some amino acids, such as lysine and proline, is not Na^+ dependent). Galactose can compete with glucose for binding and transport by the Na^+-glucose carrier so that with elevated plasma levels of galactose, such as in pregnancy, galactose can contribute to appearance of glucose in the urine.

The **proximal tubule** is also the site of reabsorption of certain **organic acids,** with the most dominant normally being **lactate** anion. Two Na^+-dependent cotransport process at the luminal membrane appear to underlie organic acid reabsorption: one specific for monocarboxylates such as lactate, pyruvate, acetoacetate, and β-hydroxybutyrate and the other for di- and tricarboxylates such as malate, succinate, and citrate. Both are Na^+-organic solute cotransporters and hence require Na^+ for uptake. Once inside the cell, the carboxylates exit the cell by means of a variety of exchange processes. Other organic acids, such as urate, an end product of purine catabolism, are both secreted and reabsorbed in the proximal tubule; both processes are Na^+-independent, with the reabsorptive mechanisms dominating. Finally, the **proximal tubule** is the site of **secretion** of numerous **organic anions** (para-aminohippurate, oxalate) and **cations** (choline, guanidine) by separate, saturable transport processes that often involve anion exchange processes that are Na^+-independent.

Filtered peptides and proteins are also **reabsorbed almost entirely** in the **proximal tubule.** However, their reabsorption is **not coupled directly to Na$^+$.** Small peptides such as angiotensin II are first hydrolyzed by brush-border peptidases to their constituent amino acids, and the amino acids then are reabsorbed via the usual Na$^+$-amino acid cotransport processes. Larger peptides and proteins such as **myoglobin and albumin** bind to the luminal membrane and enter the cell by **receptor-mediated endocytic** processes and are delivered to **lysosomes** for degradation. Some filtered inorganic anions, such as sulphate and phosphate, also are reabsorbed in the proximal tubule via a Na$^+$ cotransport process; hence, their transport can be defined by a Tm and renal plasma threshold.

COMPREHENSION QUESTIONS

[22.1] An individual has adult-onset diabetes. She has high levels of glucose in the urine and is experiencing a brisk diuresis. The appearance of glucose in the urine is a consequence of which of the following processes in the proximal tubule?

A. Inhibition of Na$^+$-K$^+$-ATPase (Na$^+$ pump)
B. Saturation of the Na$^+$-glucose cotransporter
C. Saturation of the Na$^+$-H$^+$ exchanger
D. Stimulation of glucose secretion
E. Stimulation of glycogen breakdown

[22.2] A student under stress has been feeling light-headed, especially after standing, and has developed a brisk diuresis. He has the smell of acetone on his breath. Upon admission to the emergency room, he is diagnosed with diabetic ketoacidosis, which is accompanied by extreme hypovolemia, supposedly because of the brisk diuresis. The brisk diuresis is a consequence of which of the following?

A. High levels of glucose in the tubular fluid/urine
B. Increased glomerular filtration rate
C. Suppression of arginine vasopressin secretion
D. Suppression of aldosterone secretion
E. Decreased angiotensin II plasma levels

[22.3] A 23-year-old man is brought into the emergency center because of cocaine intoxication. His urine is "tea" colored as a result of breakdown of skeletal muscle by the cocaine, so-called rhabdomyolysis. Which of the following describes the fate of myoglobin in the renal tubule?

A. Absorbed in the proximal tubule by active transport by sodium cotransport
B. Absorbed in the proximal tubule by receptor-mediated endocytosis
C. Absorbed in the distal tubule by facilitated diffusion
D. Not absorbed and excreted in the urine

Answers

[22.1]   **B.** In diabetes mellitus, in which plasma glucose levels are markedly elevated, the high glucose load being filtered (with an elevated concentration) can exceed the capacity of the luminal Na^+-glucose cotransporter to reabsorb glucose (ie, the carrier is saturated). The excess glucose that is not reabsorbed is trapped in the tubular fluid because no transport pathways are present in later nephron segments to reabsorb this hexose. Hence, glycosuria will develop.

[22.2]   **A.** In diabetic ketoacidosis, plasma levels of glucose are elevated, leading to an excess filtered load of glucose. The increased rate of filtration of glucose can exceed the capacity of the Na^+-glucose cotransporter in the proximal tubule to reabsorb all the glucose. The excess glucose that is not reabsorbed will be retained in the tubular lumen and generate a solute diuresis.

[22.3]   **B.** Larger peptides and proteins such as **myoglobin and albumin** bind to the luminal membrane and enter the cell by **receptor-mediated endocytic** processes and are delivered to **lysosomes** for degradation. Myoglobin, if crystallized in the renal tubules, can lead to a toxic effect, sometimes even renal failure. Cocaine can induce numerous toxic effects, including rhabdomyolysis. Intravenous hydration is important to increase the solubility of the myoglobin.

PHYSIOLOGY PEARLS

❖ If the filtered load of glucose exceeds the capacity of the renal tubule to reabsorb the glucose, the glucose left behind is "trapped" in the tubular lumen and acts as an osmotic solute, leading to an osmotic diuresis.

❖ The reabsorption of glucose is coupled to Na^+ via a luminal membrane Na^+-glucose cotransporter. The favorable downhill electrochemical gradient for Na^+ entry can drive influx of glucose up its chemical gradient to elevated levels inside the cell, thereby appearing to be an active influx of glucose (even though it is passive), giving rise to what is termed secondary active transport of glucose.

❖ Many amino acids are reabsorbed in the proximal tubule by Na^+-amino acid cotransport processes, whereas others are reabsorbed by Na^+-independent transport processes.

❖ Oligopeptides are reabsorbed in the proximal tubule by first being metabolized to their constitutive amino acids by luminal membrane peptidases and then being transported by Na^+-amino acid cotransporters and Na^+-independent amino acid transporters into the cell.

❖ Large peptides and proteins are reabsorbed in the proximal tubule by receptor-mediated endocytosis.

REFERENCES

Giebisch G, Windhager E. Transport of urea, glucose, phosphate, calcium, magnesium, and organic solutes. In: Boron WF, Boulpaep EL, eds. *Medical Physiology: A Cellular and Molecular Approach.* New York: Saunders; 2003:Chap 35.

Schafer JA. Reabsorption and secretion in the proximal tubule. In: Johnson LR, ed. *Essential Medical Physiology.* 3rd ed. San Diego, CA: Elsevier Academic Press; 2003:Chap 26.

A 60-year-old man with a history of heart disease is admitted to the hospital with congestive heart failure. He is stabilized and treated in the intensive care unit. His pulmonary edema and peripheral edema improve when furosemide (Lasix), a loop diuretic, is administered. The patient is discharged home with furosemide and other medications. He returns to his primary care physician 3 weeks after the hospitalization and complains of weakness, dizziness, and nausea. An electrolyte panel demonstrates hypokalemia, and he is started on supplemental potassium, with improvement of his symptoms.

◆ **How does a loop diuretic work?**

◆ **How do loop diuretics cause hypokalemia?**

◆ **What is the effect of aldosterone on sodium and potassium?**

ANSWERS TO CASE 23: LOOP OF HENLE, DISTAL TUBULE, AND COLLECTING DUCT

Summary: A 60-year-old man with congestive heart failure is treated with loop diuretics and subsequently develops hypokalemia.

◆ **Loop diuretics:** Act on the sodium-potassium-chloride cotransporter in the loop of Henle and decrease the reabsorption of sodium and water.

◆ **Hypokalemia with loop diuretics:** An increased flow rate through the late distal tubule and cortical collecting duct causes dilution of luminal potassium concentration and favors potassium secretion.

◆ **Effect of aldosterone on the reabsorption of sodium:** Increases the number of sodium channels in the luminal membrane, the number of sodium-potassium ATPase transporters, and the activity of Krebs cycle enzymes in the late distal tubule and cortical collecting duct.

CLINICAL CORRELATION

Loop diuretics such as furosemide are commonly used diuretic medications. Patients with congestive heart failure, cirrhosis, and pulmonary edema often are started on these medications. Their site of action is primarily on the sodium-potassium-chloride cotransporter (Na-K-Cl cotransporter) in the loop of Henle, hence the term loop diuretics. They ultimately decrease sodium and water reabsorption, resulting in diuresis. However, patients on loop diuretics are prone to hypokalemia. This expected side effect results because the increased flow rate through the distal tubule and cortical collecting duct causes a dilution decrease in the luminal potassium concentration and favors potassium secretion. Patients on diuretics often need to take potassium supplements. Hypokalemia presents clinically with muscle weakness, nausea, fatigue, dizziness, and intestinal ileus and, if potassium is low enough, may lead to coma and fatal cardiac arrhythmias. Not all diuretics lead to hypokalemia. Spironolactone is an antagonist of aldosterone, and amiloride acts on the sodium channel; both do not result in increased potassium loss. These two medications are examples of potassium-sparing diuretics.

APPROACH TO LOOP OF HENLE, DISTAL TUBULE, AND COLLECTING DUCT

Objectives

1. Know about reabsorption and secretion in the loop of Henle, distal tubule, and collecting duct.
2. Describe the effects of aldosterone on the distal tubule and collecting duct.

Definitions

Loop diuretic: A diuretic that inhibits the Na-K-Cl cotransporter in the thick ascending limb of the loop of Henle. An example is furosemide.

Potassium-sparing diuretic: A diuretic that acts by inhibiting sodium reabsorption and potassium secretion in the late distal tubule and cortical collecting duct, thereby inhibiting the loss of potassium.

Aldosterone: A mineralocorticoid hormone that stimulates the reabsorption of sodium from and the secretion of potassium into the late distal tubule and cortical collecting duct.

DISCUSSION

Of the **30% to 40% of the fluid filtered at the glomerulus** that is **not reabsorbed** by the **proximal tubule, most is reabsorbed by the loop of Henle, distal tubule,** and **collecting duct system,** except for a small percentage (typically <1%-2%) that normally is tightly regulated to maintain a balance of body fluids and electrolytes. The **loop of Henle** plays a particularly central role in giving the kidneys the ability to both **concentrate and dilute urine,** providing the foundation for both osmotic balance and volume balance.

The loop of Henle consists of the **thin descending limb,** the **thin ascending limb,** and the **thick ascending limb,** which ends at the **macula densa** (adjacent to its own glomerulus). The segments **reabsorb 25% to 30% of the filtered NaCl,** primarily in the **thick ascending limb,** with a smaller fraction of water, thereby rendering the medullary interstitial fluid hypertonic and the fluid leaving the thick ascending limb hypotonic, a condition that is necessary for excreting a urine with a variable osmolality. This occurs by a mechanism referred to as the **countercurrent multiplier system** that is dependent on the transport properties of the various segments: **high water permeability and low NaCl permeability of the thin descending limb, high NaCl permeability and low water permeability of the thin ascending limb, and low water permeability with active reabsorption of Na$^+$, along with Cl$^-$, of the thick ascending limb,** the segment that is the driving force for the whole process. Active reabsorption of Na$^+$, along with Cl$^-$, by the thick ascending limb renders the medullary interstitial fluid hypertonic, causing reabsorption of water from the descending limb. However, relatively more NaCl than water is transported into the interstitium, and so the medullary interstitium becomes hypertonic. With the countercurrent flow of fluid down the descending limb and up the ascending limb, a vertical amplification of the interstitial hypertonicity develops, increasing from approximately 290 mOsmol/kg at the corticomedullary junction to as high as 1200 to 1400 mOsmol/kg near the tip of the papilla (see the references at the end of this case for more detail). Conversely, fluid leaving the thick ascending limb is hypotonic (approximately 100 mOsmol/kg). An essential transport process for Na$^+$ and Cl$^-$ reabsorption in the thick ascending limb is the entry step at the luminal membrane:

a coupled cotransporter, the Na^+-K^+-Cl^- cotransporter, that transports 1 Na^+, 1 K^+, and 2 Cl^- together across the luminal cell membrane in an electroneutral fashion.

Modulating or inhibiting this cotransporter directly regulates net transport of NaCl across the cell, thereby regulating the magnitude of the medullary interstitial hypertonicity. In addition, because of this cotransporter, K^+ that enters the cell can diffuse back across the luminal membrane via a luminal membrane K^+ channel (see Figure 23-1) while Cl^- that enters diffuses across the basolateral membrane via selective Cl^- channels, leading to Cl^- reabsorption along with Na^+. The K^+ and Cl^- diffusion processes set up a lumen-positive membrane potential, as shown in the figure. Because the paracellular pathway through the tight junctions is more selective for cations, the lumen-positive potential arising from the cellular transport processes will lead to passive reabsorption of Na^+ between the cells as part of the process of NaCl reabsorption in this segment. As fluid leaves the loop of Henle, it enters the **distal convoluted tubule** in the **cortex.** Here Na^+, along with Cl^-, is reabsorbed actively, with the entry of Na^+ across the luminal membrane being coupled to Cl^- by a thiazide-sensitive NaCl cotransporter. The water permeability of the segment is relatively low so that little water is reabsorbed by this segment.

Fluid passes from the distal convoluted tubule into the late **distal tubule (connecting tubule/initial collecting tubule)** and on into the **cortical collecting duct and medullary collecting duct segments. Na^+ is actively reabsorbed** by

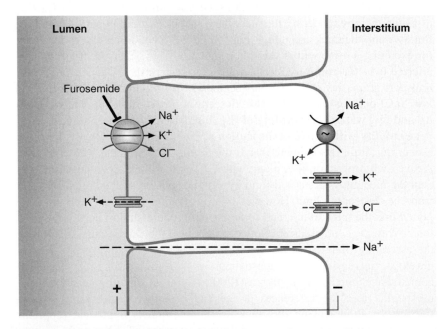

Figure 23-1. Thick ascending limb cell. Furosemide affects Na^+, K^+, and Cl^- transport.

the connecting tubule cells and by the principal cells of the initial and cortical collecting duct and, to a much lesser extent, by the principal cells of the outer medullary collecting duct. Sodium diffuses passively from the tubular fluid into the cell by a Na^+ channel and then is extruded actively across the basolateral border by the Na^+ pump (Na^+-K^+-ATPase). The same cells also contain a K^+ channel at the luminal border, and this provides for K^+ secretion across the luminal border into the tubular fluid. K^+ enters the cell across the basolateral membrane via the Na^+ pump, which maintains high intracellular K^+ concentrations, and then exits the cell either via the luminal membrane K^+ channel, giving rise to K^+ secretion, or via a basolateral membrane K^+ channel, recycling back into the interstitium. K^+ secretion by these segments is the primary determinant of K^+ excretion in the urine and hence provides regulation of K^+ balance (see Figure 23-2).

The **mineralocorticoid hormone aldosterone** regulates both **Na^+ and K^+** balance. Aldosterone secretion is stimulated by volume depletion (through the renin-angiotensin-aldosterone system), as is observed in hemorrhage and after the administration of high-ceiling loop diuretics. **Aldosterone** primarily acts in the **connecting tubule** and principal cells of the cortical collecting duct to **increase the reabsorption of Na^+ and Cl^- and the secretion of K^+.** Aldosterone acts by diffusing into the cell and binding to a cytosolic receptor. The receptor–hormone complex migrates into the nucleus, where it binds to specific sites on chromatin, which in turn induces RNA transcription and the

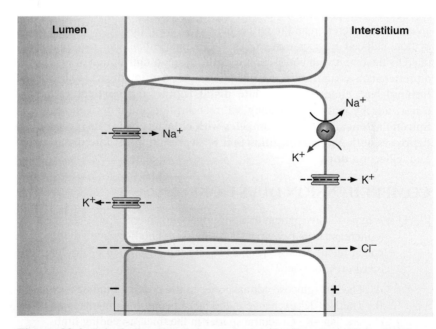

Figure 23-2. Principal cells of the cortical collecting duct. Na^+ and K^+ are actively pumped at the basolateral border by the Na^+ pump (Na^+-K^+-ATPase).

synthesis (translation) of a myriad of new proteins called **aldosterone-induced proteins (AIPs).** These proteins include new luminal membrane Na^+ channels and new Na^+ pumps (Na^+-K^+-ATPase) at the basolateral membrane. In addition, aldosterone acts by increasing the opening of existing luminal membrane Na^+ and K^+ channels. These effects require protein synthesis, and so the effects on transport are apparent only after a delay of 1 or 2 hours. Na^+ reabsorption in these cells is stimulated by enhanced Na^+ entry and Na^+ efflux after the increased opening of existing Na^+ channels, by synthesis of new Na^+ channels, and by synthesis of new Na^+ pumps. The stimulation of net Na^+ reabsorption causes a hyperpolarization of the tubule, with an increased luminal negativity (basolateral side positivity), and depolarization of the luminal membrane per se. This leads to a more favorable gradient for K^+ to diffuse from the cell into the luminal fluid by K^+ channels in the luminal cell membrane of the principal cells. Increased K^+ diffusion (secretion) into the lumen, coupled with increased K^+ uptake into the cell caused by the stimulation of the Na^+ pump (increased Na^+ efflux, increased K^+ uptake) at the basolateral membrane, leads to an enhanced rate of K^+ secretion into the tubular lumen. If the tubular flow rate does not change, the tubular fluid K^+ concentration will be elevated, ultimately reducing the electrochemical gradient for K^+ diffusion across the luminal membrane, limiting the rate of K^+ secretion.

Conversely, under conditions in which the tubular flow rate to the collecting ducts is elevated, such as after treatment with a loop diuretic, the K^+ concentration in the tubular fluid will be lower, providing a more favorable electrochemical gradient for K^+ diffusion into the lumen, thereby leading to enhanced K^+ secretion and in turn enhanced K^+ excretion. This increased rate of flow-induced K^+ secretion can lead to hypokalemia. This can be ameliorated by treatment with potassium supplements or administration of K^+-sparing diuretics such as amiloride and spironolactone. **Amiloride** acts to **block the luminal Na^+ channel** in the **late distal tubule** and **cortical collecting ducts,** thereby markedly reducing Na^+ reabsorption and in turn K^+ secretion. **Spironolactone,** in contrast, **competes with aldosterone for its receptor** and **depresses both Na^+ reabsorption and K^+ secretion in the late distal tubule and collecting duct.**

COMPREHENSION QUESTIONS

[23.1]   A hypertensive patient was prescribed the diuretic Lasix (furosemide) to increase urinary output. Furosemide, a "high-ceiling" diuretic, is a potent agent because it binds to and inhibits which of the following transport processes?

A. The Na^+-glucose cotransporter in the proximal tubule
B. The Na^+-K^+ exchange pump in all nephron segments
C. The Na^+-K^+-Cl^- cotransporter in the thick ascending limb
D. The Na^+-Cl^- cotransporter in the distal convoluted tubule
E. The Na^+ channel in the cortical collecting duct

[23.2]   A hypertensive patient is prescribed a loop diuretic such as Lasix without any supplements. One week later, the patient returns to the clinic complaining of dizziness, weakness, and nausea. The most likely cause of the patient's worsening condition is the development of which of the following?

A. Metabolic acidosis
B. Hyponatremia
C. Hypercalcemia
D. Hypokalemia
E. Hypovolemia

[23.3]   A 35-year-old female is noted to have new-onset hypertension that is thought to be due to an aldosterone-secreting adrenal tumor. Which of the following is likely to be seen in this patient?

A. Hypertension markedly improved with furosemide
B. Elevated serum sodium level
C. Elevated serum potassium level
D. Elevated urinary cortisol level

Answers

[23.1]   **C.** Furosemide inhibits the Na^+-K^+-Cl^- cotransporter in the thick ascending limb. This is a critical transporter for reabsorption of NaCl from the thick ascending limb into the medullary interstitium. This transport of NaCl is the driving force behind the establishment of the hypertonicity of the medullary interstitium that is essential for the reabsorption of water from the collecting ducts and the generation of a concentrated urine. Inhibition of the thick ascending limb cotransporter will lead to both a greater load of NaCl left behind in the tubular fluid, increasing urinary NaCl levels, and a reduced hypertonicity of the medullary interstitium (less NaCl), decreasing the gradient for water reabsorption from the collecting ducts. This leads to a rapid and sustained increase in urinary volume flow along with significant urinary levels of NaCl. Hence, furosemide is a potent diuretic.

[23.2]   **D.** Loop diuretics such as Lasix (furosemide) potently inhibit the Na^+-K^+-Cl^- cotransporter in the thick ascending limb. NaCl reabsorption in the thick ascending limb through this cotransporter is the driving force behind the operation of the countercurrent multiplier and the ability to excrete a concentrated urine (and a diluted urine). Inhibition of this cotransporter leads to a much greater load of Na^+ being delivered to the distal tubule and collecting ducts. With the increased delivery of Na^+ and fluid to the late distal tubule and cortical collecting ducts, K^+ secretion by the late distal tubule and cortical collecting ducts will be enhanced, leading to hypokalemia.

[23.3]   **B.** Aldosterone-secreting tumors may lead to hypertension, usually
          causing elevated serum sodium levels and low potassium levels
          (because of urinary reabsorption of sodium and excretion of potas-
          sium). One of the basic tests in the workup of newly diagnosed hyper-
          tension is serum electrolytes to assess for this disorder.

PHYSIOLOGY PEARLS

❖ Reabsorption of NaCl by the thick ascending limb underlies the generation of a medullary interstitial hypertonicity necessary for the
   passive reabsorption of water from the medullary collecting ducts.

❖ Loop diuretics are potent diuretics that inhibit the Na^+-K^+-Cl^-
   cotransporter at the luminal membrane of the thick ascending
   limb, thereby inhibiting NaCl reabsorption by this segment and
   water reabsorption by the medullary collecting ducts. They often
   are called high-ceiling diuretics.

❖ Administration of loop diuretics or other "upstream" diuretics can
   lead to increased tubular fluid flow to the late distal tubule and
   collecting ducts which, in turn, may stimulate K^+ secretion and
   the development of hypokalemia.

❖ Potassium-sparing diuretics such as amiloride and spironolactone
   inhibit Na^+ reabsorption and, in turn, K^+ secretion by the late distal tubule and collecting ducts.

❖ Aldosterone induces the synthesis of a myriad of new proteins in the
   late distal tubule and cortical collecting duct, including the synthesis of new Na^+ channels and Na^+ pumps.

REFERENCES

Giebisch G, Windhager E. Transport of sodium and chloride, and transport of potas-
    sium. In: Boron WF, Boulpaep EL, eds. *Medical Physiology: A Cellular and
    Molecular Approach*. New York: Saunders; 2003:Chaps 34 and 36.
Schafer JA. Regulation of sodium balance and extracellular fluid volume, and renal
    regulation of potassium, calcium, and magnesium. In: Johnson LR, ed. *Essential
    Medical Physiology*. 3rd ed. San Diego, CA: Elsevier Academic Press;
    2003:Chaps 29 and 30.

❖ CASE 24

A 27-year-old woman is being monitored in the intensive care unit after she sustained head trauma in a motor vehicle accident 3 days ago. She has undergone computed tomographic imaging of her head, which revealed cerebral swelling but no evidence of hemorrhage or brain herniation. The patient has been in critical but stable condition. The nurse calls the physician because the patient has developed hypernatremia and has had a significant increase in dilute urine output. The findings are confirmed, and it is determined that the patient has central diabetes insipidus as a result of the head trauma.

 How are antidiuretic hormone (ADH) levels affected in patients with this condition?

 What is the effect of high ADH on the late distal tubule and collecting ducts?

How does free-water clearance change in the presence of ADH?

ANSWERS TO CASE 24: REGULATION OF BODY FLUID OSMOLALITY

Summary: A 27-year-old woman who suffered head trauma has evidence of central diabetes insipidus.

◆ **Change in ADH:** Serum ADH decreased from normal values.

◆ **Effect of high ADH on distal tubule and collecting duct:** Increased permeability of the principal cells to water.

◆ **Free-water clearance with presence of ADH:** Negative free-water clearance (inability to excrete free water).

CLINICAL CORRELATION

Diabetes insipidus is a condition that results in the production of diluted urine. This can be a result of decreased ADH secretion or can occur because the kidney is no longer responsive to the hormone. When the production of ADH from the posterior pituitary is decreased, the condition is called central diabetes insipidus. Many conditions can cause central diabetes insipidus, including central nervous system (CNS) trauma or hypoxia (cerebrovascular accident [CVA]), granulomatous disease, tumor and treatment of pituitary tumors, drugs (lithium), and infections. When the ADH is normal but there is still production of dilute urine, the kidney may be resistant to ADH, a condition called nephrogenic diabetes insipidus. Signs and symptoms include polyuria and polydipsia along with the production of dilute urine (< 300 mOsmol/kg). The use of intranasal DDAVP (desmopressin), an analogue of vasopressin, helps concentrate the urine and reduces the polydipsia and polyuria.

APPROACH TO BODY FLUID OSMOLALITY

Objectives

1. Know about the regulation and secretion of ADH.
2. Describe the cellular action of ADH.
3. Know how to calculate free-water clearance.

Definitions

ADH (arginine vasopressin): A peptide hormone, secreted from the posterior pituitary, that regulates the water permeability of the kidney collecting ducts; the hormone also has vasoconstrictive properties.

Aquaporins: A family of water-permeable channels.

Diabetes insipidus: A condition in which secretion of ADH from the posterior pituitary is reduced or lacking, called central or hypothalamic diabetes insipidus, or in which the water permeability of the renal collecting ducts is not responsive to ADH, a much rarer condition called nephrogenic diabetes insipidus. Both conditions lead to the excretion of copious diluted urine.

Free-water clearance: The volume of water (urine) cleared from the plasma per unit time in excess (positive free-water clearance) or deficit (negative free-water clearance) from the volume estimated if the urine were isosmotic (with plasma) for the given amount of solute excreted in the same time. A quantitative measure of how dilute (hypotonic) or concentrated (hypertonic) the urine is (milliliters of water/time) relative to the isosmotic state.

DISCUSSION

Regulation of water balance is achieved largely through **regulation** of the **plasma/extracellular fluid osmolality.** This is accomplished by controlling the **water permeability of the collecting ducts** through the actions of **ADH,** which regulates the rate of water reabsorption and hence the free-water clearance. The binding of ADH to receptors on the **basolateral membrane** of principal cells increases the water permeability (see below) of the luminal cell membrane, allowing water to be reabsorbed passively from the tubular lumen into the hypertonic interstitium. Daily urine output is highly variable, related to water and food intake, with typical urine volumes of 1 or 2 L (osmolalities of 200-500 mOsmol/kg or so).

The **water permeability** of the **cortical and medullary collecting ducts** is **relatively low in the basal state,** primarily because of the low water permeability of the luminal (apical) cell membrane of the principal cells. In the presence of ADH, **ADH** binds to **V_2 receptors,** which **mediate the antidiuretic response** (reduced urine output). (ADH binding to **V_1 receptors** plays a major role in **vasoconstriction** of the vasculature). Binding to V_2 receptors in the collecting duct principal cells leads to activation of **adenylyl cyclase** and the production of **cyclic adenosine monophosphate (cAMP).** The subsequent activation of **protein kinase A by cAMP** leads to **phosphorylation** of water channels, namely, **aquaporin 2,** contained in cytoplasmic vesicles. After phosphorylation, the vesicles move to and fuse with the luminal cell membrane, increasing the water permeability of the luminal membrane. In the cortical collecting duct, water then can be reabsorbed passively from the hypotonic luminal fluid (typically near 100 mOsmol/kg as fluid enters the cortical collecting duct) across the luminal border into the cell.

The **basolateral membrane normally** has significant **water permeability** as a result of constitutive expression of other aquaporins (typically aquaporins 3 and 4). Hence, as water moves across the luminal border by osmosis, modestly reducing the osmolality of the cytoplasm, the water will diffuse from the cell across the basolateral membrane into the isosmotic interstitium by osmosis and be returned to the circulation. The osmotic reabsorption of water in the cortical segment of the collecting duct serves to present a smaller volume, but near isosmotic fluid, to the medullary collecting ducts so that water reabsorption in the medullary segment continues without a major reduction in the hypertonicity of the medullary interstitium. In the medullary segment, the insertion of water channels in the luminal membrane in the presence of ADH continues to allow for passive reabsorption of water from the tubular lumen into the hypertonic medullary interstitium that was set up by the countercurrent multiplier function of the loop of Henle (see Case 23). Water reabsorption continues, increasing the tubular fluid osmolarity, with the fluid approaching osmotic equilibrium with the medullary interstitium, thereby rendering a small but concentrated urine. In the presence of high levels of ADH, the urine osmolality will approach the interstitial **osmolality at the tip of the papilla,** approximately **1200 to 1400 mOsmol/kg,** with a minimal urine volume near 0.5 L/day. A defect in the water channels or in the trafficking of the channel to the luminal membrane will diminish the antidiuretic response, a condition referred to as nephrogenic diabetes insipidus.

In the **absence of ADH** (or with low levels), **few water channels are inserted** into the luminal cell membrane, and so the **water permeability of the collecting ducts is very low,** leading to little water reabsorption along the collecting ducts. Hence, the tubular **fluid entering the cortical collecting duct** (approximately 100 mOsmol/kg) remains **hypotonic,** leading to excretion of **copious but dilute urine** (a diuresis). Since NaCl is reabsorbed along the collecting ducts, in extreme cases of ADH depletion, the osmolality of the tubular fluid can decrease modestly along the collecting ducts, rendering the urine osmolality as low as 50 to 60 mOsmol/kg, but in a large volume of urine (typically several liters, with a maximum of 15 to 20 L/day).

Hyperosmolality is a major stimulus for ADH secretion, with **volume depletion** providing a secondary stimulus. **ADH is synthesized** in the **supraoptic and paraventricular nuclei** of the **hypothalamus,** where it is packaged into secretory granules. The granules migrate down the axons of the **supraopticohypophysial tract** into the **posterior pituitary** and are **stored** in the **nerve terminals,** from where they are released into the plasma. **ADH is metabolized in the liver and kidney. Osmoreceptors** in the **hypothalamus** sense the plasma osmolarity (primarily the sodium concentration). It is thought that the shrinkage of these cells with hypertonicity leads to depolarization of these cells, which in turn increases the electrical activity of the supraoptic and/or paraventricular cells, thereby inducing fusion of the secretory granules and release of ADH into the plasma. Similarly, **hypovolemia** is sensed by both **volume receptors in the left atria and pressure receptors,** primarily the **carotid sinus baroreceptors,** which control the activity of the vasomotor center in the medulla and thus the rate of ADH secretion from the paraventricular nuclei. With elevated ADH levels, water reabsorption in the collecting ducts will be increased, leading to accumulation of volume and a reduction in extracellular fluid and plasma osmolality.

Conversely, in the presence of a **hypotonic plasma,** or **volume expansion,** the **reduced stimulation of the osmoreceptors or volume/baroreceptors,** respectively, will result in a **reduced release of ADH** from the posterior pituitary. Less water will be reabsorbed from the collecting ducts, with an associated loss of extracellular fluid and plasma volume and a decrease in extracellular fluid and plasma volume back toward normal values. A **defect in the synthesis or release of ADH** also leads to a reduction in the reabsorption of water from the collecting ducts, leading to a diuresis with a hypotonic urine, a condition referred to as **hypothalamic or central diabetes insipidus.** As long as an individual has access to water, this is not a life-threatening condition. Further, an **analogue of vasopressin (DDAVP)** is available in nasal spray form that can be administered to regulate water excretion.

The ability to excrete or retain water is reflected in the osmolality of the final urine. It is the solute-free water retained or excreted that alters the osmolality of the extracellular fluids and can be calculated as the free-water clearance, CH_2O. The urine volume can be viewed as having two components: one containing all the excreted solutes in an isotonic solution, normally denoted as C_{Osm}, and one containing only **"solute-free" water,** that is, pure water, normally denoted CH_2O. For a hypotonic urine, CH_2O is the solute-free water that must be added to the theoretical isotonic urine volume, C_{Osm}, to provide for the actual urine volume per unit of time, V, and its hypotonicity. For a hypertonic urine, CH_2O is the solute-free water that must be subtracted from the theoretical isotonic urine volume to provide for the actual urine volume per unit of time, V, and its hypertonicity. That is, CH_2O is the additional water reabsorbed that will alter the osmolality of the extracellular fluids. C_{Osm} can be calculated as

$$C_{Osm} = \frac{U_{Osm} \times V}{P_{Osm}}$$

where U_{Osm} is the actual urine osmolality and V is the actual urine volume per unit time (eg, milliliters per minute or liters per day). C_{Osm} is equal to the clearance of osmotic solutes that appear in the urine per unit time. Urine volume per unit time thus can be thought of as having two components:

$$V = CH_2O + C_{Osm}$$

Hence,

$$CH_2O = V - C_{Osm}$$

For an isotonic urine, V and C_{Osm} are identical, meaning that CH_2O is zero so that there is no alteration of extracellular fluid osmolality. For hypotonic urine, V is greater than C_{Osm}, and so CH_2O is positive, meaning that an excess of water is being excreted, thereby increasing extracellular fluid osmolality. For hypertonic urine, V is less than C_{Osm}, and so CH_2O is negative, meaning that an excess of water is being retained in the body, thereby decreasing extracellular fluid osmolality. CH_2O provides a method to assess quantitatively the extent to which the kidney is either excreting or retaining free water and hence provides a measure of the degree of regulation of the osmolality of the extracellular fluid.

COMPREHENSION QUESTIONS

[24.1] A new patient is complaining about having to micturate numerous times during the day and being forced to get up multiple times throughout the night. Her diet has not changed, but she complains of being fatigued throughout the day (and frustrated with her shortened sleep periods). When she moves from a supine to an erect position, her blood pressure is observed to decrease modestly and her heart rate increases slightly. Blood chemistries reveal that she is modestly hypernatremic, and plasma arginine vasopressin and renin levels are markedly elevated. Urinalysis revealed copious diluted urine. The patient most likely has which of the following conditions?

A. Central diabetes insipidus
B. Nephrogenic diabetes insipidus
C. Psychogenic polydipsia
D. Excessive consumption of alcohol
E. Brain trauma

[24.2] If an individual becomes hypovolemic, such as during periods of diarrhea or excessive sweating, plasma ADH, or arginine vasopressin, levels are elevated rapidly and urine volume is decreased (antidiuresis). This effect of ADH on water excretion predominantly occurs in the collecting ducts by ADH-induced activation/inhibition of which of the following steps/processes?

A. Inhibition of sodium reabsorption
B. Activation of potassium secretion
C. Increased leakiness of the collecting duct to water and solute
D. Insertion of sodium channels in the luminal membrane
E. Insertion of aquaporin channels in the luminal membrane

[24.3] A 34-year-old woman feels compelled to drink water "all the time." She does not drink Gatorade or other solute drinks but takes pure water. Her serum sodium is low, as is her serum osmolality. The physician is unsure whether this patient has psychogenic water intoxication versus diabetes insipidus. Which of the following would reliably differentiate between these two disorders?

A. Urinary electrolytes compared with serum electrolytes
B. Urinary osmolality compared with serum osmolality
C. Serum ADH levels
D. Restriction from drinking water

Answers

[24.1]   **B.** Nephrogenic diabetes insipidus (nephrogenic DI) is a relatively rare disease that arises from defective water channels (aquaporins) or pathways regulating the water channels in the collecting ducts. It is characterized by high levels of ADH in the plasma and excretion of copious diluted urine. This contrasts with central diabetes insipidus, the more common form of DI, which is characterized by low synthesis and secretion of vasopressin from the posterior pituitary, giving rise to low levels of vasopressin in the plasma, but with the effect on urinary excretion being the same.

[24.2]   **E.** A key step in regulating water reabsorption in the collecting ducts is controlling the insertion and removal of aquaporins (water channels) at the luminal cell membrane. In the presence of ADH, ADH binds to a V_2 vasopressin receptor on the basolateral membrane of the cells, leading to production of cAMP and the protein kinase A-induced phosphorylation of intracellular aquaporin channels retained in cytoplasmic vesicle pools. The phosphorylation leads to the insertion of the vesicles, along with the aquaporins, into the luminal membrane, thereby increasing the water permeability of the luminal membrane.

[24.3]   **D.** Psychogenic water intoxication has the appearance of diabetes insipidus. Owing to the marked hypotonic fluid ingestion, the body attempts to excrete free water, and thus ADH secretion is inhibited. Both serum and urine sodium and osmolality are very low. However, in psychogenic water intoxication, when water is restricted, the body will produce ADH eventually, leading to normalization of the serum osmolality and concentration of urine. In diabetes insipidus, because of a problem with ADH production and secretion, even with water restriction the patient will produce very dilute urine and will not be able to concentrate the urine.

PHYSIOLOGY PEARLS

❖ Antidiuretic hormone regulates water reabsorption by the cortical and medullary collecting ducts by regulating the insertion of water channels (aquaporins) in the luminal cell membrane.

❖ Secretion of ADH from the posterior pituitary is regulated predominantly by osmoreceptors in the hypothalamus that sense plasma osmolality and secondarily by volume receptors in the left atria and pressure receptors (eg, carotid sinus baroreceptors).

❖ Diabetes insipidus is characterized by a reduction or a complete loss of secretion of ADH from the posterior pituitary (central or hypothalamic DI) or a decreased responsiveness of the collecting ducts to ADH (nephrogenic DI). Both conditions lead to excretion of copious diluted urine.

❖ Sodium chloride reabsorption from the thick ascending limb is critical for establishing a hypertonic medullary interstitium, which in turn provides the osmotic gradient for passive reabsorption of water from the medullary collecting ducts.

❖ Free-water clearance is a quantitative measure of the volume of "solute-free" water (per unit time) that is excreted (a hypotonic urine) or retained by the body (a hypertonic urine), leading to an increase or a decrease, respectively, in extracellular fluid osmolality.

REFERENCES

Giebisch G, Windhager E. Urine concentration and dilution, and transport of potassium. In: Boron WF, Boulpaep EL, eds. *Medical Physiology: A Cellular and Molecular Approach*. New York: Saunders; 2003:Chaps 37 and 36.

Schafer JA. Regulation of body fluid osmolality. In: Johnson LR, ed. *Essential Medical Physiology*. 3rd ed. San Diego, CA: Elsevier Academic Press; 2003:Chap 28.

❖ CASE 25

A 37-year-old man with a history of hepatitis C presents to the emergency center with complaints of abdominal swelling, fatigue, easy bruising, yellow eyes, and pruritus. On examination, the patient has abdominal ascites, spider angiomas, and numerous bruises on the skin, icteric sclera, and peripheral edema. Laboratory tests reveal slightly elevated liver function tests, prolongation of clotting times, hypoalbuminemia, hyperbilirubinemia, elevated ammonia, and hypokalemia. He is diagnosed with cirrhosis of the liver and admitted to the hospital for further workup.

 What is the normal effect of decreased plasma volume on sodium balance?

 Why does this patient have significant edema and continued sodium reabsorption?

 In what part of the glomerulus-tubule complex of the kidney is the majority of sodium reabsorbed?

ANSWERS TO CASE 25: REGULATION OF EXTRACELLULAR FLUID AND SODIUM BALANCE

Summary: A 37-year-old man with a history of hepatitis C has symptoms and signs of cirrhosis.

◆ **Normal response to decreased plasma volume:** Increased sodium absorption.

◆ **Continued peripheral edema and increased sodium reabsorption:** Because of the low albumin and hypoproteinemia, the colloid pressure is decreased and fluid escapes to the interstitial areas outside the vessels. Although the patient has excess retained fluid, the plasma volume (or arterial plasma volume) is low, and this causes an increase in aldosterone and sodium reabsorption.

◆ **Reabsorption of sodium:** Primarily in the proximal kidney.

CLINICAL CORRELATION

Several disease processes present with excess total body fluid but continued sodium reabsorption. Disease processes that result in diminished colloid pressure can result in interstitial fluid collection (ascites, pulmonary edema). Some examples of these disease processes are nephrotic syndrome (loss of protein in urine), cirrhosis (destruction of the liver and the proteins it makes, such as clotting factors), and malnutrition. The decreased colloid pressure causes the water to diffuse into the interstitial spaces. The plasma volume is low as a result of the fluid going to the interstitial space (and/or venous congestion—ie, venous distention—leading to accumulation of plasma volume on the venous side, reducing the arterial plasma volume perfusing the tissues), and this is recognized by volume/pressure receptors in the vasculature, resulting in sodium reabsorption and more fluid retention.

APPROACH TO EXTRACELLULAR FLUID AND SODIUM BALANCE

Objectives

1. Understand sodium regulation during hypovolemia and hypervolemia.
2. Know the sites of sodium absorption in the kidney.
3. Know the major mechanisms that control sodium excretion.

Definitions

Extracellular fluid (ECF) volume: Made up of two main components: the interstitial fluid volume and the ECF volume of the vasculature, that is, the plasma volume.

Aldosterone: A mineralocorticoid hormone that, among other actions, stimulates Na^+ reabsorption and K^+ secretion in the initial collecting tubule and cortical collecting duct.

Renin: A proteolytic enzyme secreted by the juxtaglomerular cells of the renal afferent arteriole that converts angiotensinogen to angiotensin I.

Angiotensin-converting enzyme (ACE): Converts angiotensin I to angiotensin II.

DISCUSSION

The **ECF volume** is typically **proportional to the total body sodium stores** because the sodium salts are the primary osmolytes that make up the osmolar content of the ECFs (see below). The **kidneys** play a dominant role in regulating body sodium content, and thus in regulating ECF volume, by regulating the excretion of sodium. This is accomplished by regulating sodium reabsorption by the nephron and collecting ducts (see Figure 25-1).

The **dominant site of sodium reabsorption** is the **proximal tubule,** where approximately **60% to 70% of the filtered fluid is reabsorbed.** The primary transport process underlying fluid reabsorption is **active sodium reabsorption,** with other solutes following passively. Sodium uptake across the luminal cell membrane includes a number of transport processes, with the dominant processes being **sodium-hydrogen exchange** and **sodium cotransport process,** most notably **sodium-glucose cotransport** (see Case 22). Once Na^+ enters the cells, it is extruded actively across the basolateral membrane by the Na^+ **pump (Na^+-K^+-ATPase).** Anions such as Cl^- and HCO_3^- follow passively because of the electrochemical gradients established by active Na^+ reabsorption (see the references at the end of this case). The tight junctions between the cells are also "leaky" in this tissue so that some transport of Na^+ and Cl^- ions can occur across the tight junctions through the paracellular pathway, depending on the electrochemical gradient for each ion. The tissue also has a **high water permeability** through both cellular and paracellular pathways so that as net solute is transported through the cells, water follows passively as a result of osmosis through both pathways. The reabsorbate then is taken up into the peritubular capillaries according to the Starling forces. Because this last step is in series with fluid uptake through the cellular and paracellular pathways, alterations in the Starling forces, particularly alterations in the capillary oncotic pressure and hydrostatic pressure, directly affect net fluid reabsorption in the proximal tubule. Regulation of Na^+ reabsorption by the epithelial cells and the Starling forces in the peritubular capillaries largely controls net fluid reabsorption by the proximal tubule.

The **second major site of sodium reabsorption** in the kidney is in the **thick ascending limb of the loop of Henle. The water permeability** of this segment is very **low.** Approximately 25% of the filtered NaCl is reabsorbed in the thick ascending limb. Here sodium is reabsorbed via the luminal cotransport process that **reabsorbs Na^+-K^+-$2Cl^-$ in an electroneutral fashion.** This

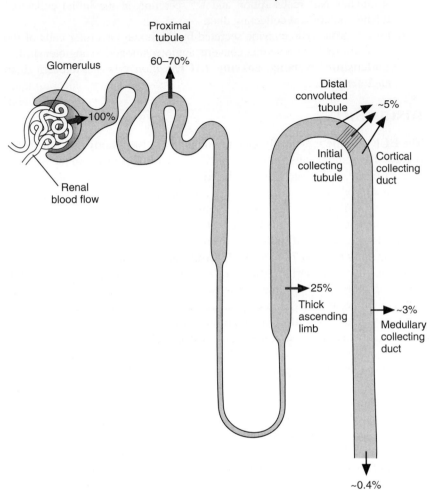

Figure 25-1. Sites of Na⁺ reabsorption along the nephron. The diagram shows approximate percentages reabsorbed relative to glomerular filtration (= 100%).

process plays a key role in the **countercurrent multiplier system** and the establishment of the **medullary interstitial hyperosmolality** that is critical for the hyperosmotic regulation of the final urine (see Case 23). Although NaCl reabsorption by this segment will be enhanced in volume depletion and reduced in volume expansion, the more distal tubular segments, particularly the late distal tubule and cortical collecting ducts, normally are considered the primary sites for controlling NaCl reabsorption, and thus sodium balance, under most states of altered volemia.

Fluid exiting from the thick ascending limb enters the **distal convoluted tubule.** Here Na⁺, **along with Cl⁻, is actively reabsorbed,** with the entry of Na⁺ across the luminal membrane being coupled to Cl⁻ by a **thiazide-sensitive NaCl cotransporter.** The water permeability of the segment is also relatively low so that little water is reabsorbed. The tubular fluid then passes from the **distal convoluted tubule** into the **late distal tubule** (connecting tubule/initial collecting tubule) and on into the **cortical collecting duct** and **medullary collecting duct** segments. In the **connecting tubule cells** and the principal cells of the **initial and cortical collecting duct, sodium is reabsorbed actively.** Sodium can continue to be reabsorbed in the medullary collecting ducts in a similar fashion, but the contribution of this segment to sodium balance is much smaller compared with that of the initial and cortical collecting duct segments. Here sodium diffuses passively from the tubular fluid into the cell by a Na⁺ channel, the epithelial Na⁺ channel (ENaC), as shown in Figure 23-2. Sodium then is extruded actively across the basolateral border by the Na⁺ pump (Na⁺-K⁺-ATPase) to give rise to Na⁺ reabsorption. The same cells also contain a K⁺ channel at the luminal border that provides for K⁺ secretion across the luminal border into the tubular fluid (see Case 23), but at a rate lower than that observed for Na⁺ reabsorption. Chloride ion is reabsorbed passively through the Cl⁻-permeable tight junctions as a result of the lumen-negative electrical potential difference set up by active sodium reabsorption. The net rate of Cl⁻ reabsorption is equal to the difference between Na⁺ reabsorption and K⁺ secretion, thus resulting in net NaCl reabsorption.

Na⁺ reabsorption and K⁺ secretion in the collecting ducts are regulated predominantly by the **mineralocorticoid hormone, aldosterone,** through the **renin-angiotensin-aldosterone system. Aldosterone** secretion is stimulated by **volume depletion** (through the renin-angiotensin-aldosterone system), as is observed in liver disease, hemorrhage, and diuretic states (see below). Aldosterone acts primarily in the connecting tubule and principal cells of the cortical collecting duct to increase the reabsorption of Na⁺ and Cl⁻ and the secretion of K⁺ by stimulating synthesis of new Na⁺ channels and Na⁺ pumps. The mechanism is discussed in Case 23 and the principal cell is shown in Figure 23-2 (also see the references).

Regulation of Na⁺ balance by the **kidneys** underlies **regulation of ECF volume.** As was noted above, the ECF volume is typically proportional to the total body sodium stores because the sodium salts are the primary osmolytes that make up the osmolar content of the ECFs. Further, the **two components of the ECF volume**—the **vascular component** (plasma volume) and the **interstitial fluid volume**—typically are regulated in parallel fashion, proportional to body sodium content. Both extracellular components normally change in a parallel fashion, increasing in hypervolemic states (volume expansion) and decreasing in hypovolemic states (volume depletion), reflecting changes in sodium retention. Alterations in the vascular volume are sensed continuously by vascular volume receptors (atria and pulmonary vessels) and baroreceptors (aortic arch, carotid sinus, and renal afferent arteriole). **Four distinct pathways** are known to respond to alterations in **vascular volume.**

First, alterations in plasma volume are communicated by afferent neurons to the medulla of the brainstem, leading to two efferent signals, one controlling the **sympathetic activity** of the autonomic nervous system and one controlling the release of **antidiuretic hormone** from the posterior pituitary. The other two pathways involved in Na^+ balance and vascular volume include the **renin-angiotensin-aldosterone system** and **atrial natriuretic peptide (ANP).** Each of these four effector pathways can modulate Na^+ excretion and water excretion to correct the primary change in vascular volume, as outlined below.

In **hypovolemic states, sympathetic activity** is increased, leading to **constriction of the renal afferent and efferent arterioles.** This **reduces renal plasma flow** and, to a relatively smaller extent, glomerular filtration, leading to a **reduction in Na^+ excretion.** The **parallel stimulation of antidiuretic hormone (ADH) release** leads to an increased **water reabsorption** by the **collecting ducts, reducing urine volume.** The reduction in renal afferent arteriole pressure directly stimulates the release of renin from the juxtaglomerular cells, leading to **increased levels of angiotensin II** as part of the renin-angiotensin-aldosterone system (renin converts angiotensinogen to angiotensin I, which in turn is converted to angiotensin II by ACE). Similarly, increased activity of sympathetic nerves terminating on the juxtaglomerular cells stimulates release of renin, leading to elevated angiotensin II levels. **Angiotensin II,** a vasoactive peptide, has multiple effects **that promote Na^+ retention.** First, it promotes a further constriction of afferent and efferent arterioles, reducing glomerular filtration and Na^+ excretion. Second, it directly **binds to receptors in the proximal tubule, stimulating Na^+-H^+ exchange** and **increased Na^+ reabsorption** by the proximal tubule (see above). Third, it **stimulates the synthesis of aldosterone** by the **zona glomerulosa** cells of the adrenal cortex. Aldosterone, a potent mineralocorticoid hormone, greatly stimulates Na^+ reabsorption (and K^+ secretion) by the initial and cortical collecting duct, markedly reducing Na^+ excretion (see above). All the responses to hypovolemia lead to retention of Na^+ and water, thereby expanding the ECF volume and correcting the defect in vascular volume.

In **hypervolemia,** the expanded vascular volume again is sensed by the **vascular volume receptors and pressure receptors,** which now respond by enhancing the excretion of Na^+ and causing a loss of ECF volume. **Sympathetic activity is depressed,** leading to dilation of the **afferent and efferent arterioles and increased renal plasma flow** and a proportionally smaller increase in the glomerular filtration rate and Na^+ excretion. **Antidiuretic hormone levels are down,** paralleled by a **decrease in water reabsorption** in the collecting ducts, leading to a diuresis. The elevated pressure in the afferent arteriole inhibits the release of renin and thus leads to **a reduction in angiotensin II** levels and synthesis of **aldosterone** by the adrenal gland. Hence, Na^+ reabsorption (and K^+ secretion) by the initial and cortical collecting duct is greatly reduced, further enhancing loss of Na^+ in the urine. Hence, all hormonal/neuronal pathways promote loss of Na^+, along with water, in the urine, correcting the defect in vascular volume and in turn the ECF volume.

However, in certain **edematous settings,** such as **hypoalbuminemia** caused by **liver disease or nephrotic syndrome, interstitial volume** may be **elevated** (edema) and the **plasma volume actually may be reduced.** In cases in which plasma protein levels are reduced, thereby reducing the plasma oncotic pressure, there will be a shift in the ECF from the plasma to the interstitial space, giving rise to edema. Such conditions, which are characterized by a reduction in plasma volume (or during venous distention and accumulation of plasma volume on the venous side), are sensed by **vascular volume** receptors and baroreceptors as if total ECF volume were **decreased,** leading to retention of sodium and water and a further expansion of ECF volume in an attempt to restore plasma volume.

COMPREHENSION QUESTIONS

[25.1]   A 24-year-old man was admitted to the emergency department and complained of abdominal pain, dizziness when standing, and nausea leading to occasional vomiting. The patient's blood pressure was low, and his heart rate was elevated. Laboratory tests revealed a reduced hematocrit, hypoalbuminemia, very modest hyponatremia, and elevated creatinine, blood urea nitrogen (BUN), and renin levels. Urine output was minimal. The patient informed the physician that he had been taking extra aspirin recently to alleviate back pain. Which of the following is the most like diagnosis?

A. Episodes of vomiting leading to hypovolemia
B. Gastrointestinal bleeding leading to hypovolemia
C. Diarrhea leading to hypovolemia
D. Cirrhosis of the liver
E. Nephrotic syndrome accompanied by excretion of protein

[25.2]   A student in a clinical study had her normal diet changed to a diet high in potassium, but everything else was unremarkable. The student noted that she had gained nearly 2 lb within a few days after starting the diet. Laboratory tests indicated a modest elevation in plasma K^+ but no change in plasma Na^+ levels. Interestingly, plasma levels of arginine vasopressin and renin were depressed, results consistent with volume expansion. What is the most likely reason for the hypervolemia?

A. Increased plasma protein oncotic pressure leading to fluid retention
B. Decreased glomerular filtration rate leading to fluid retention
C. Stimulation of the renin-angiotensin-aldosterone system leading to Na^+ and water retention
D. Stimulation of aldosterone secretion by the high-K^+ diet leading to Na^+ and water retention
E. Decreased ANP release leading to fluid retention

[25.3]   A 37-year-old man is stabbed in the arm and chest in a bar fight and
         experiences an estimated blood loss of 1000 mL. His blood pressure
         is 100/50 mm Hg, and his heart rate is 110 beats per minute. Which
         of the following describes this patient's physiologic response?

         A. β-Adrenergic stimulation of the vasculature
         B. Vasoconstriction to the renal afferent and efferent arterioles
         C. Reduction of ADH release
         D. Lowering of urine osmolality

Answers

[25.1]   **B.** This patient probably has gastrointestinal bleeding caused by sen-
         sitivity to aspirin. It is well known that aspirin can induce erosions in
         the gastrointestinal lining that can lead to bleeding ulcers. The bleed-
         ing will lead to loss of blood and hypovolemia that causes a decrease
         in capillary pressure and, as a result, a shift of fluid from the intersti-
         tial space into the vasculature. This fluid shift is apparent from the
         decrease in hematocrit and dilution of plasma proteins (hypoalbu-
         minemia).

[25.2]   **D.** The consumption of a diet high in K^+ will lead to K^+ loading,
         which is known to stimulate directly the secretion of aldosterone
         from the adrenal gland. The elevated aldosterone will stimulate the
         synthesis of new Na^+-K^+ exchange pumps and luminal membrane
         Na^+ channels in the renal cortical collecting ducts, leading to stimu-
         lation of Na^+ (and Cl^-) reabsorption and fluid retention (K^+ secretion
         also is stimulated). The salt and fluid retention will lead to volume
         expansion as made evident by a gain in weight. Secondarily, the vol-
         ume retention will be sensed by volume receptors, leading to a
         depression in the sympathetic nervous activity, a decrease in arginine
         vasopressin release, and a decrease in renin release. Hence, the K^+-
         induced stimulation of aldosterone secretion completely bypasses a
         role for the renin-angiotensin-aldosterone axis in this setting.

[25.3]   **B.** Hypovolemia triggers several responses, including sympathetic-
         mediated vasoconstriction to renal afferent and efferent arterioles,
         which decrease GFR. Meanwhile, ADH release induces more con-
         centrated urine (retention of free water), and aldosterone induces
         sodium retention.

PHYSIOLOGY PEARLS

❖ The ECF volume is typically proportional to the total body sodium stores because the sodium salts are the primary osmolytes that make up the osmolar content of the ECFs.

❖ The plasma volume is normally directly proportional to the ECF volume, decreasing during states of volume depletion and increasing during states of volume expansion.

❖ The reabsorption of fluid by the proximal tubule is proportional to the rate of glomerular filtration resulting from glomerulotubular balance.

❖ The dominant site of Na^+ reabsorption in the nephron and collecting ducts is the proximal tubule, which reabsorbs 60% to 70% of the filtered load (the amount of Na^+ filtered).

❖ Aldosterone induces Na^+ reabsorption by the initial collecting tubule and cortical collecting duct, leading to retention of Na^+ and expansion of the ECF volume.

❖ Antidiuretic hormone is secreted during hypovolemic setting, leading to water reabsorption by the collecting ducts and partial correction of volemic defect.

REFERENCES

Giebisch G, Windhager E. Integration of salt and water balance, and transport of potassium. In: Boron WF, Boulpaep EL, eds. *Medical Physiology: A Cellular and Molecular Approach.* New York: Saunders; 2003:Chaps 39 and 36.

Schafer JA. Regulation of fluid balance and extracellular fluid volume. In: Johnson LR, ed. *Essential Medical Physiology.* 3rd ed. San Diego, CA: Elsevier Academic Press; 2003:Chap 29.

❖ CASE 26

A 45-year-old woman with hypertension presents to her primary care physician for follow-up on her new blood pressure medication. She was started on an angiotensin-converting enzyme (ACE) inhibitor 1 month ago. She has been doing well other than feeling weak and fatigued. Serum electrolytes reveal that her potassium level is elevated.

◆ **How might the ACE inhibitor affect the potassium balance?**

◆ **How does acidosis affect potassium balance?**

◆ **What electrolyte competes with calcium for absorption in the ascending limb of the loop of Henle?**

ANSWERS TO CASE 26: REGULATION OF POTASSIUM, CALCIUM, AND MAGNESIUM

Summary: A 45-year-old woman with hypertension is placed on an ACE inhibitor and has developed hyperkalemia.

 Effect of an ACE inhibitor on potassium: ACE inhibitors block conversion to angiotensin II and decrease potassium secretion (resulting in hyperkalemia).

 Acidosis and potassium: Decreases potassium secretion.

 Competitive electrolyte of calcium: Magnesium.

CLINICAL CORRELATION

Potassium usually is located intracellularly. Conditions that increase the presence of potassium in the extracellular environment include inadequate renal excretion (ACE inhibitors, renal failure, potassium-sparing diuretics), increased potassium loads (crush injury, burns, excessive exercise), intracellular to extracellular shifts (acidosis, insulin deficiency), adrenal insufficiency (Addison disease), pseudohyperkalemia (hemolysis of blood sample), and hypoaldosteronism. The most important clinical effect of hyperkalemia is a change in cardiac excitability. Patients also may complain of weakness, fatigue, and paresthesias. Treatment depends on the severity of the hyperkalemia but includes sodium bicarbonate (alkalinizes the blood, causing potassium to move from the outside of the cell to the inside), insulin, cation-exchange resins (Kayexalate removes potassium from the body by binding to it in the gastrointestinal tract), potassium restriction, dialysis, and aerosolized β-agonists (drive potassium intracellularly). Continuous electrocardiograph (ECG) monitoring may be warranted with significantly elevated levels, and calcium gluconate can be administered to stabilize the myocardium and cardiac conduction system.

APPROACH TO POTASSIUM, CALCIUM, AND MAGNESIUM REGULATION

Objectives

1. Describe the regulation of potassium.
2. Understand the regulation of calcium.
3. Understand the regulation of magnesium.

Definitions

Hyperkalemia: An elevation in plasma K^+ above normal (> 5.5 mEq/L).
Hypokalemia: A decrease in plasma K^+ below normal (< 3.5 mEq/L).

ACE: Converts angiotensin I to angiotensin II.

Aldosterone: A mineralocorticoid hormone that, among other things, stimulates Na⁺ reabsorption and K⁺ secretion in the initial collecting tubule and cortical collecting duct.

Parathyroid hormone (PTH): Plays a critical role in controlling calcium, phosphate, and magnesium metabolism

DISCUSSION

Potassium

The **regulation of extracellular K⁺ levels** is closely associated with **intracellular K⁺** levels. This relates to the fact that **K⁺ is primarily an intracellular cation,** with 98% (3000-4000 mEq) of body K⁺ stores being located within the cells and only 2% (30-40 mEq) within the extracellular fluid (ECF). The intracellular concentration is normally 130 to 140 mEq/L, whereas the concentration in the ECF normally is tightly regulated to between 3.5 and 5.0 mEq/L. The distribution between the two compartments is maintained primarily by the activity of the **Na⁺-K⁺ exchange pumps (Na⁺-K⁺-ATPase), which actively pump Na⁺ out of the cell and K⁺ into the cell.** In addition, there is an **exchange process between H⁺ and K⁺,** the mechanism of which is poorly understood, in which **elevation of the pH in the ECF (alkalosis)** will lead to a loss of H⁺ from the cell in exchange for K⁺ uptake **(decreasing ECF K⁺ levels)** and a **decrease in the pH of the ECF (acidosis)** will lead to an uptake of H⁺ in the cell in exchange for **loss of K⁺ to the ECF** (increasing ECF K⁺ levels).

Potassium ion has a number of important physiologic effects, including **regulation of protein and glycogen synthesis, cell volume, intracellular pH, and resting membrane potential and thus muscle excitability and cardiac function.** The **regulation of K⁺ balance** is controlled primarily by the **regulation of urinary excretion of K⁺,** reflecting dietary intake that is first added to the ECF and then distributed between the intracellular compartment and the ECF. Dietary intake of K⁺ is typically 80 to 120 mEq/day, although this can vary widely. The kidney must excrete this intake of K⁺, by tightly regulated processes, to maintain a relative constancy of ECF K⁺ levels. **Approximately 80% of the ingested K⁺ temporarily moves into the cells,** thereby preventing dangerous, rapid fluctuations in ECF K⁺ levels during ingestion of food with high K⁺ content (eg, bananas, orange juice). This uptake normally occurs through the operation of the **Na⁺-K⁺ exchange pump,** which itself is modulated by the effects of a number of hormones, including **insulin, β-adrenergic agonists, and aldosterone,** all of which **promote K⁺ uptake into cells.** Hence, the redistribution of K⁺ into and out of cells represents a major process for modulating ECF K⁺ levels.

The other dominant process for controlling body K⁺ balance is regulation of K⁺ **excretion** by the **kidneys.** This involves both reabsorption and secretion of the filtered K⁺ by the nephron and collecting duct segments. Typically,

almost all the filtered K$^+$ is reabsorbed in the proximal tubule and the loop of Henle (in the **thick ascending limb**), with less than 10% reaching the distal convoluted tubule. In the proximal tubule, approximately 80% of the filtered K$^+$ is reabsorbed. The mechanism appears to be **passive, with K$^+$ reabsorption following NaCl and water reabsorption.** As fluid moves along the **thick ascending limb,** approximately another 10% of the filtered K$^+$ is reabsorbed and appears to be mediated by the **Na$^+$-K$^+$-Cl$^-$ cotransporter** in the luminal membrane. It is the more distal sites, particularly the connecting tubule and collecting duct segments, which appear predominantly to control the amount of K$^+$ appearing in the urine.

During periods of normal or high dietary K$^+$ intake, the principal cells of the **initial collecting duct, the cortical collecting duct,** and even the early part of the medullary collecting duct all **secrete potassium,** which accounts for the majority of K$^+$ excreted in the urine. **Secretion of K$^+$** by these segments is considered to be the **distal K$^+$-secretory system and is very tightly controlled,** ranging from 2% to over 180% of the filtered load. The K$^+$ secretory cells are characterized by a luminal membrane K$^+$ channel. K$^+$ first is taken up across the basolateral membrane via the **Na$^+$-K$^+$ exchange pump (Na$^+$-K$^+$-ATPase)** and then is secreted into the tubule lumen via a luminal membrane K$^+$ channel (see Case 23) down a favorable electrochemical gradient. Critical to this process is active Na$^+$ reabsorption in the same cells where Na$^+$ enters the cell passively via a luminal membrane Na$^+$ channel, but then is extruded across the basolateral membrane via the Na$^+$-K$^+$ exchange pump into the interstitium. Hence, **K$^+$ secretion is closely tied to Na$^+$ reabsorption in these segments.**

The main factors regulating K$^+$ secretion are **aldosterone, plasma K$^+$ concentration, and luminal flow rate. Aldosterone induces K$^+$ secretion,** particularly in the principal cells of the initial collecting tubule and cortical collecting duct (see Case 23), through enhanced synthesis of new Na$^+$-K$^+$ exchange pumps, increasing K$^+$ uptake and the synthesis of new luminal membrane Na$^+$ channels and thus stimulating Na$^+$ reabsorption and depolarization of the luminal membrane, which in turn favor K$^+$ secretion into the tubule lumen. Under conditions of **hypovolemia,** such as with **dehydration** or the administration of **loop diuretics, renin secretion** is enhanced, leading to stimulation of aldosterone secretion via the adrenal gland through the renin-angiotensin-aldosterone system. In addition, elevated plasma K$^+$ concentrations are also a potent stimulus of aldosterone secretion by the adrenal gland, **inducing K$^+$ secretion.**

Dietary K$^+$ loading also can stimulate the Na$^+$-K$^+$ exchange pump independently of aldosterone, **leading to increased K$^+$ secretion.** Chronic K$^+$ loading can induce the synthesis of new Na$^+$-K$^+$ exchange pumps, further enhancing K$^+$ secretion. Chronic K$^+$ loading or elevated plasma K$^+$ levels therefore potently regulate K$^+$ secretion through direct actions on the K$^+$ transport process and through the actions of aldosterone. Finally, increased flow rates to the collecting ducts lead to increased delivery of NaCl to the distal K$^+$ secretory segments and a stimulation of net Na$^+$ reabsorption. This leads to enhanced K$^+$ uptake after stimulation of the Na$^+$-K$^+$ exchange pump and a favorable gradient for diffusion of K^+ into the tubule lumen after enhanced Na^+ entry and depolarization of the luminal membrane. As a consequence, K^+ secretion by the principal cells is flow-dependent: Increased fluid delivery to the late distal tubule, as with the administration of loop diuretics or an increased glomerular filtration rate, will lead to enhanced K^+ secretion, whereas decreases in fluid delivery rates, such as with hypovolemia, will tend to retard K^+ secretion even though the transport processes may be stimulated by other processes, such as elevated aldosterone levels (see Case 23).

Calcium

Calcium plays an essential role in many cellular processes, including **muscle contraction, hormone secretion, proliferation, and gene expression.** Hence, calcium balance is critical for the maintenance of normal body functions. Calcium balance is a dynamic process that reflects a balance among **calcium absorption by the intestinal tract, calcium excretion by the kidney, and release and uptake of calcium by bone during bone formation/resorption** (see the references at the end of this case). Most body calcium is stored in bone (~1000 g), which is a very dynamic site as bone is being remodeled continuously, with only approximately 0.1% in the ECF (~1 g). Each of the processes contributing to calcium homeostasis is regulated predominantly by **parathyroid hormone, vitamin D_3, calcitonin, and plasma calcium levels.**

The **kidney** plays a critical role in calcium homeostasis by tightly regulating loss of calcium to the urine. Typically more than **99% of the filtered calcium is reabsorbed.** The **proximal tubule** reabsorbs the majority of the filtered calcium, approaching 65%, mostly via **passive mechanisms** after reabsorption of NaCl and water, which creates a favorable gradient for calcium reabsorption. The next site of significant calcium reabsorption is the thick **ascending limb,** which reabsorbs approximately 25% of the filtered load. Although 50% of this calcium is reabsorbed passively, between the cells, the remaining 50% is reabsorbed by a transcellular route under the control of PTH, although the mechanism is not well understood. The paracellular reabsorption is driven by the lumen-positive electrical potential difference typically present in this segment. Hence, some hormones, such as antidiuretic hormone, which stimulates NaCl reabsorption via the Na^+-K^+-Cl^- cotransporter, lead to an increase in the lumen-positive voltage and stimulation of calcium reabsorption. The **distal convoluted tubule** and **connecting tubule** reabsorb another 8% or so of the filtered calcium via active transcellular mechanisms that are tightly regulated. Calcium entry occurs via a luminal membrane calcium channel down a favorable electrochemical gradient and then is extruded across the basolateral membrane via a Ca^{2+}-ATPase pump or an electrogenic 3 Na^+-1 Ca^{2+} exchange process. Regulation of **calcium reabsorption in the distal convoluted tubule/connecting tubule** is the predominant process controlling **excretion of calcium.** Finally, the initial collecting tubule and cortical collecting duct are the last segments thought to reabsorb calcium, accounting for 1% to 1.5% of the filtered load, although the mechanisms of reabsorption and regulation in the collecting duct segments are not well understood.

Calcium reabsorption is regulated predominantly by **PTH,** which stimulates calcium reabsorption in the **thick ascending limb, distal convoluted tubule, and connecting tubule.** Similarly, **calcitonin** at low concentrations can stimulate calcium reabsorption. Both hormones appear to act through coupling to **adenylyl cyclase** and the **production of cyclic adenosine monophosphate (cAMP)** to induce the calcium reabsorptive processes. Vitamin D_3 also **increases calcium reabsorption in the distal nephron,** but it does so by acting on gene transcription of a calcium-binding hormone that contributes to transcellular calcium movement. Low plasma calcium levels also enhance calcium reabsorption. The low plasma calcium is sensed by the parathyroid gland, stimulating PTH release and in turn calcium reabsorption. High plasma calcium has the opposite effect, reducing PTH release and in turn calcium reabsorption. In addition, high plasma calcium is sensed by a basolateral calcium receptor in the thick ascending limb that responds by indirect inhibition of calcium reabsorption in this segment. The net result is decreased excretion of calcium.

Magnesium

Renal magnesium excretion plays an important role in **maintaining plasma magnesium levels.** Total body stores of magnesium are distributed among **bone** (54%) and the **intracellular compartment** (45%), with the remaining **1%** residing in the **plasma.** Typical plasma magnesium concentrations are tightly regulated between 0.8 and 1.0 mM, with about 70% of this magnesium being filterable (the remaining 30% is bound to plasma proteins). Of the filtered magnesium, typically 5% or less is excreted in the urine; the rest is reabsorbed. In contrast to most of the filtered solutes, which are reabsorbed predominantly in the proximal tubule, **only 15%** or so of the filtered magnesium is **reabsorbed in the proximal tubule,** apparently passively through the paracellular pathway. **Most of the magnesium is reabsorbed in the thick ascending limb,** accounting for nearly 70% of the filtered load. Magnesium is reabsorbed via the para-cellular pathway driven by the lumen-positive potential in this segment. As such, it is closely tied to NaCl reabsorption, which sets the lumen-positive potential (see Case 23). An additional 10% or so of the filtered magnesium is reabsorbed in the distal convoluted tubule, connecting tubule, and collecting ducts, apparently by an active transcellular process. Magnesium reabsorption in the thick ascending limb is influenced by variations in plasma magnesium and/or calcium concentrations.

Hypermagnesemia and hypercalcemia both lead to inhibition of reabsorption of magnesium and calcium, leading to **increased urinary excretion.** This effect is thought to be mediated by a calcium-sensing receptor on the basolateral membrane of thick ascending limb cells that binds either magnesium or calcium, apparently in a competitive fashion. Hence, upon the binding of either magnesium or calcium, cellular processes are activated that lead to inhibition of NaCl reabsorption and a decrease in the lumen-positive voltage that drives magnesium and calcium transport. Thus, the transport of both cations is diminished, resulting in increased excretion. In addition, magnesium reabsorption can be modulated by hormonal influences, with PTH being the most significant. Increased PTH levels lead to stimulation of magnesium reabsorption in both the proximal tubule and the thick ascending limb, although the mechanism is still poorly understood.

COMPREHENSION QUESTIONS

[26.1]   A 56-year-old patient has chronic renal failure that results in fewer functioning nephrons. The patient's dietary intake of potassium has not changed, and this could lead to dangerous hyperkalemia in the face of fewer functioning nephrons. However, because of adaptive responses to the potassium load, plasma potassium is noted to rise only slightly (< 0.5 mEq/L). Although numerous renal and extrarenal responses may underlie this K^+ adaptation, what is the dominant adaptive response of the kidney to maintain plasma K^+ levels in this chronic condition?

A. Increased glomerular filtration leading to increased filtration of K^+
B. Increased expression of Na^+-K^+ exchange pumps in the proximal tubule leading to enhanced K^+ secretion
C. Decreased expression of the Na^+-K^+-Cl^- cotransporter in the thick ascending limb leading to reduced K^+ reabsorption
D. Increased expression of Na^+-K^+ exchange pumps in the cortical collecting tubule leading to enhanced K^+ secretion
E. Decreased recycling of K^+ from the outer medullary collecting duct to the thin descending limb giving rise to enhanced K^+ excretion

[26.2]   The occurrence of hypocalcemia can have dire consequences for numerous physiologic processes. The kidney plays a major role in maintaining calcium balance during hypocalcemic states by decreasing calcium excretion. The major mechanism underlying the response of the kidney during hypocalcemia is which of the following?

A. Parathyroid hormone-induced stimulation of calcium reabsorption by the thick ascending limb
B. Fluid flow-induced stimulation of calcium reabsorption by the collecting duct
C. Calcitonin-induced inhibition of calcium secretion by the distal convoluted tubule
D. Vitamin D-induced activation of calcium reabsorption by the proximal tubule

[26.3] A 56-year-old woman receives chemotherapy for ovarian cancer and develops hypomagnesemia as a result. Urine chemistries reveal a large amount of magnesium in the urine. Which of the following areas most likely was affected by the chemotherapeutic agent?

A. Proximal tubule
B. Descending loop
C. Ascending loop
D. Convoluted distal tubule
E. Collecting duct

Answers

[26.1] **D.** The continuous ingestion of a constant potassium load in the face of a reduced number of functioning nephrons leads to a chronic overload of K^+, but without the development of extreme hyperkalemia. The kidney slowly adapts to the increased potassium load in a process called K^+ adaptation, which leads to a kaliuresis caused by an enhanced rate of K^+ secretion by the late distal tubule and cortical collecting tubule (the early part of the outer medullary collecting duct also may participate). This enhanced K^+ secretion arises from both a direct effect of the elevated plasma K^+ on the expression of new Na^+-K^+ exchange pumps at the basolateral membrane in these segments and an indirect effect through K^+-induced stimulation of aldosterone secretion from the adrenal gland.

[26.2] **A.** The occurrence of low plasma calcium levels is sensed by a calcium receptor on the surface of the parathyroid gland, leading to stimulation of synthesis and secretion of parathyroid hormone. PTH, along with vitamin D and to a lesser extent calcitonin, plays a dominant role in regulating calcium balance. In the kidney, PTH has diverse actions, but its key action appears to be to promote calcium reabsorption. The key sites regulating calcium reabsorption are the thick ascending limb and the distal convoluted tubule.

[26.3] **C.** The majority of magnesium is resorbed in the thick ascending limb of the renal tubule.

PHYSIOLOGY PEARLS

❖ The initial collecting tubule and the cortical collecting duct are the primary sites for K^+ secretion and as a consequence are the dominant sites regulating urinary K^+ excretion and K^+ balance.

❖ Aldosterone secretion by the adrenal gland is stimulated by high plasma K^+ levels and by angiotensin II.

❖ The distal convoluted tubule and connecting tubule actively reabsorb only a small amount of the filtered load of calcium but represent the dominant sites for controlling urinary calcium excretion.

❖ Parathyroid hormone secretion is stimulated by a reduction in plasma calcium levels.

❖ Magnesium excretion is controlled primarily by regulating passive magnesium reabsorption in the cortical thick ascending limb.

REFERENCES

Barrett EJ, Barratt P. The parathyroid glands and vitamin D. In: Boron WF, Boulpaep EL, eds. *Medical Physiology: A Cellular and Molecular Approach.* New York: Saunders; 2003:Chap 51.

Giebisch G, Windhager E. Transport of urea, glucose, phosphate, calcium, magnesium, and organic solutes. In: Boron WF, Boulpaep EL, eds. *Medical Physiology: A Cellular and Molecular Approach.* New York: Saunders; 2003: Chap 35.

Schafer JA. Renal regulation of potassium, calcium, and magnesium. In: Johnson LR, ed. *Essential Medical Physiology.* 3rd ed. San Diego, CA: Elsevier Academic Press; 2003:Chap 30.

❖ CASE 27

A 21-year-old man with insulin-dependent diabetes presents to the emergency center with mental status changes, nausea, vomiting, abdominal pain, and rapid respirations. On examination, the patient is noted to be hypotensive, breathing rapidly (tachypneic), and febrile. A fruity odor is detected on his breath. A random blood sugar is significantly elevated at 600 mg/dL. The patient also has hyperkalemia, hypomagnesemia, and elevated serum ketones. An arterial blood gas reveals a metabolic acidosis. The patient is diagnosed with diabetic ketoacidosis (DKA) and is admitted to the intensive care unit for intravenous (IV) hydration, glucose control, and correction of metabolic abnormalities.

◆ **What is the response of the kidney to metabolic acidosis?**

◆ **What is the response of the kidney to a respiratory alkalosis?**

◆ **What is the predicted compensatory response to metabolic acidosis?**

ANSWERS TO CASE 27: ACID–BASE PHYSIOLOGY

Summary: A 21-year-old man with type I diabetes develops DKA and metabolic acidosis.

 Response of the kidney to metabolic acidosis: Increased excretion of the excess fixed hydrogen as ammonia and increased reabsorption of bicarbonate

 Response of the kidney to respiratory alkalosis: Decreased hydrogen excretion and decreased bicarbonate absorption

 Compensatory response to metabolic acidosis: Decrease in bicarbonate and in PCO_2

CLINICAL CORRELATION

This 21-year-old man with type I diabetes (insulin deficiency) has the clinical manifestations of DKA. The first priorities are always the ABCs: Because the airways and breathing are normal, the focus in this case is on the circulation. Two large-bore IV lines should be placed, and the patient should receive 2 L of isotonic solution. The cornerstones of therapy are insulin in an IV drip, correction of metabolic abnormalities, and detection of the underlying etiology of the DKA (such as an infection).

Understanding how the body manages acid–base changes is critical to make the correct diagnosis, develop a treatment plan, and monitor the effectiveness of the treatment. Respiratory acidosis and alkalosis primarily begin in the lungs, whereas metabolic acidosis and alkalosis begin with abnormalities of bicarbonate in the blood. An arterial blood gas can be done to help determine which type of acid–base abnormality may be present. Metabolic acidosis can be differentiated into two groups: anion gap and non-anion gap. Examples of normal anion gap acidosis include renal tubular acidosis and gastrointestinal (GI) bicarbonate losses (diarrhea). Examples of increased anion gap acidosis include ingestion of methanol, ethanol or ethylene glycol (antifreeze), salicylates, cyanide, or paraldehyde; uremia or renal failure; lactic acidosis; and diabetic or alcoholic ketoacidosis. The serum anion gap can be calculated by determining the concentration of sodium minus the sum of the chloride and bicarbonate concentrations. The serum anion gap is increased if the concentration of an unmeasured anion is present and is normal if the concentration of chloride is increased to replace the bicarbonate. Treatment is based on diagnosing and treating the underlying disease process.

In this example of DKA, the patient will be started on IV fluids, insulin to correct the DKA, and supportive care, depending on the severity of the symptoms. The potassium level will be monitored closely as the hyperkalemia will resolve with treatment of the acidosis and the addition of insulin.

APPROACH TO ACID–BASE PHYSIOLOGY

Objectives

1. Understand the role of the kidney in acid–base balance.
2. Know how to calculate the anion gap and be able to list examples of disorders that cause anion gap acidosis.
3. Understand volatile and nonvolatile acids and buffers.
4. Understand the significance of the Henderson-Hasselbalch equation.

Definitions

1. **Hydrogen ion homeostasis:** The process of maintaining the pH of the plasma at a constant value of 7.4.
2. **Acid-base balance:** Matching the daily intake or production of acids and bases with an equivalent daily excretion.
3. **Carbonic acids:** Substances such as fatty acids or carbohydrates whose end products of metabolism are CO_2 and H_2O.
4. **Noncarbonic acids:** Also known as fixed acids are substances such as phospholipids or sulfur containing amino acids whose end product of metabolism is a nonvolatile acid.

DISCUSSION

Acid–base physiology includes **H^+ ion homeostasis** (maintaining the arterial pH at 7.4) and acid–base balance: the ability to match the daily production of acids and bases with an equivalent excretion. A disturbance or change in the rates of ingestion, production, and excretion of acids or bases can alter the balance and cause a change in pH. The body **has four lines of defense against an acid or base challenge** to minimize the change in pH and restore acid–base balance:

1. **Simple chemical buffers** in the blood (eg, the CO_2-bicarbonate buffer system, proteins such as hemoglobin and albumen) minimize a change in pH by reacting with an acid or base upon contact.
2. **Intracellular buffering** is afforded by the **protein mass** contained within the cells. This process requires the movement of protons (H^+) into the cell largely in exchange for potassium ions and is slower reacting than is the extracellular buffer pool.
3. **Pulmonary compensation** for a change in arterial pH or CO_2 is effected by a neural feedback loop involving central and peripheral chemoreceptors that control the rate of ventilation. The CO_2-bicarbonate buffer system is unique in that one of its components, CO_2, is gaseous and is controlled by pulmonary ventilation. Changes in the rate of ventilation can increase or decrease the alveolar and thus the arterial CO_2 concentration, compensating for changes in bicarbonate in response to a metabolic acidosis or alkalosis. The pulmonary response to changes in arterial pH or PCO_2 is almost immediate.

4. The **kidney** responds to an acidosis or alkalosis by excreting non-volatile acids or bases and controlling the rate of bicarbonate reabsorption. Unlike pulmonary ventilation, which is under the control of a neural feedback loop involving chemoreceptors that are sensitive to H^+, CO_2, and O_2, renal function is controlled by mass action and the relative rates of H^+ secretion and bicarbonate filtration. Because the renal response is dependent on glomerular filtration and the transport of large amounts of electrolytes, it is somewhat slower responding than are the other buffer systems. It is worth noting that renal and pulmonary functions are coupled to each other because one of the main factors determining the rate of renal bicarbonate reabsorption is the arterial PCO_2.

Many substances in the blood can serve as effective buffers; however, identifying each chemically distinct component is a monumental task. The task is simplified by the use of the **isohydric principle,** which states that in a **mixed solution all acid–base pairs are in equilibrium with each other.** Thus, to assess the acid–base status of a patient, it is not necessary to measure a hundred different species, but simply **one representative pair.** The most convenient and informative representative is the CO_2-HCO_3^--**buffer system.** The dissociation of an acid is governed by the physical chemical properties of acids and bases, and their behavior can be predicted from the **Henderson-Hasselbalch equation:**

$$pH = pK_a + \log \frac{[\text{base}]}{[\text{acid}]}$$

The pK_a or dissociation constant is characteristic for a specific acid–base pair; thus, knowing any two of the three variables allows the calculation of the third. Physiologically, the most important pair is the CO_2 and HCO_3^-:

$$CO_2 + H_2O \rightarrow H_2CO_3 \rightarrow H^+ + HCO_3^-$$

This expression can be simplified by assuming that CO_2 represents the free acid pool and HCO_3^- is the conjugate base. The Henderson-Hasselbalch expression for the CO_2-HCO_3^- buffer is

$$pH = pK_a + \log \frac{[HCO_3^-]}{[CO_2]_{dis}}$$

where the $pK_a = 6.1$ and the $[CO_2]_{dis} = 0.03$ mmol/L_mm Hg CO_2. Under normal physiologic conditions,

$$pH = pK_a + \log \frac{[24 \text{ mEq / L}]}{[1.2 \text{ mEq / L}]}$$

Perhaps one of the *most important features* of this expression is that the **pH** is not determined by the absolute concentration of either component, but is determined solely by the **ratio $[HCO_3^-]/[CO_2]$.** If the ratio gets larger (more **HCO_3^-** or less **CO_2**), the pH is more alkaline. If the ratio gets smaller (less **HCO_3^-** or more **CO_2**), the pH is more acidic. This greatly simplifies the understanding of the physiologic response to an acid–base disturbance. For example, if the disturbance is of metabolic origin, there will be an initial change in $[HCO_3^-]$. A metabolic acidosis will decrease $[HCO_3^-]$, and the ratio $[HCO_3^-]/[CO_2]$ will shrink. To compensate for the change, there are two options: The $[HCO_3^-]$ could be restored to normal, or the $[CO_2]$ could be reduced. The pulmonary response to an acid–base disturbance is mediated by central and peripheral chemoreceptors and is almost immediate. The **initial response to a metabolic acidosis (fall in $[HCO_3^-]$)** would be an **increase in pulmonary ventilation (hyperventilation) to lower the PCO_2,** thereby restoring the ratio $[HCO_3^-]/[CO_2]$ more closely to normal. In this instance, the pH has been corrected, yet the acid–base balance has been disturbed. To restore balance, the $[HCO_3^-]$ must be restored to normal. The kidney will excrete the acid that caused the disturbance and generate bicarbonate at the same time to restore $[HCO_3^-]$. Because the lungs control the $[CO_2]$ and the kidney controls the $[HCO_3^-]$, one may view the Henderson-Hasselbalch equation metaphorically as follows:

$$pH = pK_a + \log \frac{[kidney]}{[lung]}$$

Physiologically, acids can be divided into two groups. The distinction is made on the basis of their routes of production, the rates of production, and the routes of excretion. Carbonic acids often are referred to as volatile acids:

1. **Carbonic acids** are substances whose **end product of metabolism is CO_2 and water.** CO_2 is a volatile gas that is excreted by the lungs. Substances such as fats and carbohydrates are not acids or bases per se, but their metabolism yields CO_2 and water. They are considered to be acids because the end product of their metabolism, CO_2, reacts with water to form carbonic acid:

$$CO_2 + H_2O \rightarrow H_2CO_3 \rightarrow H^+ + HCO_3^-$$

2. **Noncarbonic or fixed acids** are substances whose end products of metabolism are **nonvolatile acids.** For example, metabolism of phospholipids or proteins results in the production of H_3PO_4 and H_2SO_4. These are strong acids that readily dissociate in the blood and are nonvolatile substances that have to be excreted by the kidney.

To understand the role of the kidney in acid–base disturbances, it is necessary to understand the mechanism of bicarbonate reabsorption. In the tubular cells, secreted H^+ is formed by the dissociation of carbonic acid as follows:

$$CO_2 + H_2O \rightarrow H_2CO_3 \rightarrow H^+ + HCO_3^-$$

For each H$^+$ that is formed and secreted, a bicarbonate ion is formed and transported into the blood. The **secreted H$^+$** has several available fates. If it reacts with filtered bicarbonate, it is neutralized and there is no net gain or loss of bicarbonate. The secreted H$^+$ also can react with a titratable acid or NH$_3$. A bicarbonate is added to the blood, but the H$^+$ is excreted in the urine as titratable acidity (TA) or ammonium ion. In either case, there is a net gain of one bicarbonate and the excretion of one fixed acid. Titratable acids are weak acids in the glomerular filtrate, such as uric acid, which can react with secreted H$^+$. They are formed at a steady rate and are of limited availability during an acid–base disturbance. However, the **primary adaptive response of the kidney** to a **chronic acidosis is ammoniagenesis,** the increased production of NH$_3$ from glutamine. The maximal adaptive response may take several days and can augment the daily excretion of H$^+$ by twofold to threefold.

In the case of an alkalosis, the situation is reversed. If the rate of bicarbonate filtration exceeds the rate of H$^+$ secretion, excess bicarbonate is not reabsorbed but simply is excreted in an alkaline urine.

What factors control the rate of H$^+$ secretion? The bulk (~90%) of **bicarbonate reabsorption and H$^+$ secretion occurs in the proximal tubule.** The mechanism of H$^+$ secretion is via a Na$^+$-H$^+$ exchanger in the apical membrane of the tubular cells. This exchanger is regulated by the intracellular pH, with activation occurring at more acidic cytosolic pH. In the present discussion, the key factors that will influence the intracellular pH are the arterial H$^+$ and the arterial PCO$_2$. An increase in either of those two factors will cause an increase in intracellular H$^+$ and activation of the Na$^+$-H$^+$ exchanger.

In the present case, there was an **uncontrolled overproduction of ketoacids** as a consequence of the insulin insufficiency. Normally, ketoacids are oxidized to CO$_2$ and water and eliminated as CO$_2$ through pulmonary ventilation. In a **DKA, their production exceeds the oxidative capacity, with their accumulation in the blood.** These ketoacids dissociate in the blood, yielding the **carboxylate anion and H$^+$** that were buffered by the chemical buffers in the blood and the intracellular compartment. The H$^+$ reacted with bicarbonate, reducing its concentration with the production of CO$_2$, which was eliminated through pulmonary ventilation. This reaction created the **anion gap.** The fall in bicarbonate also resulted in a fall in the arterial pH that would stimulate peripheral chemoreceptors. Increased peripheral chemoreceptor activity would stimulate ventilation to initiate a compensatory fall in PCO$_2$.

The function of the **kidney** in this circumstance is to restore acid–base balance by **eliminating all the excess fixed (or noncarbonic) acid** that was generated in the episode and at the same time restore bicarbonate back to normal levels. Although the PCO$_2$ is reduced, the arterial H$^+$ is elevated, and this will lead to a parallel rise in the intracellular H$^+$ concentration to ensure the activity of the Na$^+$-H$^+$ exchanger. The plasma [HCO$_3^-$] is reduced; therefore, the filtered load of HCO$_3^-$ is reduced, and thus all filtered HCO$_3^-$ will be reabsorbed. The generation of additional HCO$_3^-$ requires that H$^+$ be excreted. In fact, under these conditions the rate-limiting factor for HCO$_3^-$ reabsorption is not H$^+$

secretion but H^+ excretion. The availability of TA and NH_3 is limiting for binding to the secreted H^+. In a chronic state, the kidney will increase production of NH_3, but this may take several days. Over a period of days, the fixed acid generated during the acidosis will be excreted with the addition of an equivalent amount of HCO_3^- to the blood. As the HCO_3^- levels in the blood are restored, there will be a gradual rise in the pH toward a normal 7.4, and as the pH rises, the hyperventilation will abate. When the entire acid load is excreted, HCO_3^- will be restored to normal and acid–base balance will be restored.

COMPREHENSION QUESTIONS

[27.1] Recovery from a severe metabolic acidosis is most dependent on which of the following?

A. The rate of ventilation to blow off excess CO_2
B. The rate of H^+ secretion by the kidney
C. The rate of H^+ excretion by the kidney
D. The arterial pH
E. The arterial PCO_2

[27.2] After a rapid ascent to very high altitude, one begins to hyperventilate because of hypoxic drive. The hyperventilation will cause a decrease in the arterial PCO_2. What is the renal response to this condition?

A. Increased rate of acid excretion
B. Decreased rate of acid excretion
C. Increased rate of bicarbonate reabsorption
D. Diuresis to eliminate excess fluid
E. Increased ammoniagenesis

[27.3] A 21-year-old man with gastroenteritis developed severe vomiting with a loss of stomach acids. A metabolic alkalosis is present. Which of the following is most likely to occur?

A. The plasma bicarbonate concentration will decrease.
B. H^+ will move from the plasma into the cells.
C. Peripheral chemoreceptors will stimulate pulmonary ventilation.
D. Renal H^+ excretion will decrease.

Answers

[27.1] **C.** The rate of recovery from a severe metabolic acidosis is most dependent on the rate of H^+ excretion. Pulmonary compensation occurs rapidly; however, it can only minimize the change in pH. Pulmonary compensation cannot restore the balance after a metabolic disturbance. Recovery necessitates the excretion of the entire acid load to the system. Renal acid excretion is limited by the availability of titratable acids and ammonia for ammonium ion formation from secreted H^+. The primary adaptive response of the kidney to an acidosis is ammoniagenesis. Ammoniagenesis can augment the daily excretion of acids as much as threefold. When an equivalent amount of acid is excreted, acid–base balance will be restored.

[27.2]   **B.** The two most important drivers of renal bicarbonate reabsorption are CO_2 and H^+. The hyperventilation experienced at high altitude decreases the PCO_2, which generates a respiratory alkalosis. Reducing both CO_2 and H^+ will decrease renal H^+ secretion and thus bicarbonate reabsorption. The filtered bicarbonate load will exceed the rate of H^+ secretion with a loss of excess bicarbonate in the urine.

[27.3]   **D.** The loss of gastric (hydrochloric) acid leads to an increase in the plasma bicarbonate concentration and a metabolic alkalosis. The increase in the pH will depress peripheral chemoreceptors to slow ventilation and increase the PCO_2 to compensate for the increased bicarbonate. The increase in PCO_2 will bring the pH nearer to 7.4 and at the same time increase renal H^+ secretion. Because there is an increased level of bicarbonate in the glomerular filtrate, there will be an increase in bicarbonate reabsorption. The rate of filtration will exceed the rate of H^+ secretion, and there will be a continuous loss of bicarbonate. As the plasma bicarbonate falls, the pH will continue to approach the normal of 7.4 and the ventilatory rate will increase gradually. When all the excess bicarbonate has been excreted, the plasma bicarbonate and pH will have returned to normal with a normal respiratory rate.

PHYSIOLOGY PEARLS

❖ Carbonic acids are substances whose end products of metabolism are CO_2 and water, such as triglycerides and carbohydrates.

❖ Noncarbonic or fixed acids are substances whose end products of metabolism are nonvolatile, such as phosphoric acid and sulfuric acid produced from phospholipids and protein breakdown.

❖ The rate of bicarbonate reabsorption is dependent on the relative rates of bicarbonate filtration and H^+ secretion.

❖ The rate of urinary acid excretion is limited by the availability of titratable acids and NH_3.

❖ Ammoniagenesis is the primary adaptive response of the kidney to a chronic acidosis.

❖ The isohydric principle states that in a mixed solution all the acid–base pairs are in equilibrium with each other.

❖ The Henderson-Hasselbalch equation relates the pH of the plasma to the concentrations of HCO_3^- and CO_2. The ratio $[HCO_3^-]/[CO_2]$ determines the pH. Respiratory function controls CO_2, and renal function controls $[HCO_3^-]$.

REFERENCES

Goodman HM. The pancreatic islets. In: Johnson LR, ed. *Essential Medical Physiology*. 3rd ed. San Diego, CA: Elsevier Academic Press; 2003:637-658.

Rose BD, Post TW. *Clinical Physiology of Acid-Base Disorders*. 5th ed. New York: McGraw-Hill; 2001:578-646.

A 43-year-old woman presents to the emergency department with the acute onset of abdominal pain. Her pain is located to the right upper quadrant (RUQ) and radiates to the right shoulder. She reports nausea and vomiting but no fever or chills. The RUQ pain is worse after she eats fatty meals. On examination, the patient has severe RUQ tenderness. Her white blood cell count is elevated, as are her liver function tests and alkaline phosphatase level. The amylase and lipase levels are normal. An abdominal ultrasound reveals an enlarged gallbladder with multiple stones and gallbladder wall thickening. She subsequently is admitted to the hospital and undergoes a cholecystectomy.

◆ **Why would fatty foods aggravate the patient's RUQ pain?**

◆ **What effect does cholecystokinin (CCK) have on gastric emptying?**

◆ **Why does CCK have some gastrin-like properties?**

ANSWERS TO CASE 28: GASTROINTESTINAL REGULATION

Summary: A 43-year-old woman has acute-onset RUQ pain that worsens with fatty foods and an ultrasound demonstrating signs of gallstones and acute cholecystitis.

◆ **Effect of fatty foods on gallstones:** Fatty foods cause secretion of CCK, which causes contraction of the gallbladder and relaxation of the sphincter of Oddi. Because gallstones are blocking the outflow of bile, when the gallbladder is stimulated to contract, the obstruction leads to increased pain.

◆ **CCK and gastric emptying:** Delays gastric emptying to allow for a longer period of time to digest the fatty meal.

◆ **CCK and gastrin:** Five *C*-terminal amino acids the same as gastrin, and this terminal heptapeptide is where the biologic activity resides.

CLINICAL CORRELATION

The incidence of cholelithiasis increases with age, and this condition is more common in females. Most gallstones are not symptomatic and do not require treatment. However, when acute cholecystitis develops, surgery often is required. Typical symptoms include biliary colic and RUQ pain with radiation to the right shoulder, nausea, vomiting, fever, leukocytosis, and elevated alkaline phosphatase. The gallstones can be visualized without difficulty with an abdominal ultrasound. Immediate consultation with a surgeon is indicated when acute cholecystitis develops. The patient is immediately made nothing by mouth (NPO). Antibiotics often are begun. Pain medication can be given, but morphine should not be used because it will cause constriction of the sphincter of Oddi and increase the biliary pressure. When the patient is made NPO, the CCK level is decreased and contractions of the gallbladder will begin to diminish. Patients with asymptomatic gallstones are instructed to follow low-fat diets to try to diminish the secretion of CCK.

APPROACH TO GASTROINTESTINAL REGULATION

Objectives

1. Understand the difference between the mechanisms of stimulation of hormones (endocrines), paracrines, and neurocrines.
2. Know and understand the role of various gastrointestinal (GI) hormones (gastrin, CCK, secretin, glucose-dependent insulinotropic peptide [GIP]).

3. Know and understand the role of various paracrines (somatostatin, histamine).

4. Know and understand the role of various neurocrines (vasoactive intestinal peptide [VIP], serotonin, nitric oxide [NO]).

Definitions

Neurocrine: An endogenous chemical released from nerve endings to act on cells innervated by those nerves.

Endocrine: An endogenous chemical released from endocrine cells into the circulation to act on distant cells that possess receptors for that chemical

Paracrine: An endogenous chemical released from one cell to act on adjacent cells that possess receptors for that chemical

DISCUSSION

The **GI tract** can be viewed as a food-processing line in which the complex foodstuffs that are ingested are broken down into simpler molecules that can be absorbed and utilized in the body. Each organ in the tract plays a role in this processing as the ingested material is propelled aborally. The overall chemical and mechanical processes involved are divided into **secretory, digestive, absorptive, and motility processes.**

For the processes to proceed in an orderly fashion, numerous control mechanisms come in to play. There are chemical and mechanical receptors within the organs of the tract that, when stimulated, initiate regulatory events that are mediated by chemicals that in turn modulate the secretory, absorptive, and motility functions of the effector cells. The manner by which these chemicals are delivered to the effector cells can be **neurocrine** (released from nerve endings innervating the effector cells), **endocrine** (released from distant cells and delivered to the effector cells by the circulation), and **paracrine** (released from neighboring cells and diffuses to the effector cells).

The secretory, digestive, absorptive, and motility processes of the GI tract and their regulation can be divided into stages: **cephalic, gastric, and intestinal.** The **cephalic phase begins before any food is ingested,** is reinforced during the act of chewing, and ends shortly after the meal is finished. The **gastric phase** begins when food arrives in the stomach and continues as long as nutrients remain in the stomach. The **intestinal phase** begins with the first emptying of contents from the stomach. It is the longest and perhaps the most important phase, lasting as long as nutrients and undigested residue are present in the intestinal lumen. Although regulatory events are more numerous during digestion of a meal, they also are important during the time when no digestion and absorption of nutrients are taking place: the interdigestive state.

Regulation during the **cephalic** phase is mostly **neurocrine.** Reflexes initiated by the sight and smell of food as well as the presence of material in the mouth bring about the **release of acetylcholine (ACh) at the salivary glands,** at **acid-secreting (parietal) and pepsin-secreting (chief) cells in the body of the stomach,** and at enzyme-secreting **(acinar) cells of the pancreas. Vagal neural pathways** also initiate the release from **antral G cells of the hormone gastrin,** which reaches **parietal cells** through the circulation. Thus, salivary (large volume), gastric acid and pepsin (small volumes), and pancreatic enzyme (small volume) secretions are stimulated during this phase.

The voluntary act of swallowing initiates a neural reflex that elicits a **peristaltic contraction** of the **pharynx and esophagus** that propels material into the stomach to begin the gastric phase. During this phase, nerves intrinsic to the stomach as well as vagal reflexes respond to mechanical stimulation of the gastric mucosa and release **ACh near parietal and chief cells** and **gastrin-releasing peptide (GRP) near antral G cells.** Gastrin also is released in response to stimulation by products of digestion, especially small peptides and amines. **ACh and gastrin** do stimulate parietal cells directly, but more important, they act on **enterochromaffin-like (ECL) cells to release histamine, which in turn stimulates the parietal cells.** The gastric phase accounts for 60% to 70% of the acid secretory response to a meal. Neural reflexes also bring about **receptive relaxation** of the orad region of the stomach to accommodate the ingested food, and they modulate electrical events of the muscle that constitutes the body and antrum to regulate gastric contractions that accomplish mixing and emptying. Pancreatic secretion, which begins during the cephalic phase, also is enhanced by local reflexes elicited during the gastric phase, though not to a great extent. Not all events of the gastric phase are stimulatory. When acid secretion is sufficient to lower the pH of the antral contents to 3 or so, somatostatin is released from cells close to antral G cells and acts in a paracrine manner to inhibit gastrin secretion.

The **emptying of gastric contents into the duodenum** initiates and perpetuates the **intestinal phase.** Products of digestion as well as acid stimulate intestinal mucosal receptors to initiate neural reflexes and the secretion of many hormones, including **secretin, CCK, GIP, and glucagon-like peptide (GLP, or enteroglucagon).** When the contents emptied from the stomach lower duodenal pH to about 4.5 or less, **S cells release secretin,** which circulates to the pancreas to stimulate HCO_3^- **secretion.** The HCO_3^- neutralizes the acid to allow for more optimal activity of the pancreatic enzymes. **Protein and lipid breakdown products** in the contents induce I cells to release CCK, which acts as an endocrine to induce pancreatic enzyme secretion, contraction of the gallbladder, and relaxation of the sphincter of Oddi (perhaps through a neural reflex as well). The enzymes and bile secreted effect the digestion and absorption of protein, fat, and carbohydrate moieties. **CCK also induces relaxation of smooth muscle of the orad stomach to lead to slow gastric emptying.** The release and absorption of glucose induce the release of both GIP and GLP, which act in an endocrine fashion to enhance the release of insulin, another hormone, from the endocrine pancreas. Neural reflexes, and perhaps CCK and other hormones, regulate contractions of the intestine to induce mixing of contents (**segmenting contractions**). The contractions also effect the slow aboral progression of contents toward the colon. In the colon, neural reflexes, and perhaps endocrine influences, control segmenting contractions (haustral contractions) that aid in the absorption of electrolytes and water and peristaltic contractions (mass movements) that ultimately lead to the evacuation of feces.

If the interval between ingestion of foodstuffs is long enough (roughly 6 hours or more), the GI tract enters an **interdigestive state.** The activity characteristic of this state, described in Case 29, is regulated by both endocrine and neurocrine pathways. The hormone **motilin** is released periodically during the interdigestive state and appears to initiate the increasing and burst of contractile activity in the stomach and duodenum. The migration of the intense contractile activity aborally along the intestine is coordinated by enteric nerves.

In addition to the neurocrines, endocrines, and paracrines mentioned above, there are many others whose roles in the GI tract are not as clear. **Vasoactive intestinal polypeptide,** although a peptide, normally acts mainly as a **neurocrine.** It is found in nerve endings and, when released, **induces relaxation of GI smooth muscle.** However, there are tumors that secrete VIP into the blood, where it acts as an endocrine to induce voluminous pancreatic secretion. Peptides such as leptin, ghrelin, and peptide YY are being evaluated for their possible roles in regulating appetite and satiety. Serotonin, which is found in many enteric nerves and in enterochromaffin cells, plays a major role in regulating motility and the secretory and absorptive functions of the GI tract. Finally, both nitric oxide and carbon monoxide (CO) are two neurocrines/paracrines that appear to be responsible for the inhibition of GI smooth muscle that occurs in many physiologic reflexes and pathologic states.

COMPREHENSION QUESTIONS

[28.1]   During the chewing of a bolus of food, but before swallowing, salivary secretion, gastric secretion, and pancreatic secretion are stimulated by which of the following neurocrine, endocrine, and paracrine mediators?

A. ACh, gastrin, histamine
B. ACh, CCK, nitric oxide
C. Nitric oxide, vasoactive intestinal polypeptide, histamine
D. Vasoactive intestinal polypeptide, gastrin, somatostatin
E. Nitric oxide, CCK, serotonin

[28.2]   A 31-year-old woman takes antacids with and after a meal so that gastric pH does not decrease below pH 6, for peptic ulcer disease. This agent will cause a greater than normal secretion of which of the following?

A. Gastrin
B. Secretin
C. Pancreatic bicarbonate
D. CCK
E. Somatostatin

[28.3] Motility recordings in a patient with signs of bacterial overgrowth of
        the small intestine indicate an abnormal pattern of motility in the fast-
        ing state that is characterized by a lack of the normal periodic bursts
        of gastric and intestinal contractions. This patient is likely to demon-
        strate abnormal secretion of which of the following hormones?

        A. CCK
        B. Gastrin
        C. Motilin
        D. Secretin
        E. Vasoactive intestinal polypeptide

Answers

[28.1] **A.** During the cephalic phase of digestion, the presence of food in the
        mouth induces local and vagal neural reflexes, culminating in the
        release of the neurocrine ACh at the salivary glands, gastric parietal
        cells, antral gastrin cells, and pancreatic acinar cells. This results in
        secretion of saliva, gastric acid, gastrin, and pancreatic enzymes. The
        hormone gastrin in turn stimulates gastric parietal cells directly and
        also induces gastric enterochromaffin cells to release histamine,
        which also stimulates gastric parietal cells in a paracrine manner.

[28.2] **A.** The ingestion of a meal results in local and vagal reflexes, result-
        ing in the secretion of gastric acid by neurocrine, endocrine, and
        paracrine pathways. The major endocrine involved is gastrin released
        from G cells in the antrum. Normally, as gastric acid lowers gastric
        pH to around 3, somatostatin is secreted by cells located next to the
        G cells to inhibit further gastrin release. If pH is not allowed to fall,
        this does not occur and gastrin secretion continues. Normally, gastric
        contents emptying from the stomach lower intraduodenal pH to lev-
        els that result in the secretion of secretin (around 4.5 and less). If gas-
        tric acid is buffered, this does not occur, and so both secretin and
        pancreatic bicarbonate secretion are decreased.

[28.3] **C.** The motility pattern that is disorganized is the migrating motor
        complex (MMC), which is highly propulsive. Data indicate that the
        phase of intense contractions in the stomach and duodenum is asso-
        ciated with and perhaps initiated by the hormone motilin.

PHYSIOLOGY PEARLS

❖ ACh is the major excitatory neurocrine; and NO and VIP are the major inhibitory neurocrines. Serotonin is an important neurocrine modulator.

❖ Gastrin, secretin, GIP, CCK, and motilin are the major GI hormones (endocrines).

❖ Histamine and somatostatin are the major paracrines.

❖ The cephalic phase of digestion is mediated primarily by neural (vagal) reflexes and consists of salivary secretion, gastric acid and pepsin secretion, pancreatic secretion, and gastrin secretion.

❖ The gastric phase of digestion is mediated by neural (vagal and enteric) reflexes and gastrin.

❖ The intestinal phase of digestion is mediated by neural (vagal and enteric) reflexes and the hormones secretin, CCK, and GIP.

❖ The interdigestive state is characterized by MMCs initiated by motilin and regulated by local nerves.

❖ VIP and NO are major neurocrines that are important for relaxation of GI smooth muscle, especially sphincteric smooth muscle.

REFERENCES

Johnson LR. Gastrointestinal physiology. In: Johnson LR, ed. *Essential Medical Physiology*. 3rd ed. San Diego, CA: Elsevier Academic Press; 2003:465-558.

Johnson LR. Regulation: Peptides of the gastrointestinal tract. In: Johnson LR, ed. *Gastrointestinal Physiology,* 7th ed. Philadelphia, PA: Mosby: 2007:1-11.

Kutchai IIC. Digestive system. In: Levy MN, Koeppen BM, and Stanton BA, eds. *Berne & Levy, Principles of Physiology* 4th ed. Philadelphia, PA: Mosby: 2006:429-494.

A 34-year-old man presents to his primary care physician with the complaint of increased difficulty swallowing both solid and liquid foods. He notices that he sometimes has more difficulty when he is under stress. He often has chest pain and regurgitation and reports difficulty with belching. After a thorough examination, he is diagnosed with achalasia (disorder of the lower esophageal sphincter).

◆ **What part of the gastrointestinal (GI) tract is composed of striated muscle and smooth muscle?**

◆ **What factors are responsible for the tonic contraction of the lower esophageal sphincter (LES) between swallows?**

◆ **What are the major neurotransmitters responsible for regulating contraction and relaxation of the LES?**

ANSWERS TO CASE 29: GI MOTILITY

Summary: A 34-year-old man is diagnosed with achalasia. He has difficulty swallowing solids and liquids.

◆ **Striated and smooth muscles in GI tract:** Striated muscle found in pharynx, upper third of the esophagus, and external anal sphincter. Smooth muscle found in all areas in between, including the LES.

◆ **Tone of the LES:** Inherent to the LES smooth muscle and augmented by cholinergic nerves.

◆ **Neurotransmitters in LES:** Acetylcholine (ACh), vasoactive intestinal peptide (VIP), nitric oxide (NO), adenosine triphosphate (ATP).

CLINICAL CORRELATION

Achalasia is a motor disorder of the esophageal smooth muscle in which the LES does not relax normally with swallowing. Patients present with difficulties swallowing both solid and liquid food. They also may experience chest pain and difficulty with belching. The pathophysiology is thought to be a loss of enteric inhibitory nerves. The diagnosis may be confirmed with a barium swallow that shows esophageal dilation and a beaklike narrowing in the terminal portion of the esophagus. Treatment options include medications (nitroglycerin, isosorbide dinitrate, calcium channel blockers), esophageal dilation, and surgery. Other clinical disorders characterized by disordered neuromuscular activity of the GI tract include Hirschsprung disease, which is caused by a developmental lack of inhibitory enteric nerves in the colon; gastroparesis usually resulting from an autonomic neuropathy, often diabetic; ileus caused by trauma or infection; intestinal pseudoobstruction caused by an enteric neuropathy and/or muscle atrophy; and irritable bowel syndrome resulting from altered sensory nerve function and/or altered motility, usually of the colon.

APPROACH TO GI MOTILITY

Objectives

1. Describe phasic and tonic contractions.
2. Understand the mechanisms of chewing, swallowing, and esophageal motility.
3. Know about gastric motility and small and large intestine motility.
4. Describe regulation of motility.

Definitions

Segmenting contractions: Contractions of the small and large intestine (where they are called haustral contractions) that serve to mix and locally circulate intestinal contents.

Peristaltic contractions: Contractions occurring in all areas of the gastrointestinal tract that serve to propel intestinal contents, usually forward.

MMC: The pattern of contractions in the stomach and small intestine that occurs during the interdigestive state.

DISCUSSION

Digestion and absorption of ingested food and drink require an **orderly movement** of material **through the GI tract.** This is accomplished by **contractions of the musculature** that in part constitutes the walls of the tract. In the esophagus, small intestine, and large intestine, this muscle is arranged in **two layers:** an **outer longitudinal** muscle layer and an **inner circular layer.** In the **stomach,** an **incomplete oblique layer** also is present. The muscle in the pharynx, the upper esophageal sphincter (UES), the upper third or so of the esophagus, and the external anal sphincter is **visceral striated muscle.** The **muscle in all other areas is smooth muscle.**

The major regulation of contractions of the striated muscle is accomplished by **extrinsic special efferent nerves that innervate the muscle cells directly.** The major regulation of contractions of the smooth muscle is accomplished by **enteric nerves** located mainly in the **myenteric, or Auerbach, plexus.** Activity of these nerves in turn is influenced by extrinsic sympathetic and parasympathetic nerves. Muscles in certain regions also are influenced by endocrine and paracrine mediators.

There are regions of the GI tract, usually between two organs, where the musculature is in a state of fairly stable contraction to partially or totally occlude the lumen. Such **tonic contractile activity** is found in the **UES,** the **LES,** the **ileocecal sphincter,** and the **internal anal sphincter.** The orad, or proximal, portion of the stomach is in a state of tonic contraction, but rather than occluding the lumen, it contracts tonically to shift ingested material into the antrum. The pylorus, rather than acting as a true sphincter to maintain closure of the lumen, contracts tonically and phasically to alter resistance to gastric emptying. The external anal sphincter exhibits little to no tone unless the internal anal sphincter relaxes at a time when the act of defecation is not desired. Although the musculature of the esophagus, antrum, small intestine, and colon exhibits tone, it is characterized mostly by **periodic contractions lasting a few seconds,** followed by relaxations, often in a cyclical pattern. Thus, these muscles are said to exhibit **phasic contractile activity.**

The process of **digestion** begins with the **chewing and swallowing of ingested food.** Chewing effectively reduces the size of the food and mixes it with **saliva** that contains **salivary amylase and lingual lipase** to begin digestion and mucus to aid in swallowing. Swallowing begins with the voluntary act of manipulating the portion to be swallowed to the oropharynx, using mainly the tongue. The bolus then stimulates receptors in the pharynx to initiate the **swallowing reflex.** This reflex involves **coordinated contractions and relaxations of the striated and smooth muscle** that constitute the **pharynx and esophagus.** The reflex begins with contraction of the pharyngeal muscles to propel the bolus toward the esophagus. Between swallows, the entrance to the esophagus, the **UES,** is closed to form a barrier between the pharynx, where the pressure is atmospheric, and the intrathoracic esophagus, where the pressure is subatmospheric. With swallowing, the UES relaxes as the bolus approaches to allow easy entry. The UES then regains tone and the muscle of the body of the **esophagus contracts in a peristaltic sequence to propel the bolus toward the stomach.** The junction between the esophagus and the stomach, the **LES,** also remains closed between swallows to prevent reflux of gastric contents. During swallowing and before the arrival of the bolus, the LES relaxes to allow passage into the stomach. The LES then regains tone.

Movement of the swallowed bolus into the stomach is facilitated by a decrease in tone of the proximal stomach that is called **receptive relaxation** with each swallow. Thus, the orad stomach accommodates to maintain a relatively constant pressure as the food is swallowed much faster than it empties into the small intestine. Beginning almost immediately and during the time of gastric emptying of the meal, material moves from the orad stomach into the distal stomach in an orderly fashion. There it is acted on by **peristaltic contractions that begin about midstomach and progress toward the pylorus.** These contractions usually are not lumen occluding, and they mix contents with gastric secretions as well as propel the contents forward. Indeed, during a single contraction, more material is "retropelled" back into the stomach, causing mixing and mechanical breakdown of the food, than is emptied into the small intestine. Also, this contractile activity, along with tonic and phasic contractions of the pylorus, somehow sieves the material so that only liquids and particles less than about 2 mm^3 empty into the small bowel.

The material that enters the small intestine is acted on by phasic contractions of varying strength. **Most of the contractions** are **segmenting** and serve to **mix contents with secretions of the pancreas and liver** and bring the contents into contact with the mucosa, where they can be digested and absorbed further. Some contractions, however, are organized into short peristaltic sequences that serve to propel the contents in a net aboral direction. Thus, meal components, electrolytes, and water that are not absorbed in the small intestine are delivered to the colon.

To **access the colon,** material must pass through the **ileocecal sphincter,** a band of muscle that is tonically contracted, but relaxes with ileal distention. Material in the colon is acted on by **phasic contractions of long duration** that are called **haustral contractions.** These contractions serve to bring contents into contact with the mucosa so that electrolytes and water can be absorbed. Net aboral propulsion of the remaining contents is accomplished by infrequent peristaltic contractions called mass movements. Once in the rectum, the contents elicit the rectosphincteric reflex, which is characterized by relaxation of the internal anal sphincter and the sensation of the urge to defecate. Defecation can be prevented, and the reflex accommodated, by contraction of the external anal sphincter. Alternatively, **defecation** can ensue through **voluntary relaxation of the external anal sphincter** and increases in **intraabdominal pressure.**

During interdigestive periods when no nutrients are in the stomach or small intestine, contractions of the stomach and small intestine occur, but their pattern of occurrence changes to one that has been referred to as the **migrating motor complex (MMC).** This complex consists of three phases, and the transition from the digestive to the MMC pattern can begin with any of the phases. **Phase 1** is a period of time lasting 20 to 60 minutes during which no gastric contractions occur. This is followed by a 10- to 30-minute period of intermittent peristaltic contractions of variable amplitude (**phase 2**). This is followed by a period of 5 to 10 minutes of strong peristaltic contractions (**phase 3**) that begin in the orad stomach and sweep the length of the stomach, pushing the contents through a relaxed pylorus into the small intestine. As each peristaltic contraction approaches the duodenum, the duodenum relaxes to accommodate the material being emptied from the stomach. The timing of the various phases of the complex is almost identical in the duodenum and the stomach. However, each phase occurs at progressively more distal sites of the small intestine, with a lag in time giving the impression of a slow migration of the phases toward the colon. Phases 2 and 3 move undigested material toward the colon, reaching the distal ileum about the time the cycle is repeating in the stomach. The MMC pattern recurs until ingestion of the next nutrients.

The **act of swallowing** is under **neural regulation. Sensory nerves from the pharynx and esophagus** project to regions of the medulla referred to collectively as the **swallowing center.** This "center" then **initiates a sequence of motor events** consisting of (1) **sequential activation of vagal nerves** innervating striated muscle of the **pharynx,** causing a **peristaltic contraction,** (2) **inhibition of vagal nerves** innervating the **UES,** causing relaxation, (3) **activation of vagal nerves** innervating visceral striated muscle of the **esophagus,** causing a **peristaltic contraction,** and (4) activation of **vagal nerves innervating the enteric nerves** in smooth muscle regions of the **esophagus and stomach.** Activation of the enteric nerves leads to a continuation of the peristaltic contraction in the body of the esophagus and to relaxation of the LES and orad region of the stomach. The **excitatory neurotransmitter** released by the vagal nerves innervating the **striated muscle and enteric nerves is acetylcholine.** The excitatory and inhibitory neurotransmitters released by the enteric nerves innervating the smooth muscle are less well characterized.

There is evidence for ACh and the tachykinins serving as excitatory transmitters and for nitric oxide, VIP, and ATP, serving as inhibitory transmitters.

Contractions of the distal stomach, the small intestine, and the large intestine are regulated by inhibitory and excitatory enteric nerves that modulate intrinsic electrical activities of the smooth muscle cells. The enteric nerves and/or muscles are influenced by excitatory and inhibitory extrinsic nerves and hormones. Also in this region, smooth muscle cells and associated **interstitial cells of Cajal** generate omnipresent **cyclical membrane depolarizations and repolarizations that are called slow waves.** In the antrum, their frequency is about 3 cycles per minute (cpm). In the small intestine, the frequency is about 12 cpm in the duodenum and decreases to about 8 cpm in the ileum. Frequencies in the colon are more complex but also usually are about 3 cpm. Although frequencies at two adjacent sites in any area will be the same, there will be a phase lag so that there appears to be a wave of depolarization spreading aborally. Slow waves themselves do not initiate significant contractions. However, the electrical events leading to contraction (spike or action potentials) occur only during the depolarization phase of a slow wave. Thus, slow waves ensure that contractions are phasic, set the maximum frequency of contraction, and help establish the peristaltic nature of contraction, especially in the stomach.

Regulation by enteric nerves is critical for normal motility of smooth muscle regions of the GI tract. This is best exemplified, as in this case, by the consequences of their being absent or damaged. Although the neurotransmitters involved have not been identified precisely, the ones mentioned above play major roles. In addition, **serotonin (5-hydroxytryptamine [5-HT])** appears to be involved in many of the enteric nerve reflexes that control **motility.** A few of the GI hormones appear to play physiologic roles in regulating motility. **CCK relaxes the orad stomach, relaxes the sphincter of Oddi, and contracts the gallbladder. Gastrin** and other digestive hormones may play a role in the **gastrocolic reflex,** which is the increase in colonic motility often seen upon the initial ingestion of a meal. Finally, **motilin** may be the hormone that initiates the migrating motor complex seen in the fasting state.

COMPREHENSION QUESTIONS

[29.1]   During the ingestion and digestion of a meal, peristaltic contractions are the primary type of contractions occurring in which of the following regions of the GI tract?

A. Esophagus
B. Proximal stomach
C. Jejunum
D. Ileum
E. Colon

[29.2]   Which of the following regions of the GI tract are the most dependent on extrinsic nerves for regulation?

A. Lower esophagus and distal stomach
B. Lower esophagus and proximal stomach
C. Small intestine and large intestine
D. Upper esophagus and distal stomach
E. Upper esophagus and external anal sphincter

[29.3]   Esophageal manometry is performed on a patient who is experiencing
difficulty swallowing. Between swallows, pressures above atmospheric pressure are recorded in the UES and LES and pressures below
atmospheric pressure are recorded in the thoracic esophageal body.
Upon swallowing, the UES relaxes and a normal peristaltic contraction occurs in the upper esophagus. The peristaltic contraction occurring in the lower esophagus is slightly abnormal, but there is no
relaxation of the LES. The defect in this patient most likely lies in
which of the following structures?

A. Extrinsic nerves innervating the esophagus
B. Intrinsic nerves of the esophagus
C. Smooth muscle of the esophagus
D. Striated muscle of the esophagus
E. Swallowing center

Answers

[29.1]   **A.** Peristaltic contractions are the primary, if not the only, contractions of the esophagus that result in the rapid transfer of material from
the mouth to the stomach. The proximal stomach undergoes mainly
receptive relaxation and tonic contraction during the ingestion and
digestion of a meal. In both the small and the large intestine, segmenting (phasic) contractions are most numerous.

[29.2]   **E.** The upper esophagus and the external anal sphincters are composed
of striated muscle that has no intrinsic activity and depends on extrinsic
innervation to regulate its contractions. The lower esophagus, distal
stomach, small intestine, and colon are composed of smooth muscle and
are innervated by enteric nerves that impart a high degree of independ-
ence from extrinsic nerves. The proximal stomach is intermediate in its
dependence, with receptive relaxation being impaired by vagotomy.

[29.3]   **B.** Normal resting pressures in the UES and LES and normal peri-
stalsis in the upper esophagus with swallowing indicate that the muscle, extrinsic nerves, and swallowing center are intact. The slightly
abnormal peristaltic contractions of the lower esophagus and especially the lack of relaxation of the LES upon swallowing indicate a
defect in the intrinsic nerves.

PHYSIOLOGY PEARLS

❖ Contractions of the pharynx, UES, and striated portion of the esophagus are coordinated by a central nervous system (CNS) center
and are mediated by direct vagal innervation of the muscle.
Events in the smooth muscle portion of the esophagus, LES, and
orad stomach are coordinated by both central and enteric nerves
acting on the muscle.

❖ Tonic contraction of the orad stomach is regulated by enteric and
extrinsic nerve reflexes and by CCK. Antral contractions are regulated by slow waves and enteric neural reflexes. Tonic and phasic contractions of the pylorus are regulated by enteric neural
reflexes.

❖ Segmenting and peristaltic contractions of the small intestine and
segmenting (haustral) contractions and mass movements of the
colon are regulated by slow waves, enteric and extrinsic nerve
reflexes, and perhaps GI hormones.

❖ In smooth muscle areas of the GI tract, enteric nerves are vital for
normal motility. Their lack or damage can result in achalasia,
pseudoobstruction, Hirschsprung disease, and other motility
disorders.

REFERENCES

Johnson LR. Gastrointestinal physiology. In: Johnson LR, ed. *Essential Medical Physiology*. 3rd ed. San Diego: Elsevier Academic Press; 2003:465-558.

Kutchai HC. Digestive system. In: Levy MN, Koeppen BM, Stanton BA, eds. *Berne & Levy, Principles of Physiology*. 4th ed. Philadelphia, PA : Mosby; 2006:429-450.

Weisbrodt NW. Swallowing, gastric emptying, motility of the small intestine, motility of the large intestine. In Johnson LR, ed. *Gastrointestinal Physiology*. 7th ed. Philadelphia, PA: Mosby; 2007:23-55.

❖ CASE 30

A 43-year-old man presents to his gastroenterologist with symptoms of peptic ulcer disease. He states that he has a midepigastric burning pain that is relieved by eating food and worse on an empty stomach. The patient has been on numerous antacid medications without relief. He has had recurrent peptic ulcers for the last 5 years, and has had minimal relief with the usual treatments. A fasting serum gastrin level is drawn and found to be extremely elevated. After further tests are done, the patient is diagnosed with a gastrin-secreting tumor in the pancreas.

◆ **By what mechanism might elevated gastrin levels cause ulcers?**

◆ **What cells are stimulated to secrete acid by gastrin?**

◆ **What cells are responsible for secretion of intrinsic factor?**

ANSWERS TO CASE 30: GASTRIC SECRETION

Summary: A 43-year-old man has recurrent peptic ulcers that are not responsive to normal therapy. He has elevated fasting gastrin levels and is diagnosed with a gastrin-secreting pancreatic tumor (Zollinger-Ellison syndrome).

 Mechanism that might lead to peptic ulcers: Continuous acid secretion that is not subject to negative feedback and injures the gastric mucosa.

 Cells that secrete acid in response to gastrin: Parietal cells.

 Cells that are responsible for secretion of intrinsic factor: Parietal cells.

CLINICAL CORRELATION

Peptic ulcer disease is seen commonly in the primary care physician's office. Peptic ulcers result when there is a disruption of the mucosal integrity of the stomach and/or the duodenum that leads to inflammation and pain. A patient's pain usually is described as epigastric in location and burning in nature, with aggravation when fasting and relief with food. The use of nonsteroidal anti-inflammatory drugs (NSAIDs) and *Helicobacter pylori* infection are the two major causes of peptic ulcer disease. Gastric acid contributes to mucosal injury but does not always play a primary role. Gastric acid production in the stomach is controlled by a variety of mechanisms, including the hormone gastrin, the paracrine histamine, and the neurocrine acetylcholine (ACh). The production of gastrin usually is closely controlled; however, for patients with Zollinger-Ellison syndrome, severe peptic ulcer disease results from hypersecretion of gastric acid from an unregulated gastrin release from a non-β-cell endocrine tumor. Patients with Zollinger-Ellison often present with symptoms of peptic ulcer disease. Suspicion for this disorder should be present when patients have ulcers in unusual locations, ulcers refractory to standard medical therapy, ulcer recurrence after acid-reducing surgery, or ulcers with frank complications. A fasting gastrin level will help confirm the diagnosis, although further studies are needed.

APPROACH TO GASTRIC SECRETION

Objectives

1. Know about salivary secretion, gastric secretion, and pancreatic secretion.
2. Be able to describe bile secretion.
3. Understand the function of the gallbladder.

Definitions

Amylase: An enzyme secreted by salivary glands and the pancreas that takes part in starch digestion.

Pepsinogen: A pro-enzyme secreted by the stomach that is converted to pepsin that takes part in protein digestion.

Trypsinogen, chymotrypsinogen, and prophospholipases: Proenzymes secreted by the pancreas which when activated take part in protein and fat digestion.

Lipase: An enzyme secreted by the pancreas that takes part in fat digestion.

DISCUSSION

Specialized epithelial cells that **line the acini and ducts of the organs** that constitute the gastrointestinal system **secrete the organic and inorganic components** that affect the digestion and absorption of the materials that people ingest and protect the organs from possible deleterious effects of many of the secretions. The chemical makeup of the secretion, as well as the regulation of the secretion, varies remarkably from organ to organ.

In the oral cavity, **secretory and absorptive activities of the acinar and ductule cells of the salivary glands** result in the production of a large volume, compared with glandular weight, of **hypotonic solution that is rich in potassium and bicarbonate** compared with plasma. Through a **secondary active transport system** involving apical membrane **chloride channels,** acinar cells secrete a solution similar in inorganic composition to that of plasma. As this fluid passes through the ducts, sodium and chloride are absorbed in partial exchange for potassium and bicarbonate to result in the final secretion. In addition to the inorganic components, several of the **salivary glands** contain cells that secrete **amylase and lipase,** which begin the process of digestion; **lysozyme and lactoferrin,** which have antimicrobial activity; and mucus. These components are synthesized in the endoplasmic reticulum and stored in secretory granules until they are released. Regulation of salivary secretion is done almost entirely through neurocrine pathways, primarily parasympathetic. However, salivary glands are among the few organs whose secretions are stimulated by both parasympathetic and sympathetic divisions of the autonomic nervous system.

In the body of the stomach, **parietal (oxyntic), chief (peptic), and mucus neck cells** secrete **hydrochloric acid, pepsin, and soluble mucus,** respectively. In addition, surface epithelial cells in all regions secrete a more viscous **mucus in an alkaline fluid.** All of these products are secreted into the gastric lumen to take part in digestion of ingested foodstuffs, and in **protection** of the stomach. In addition to these digestive and protective secretions, the parietal cells secrete **intrinsic factor which** is necessary for the absorption of **vitamin B$_{12}$.** In the antrum, there are **endocrine (G) cells** that secrete **gastrin** in an endocrine fashion to stimulate parietal cells, and endocrine cells that secrete **somatostatin** in a paracrine fashion to inhibit G cell secretion of gastrin. The secretion of acid by parietal cells is accomplished by a primary active transport process involving a **hydrogen-potassium-ATPase (H$^+$-K$^+$-ATPase).** In resting cells, this enzyme is localized to a system of membranes (tubulovesicles) residing just below the surface of the cells' apical membrane. In this location, the enzyme is inactive. Upon stimulation of the parietal cell, the tubulovesicles fuse with the apical cell membrane, which contains potassium channels. In the presence of these channels, the H$^+$-K$^+$-ATPase becomes active, resulting in the secretion of HCl in a concentration of 150 mmol/L. During the secretion of this acid into the gastric lumen, bicarbonate is produced and released into the venous blood, producing an alkaline tide. Secretion of the **pepsin precursor pepsinogen by** chief cells is via exocytosis of protein that has been synthesized in the endoplasmic reticulum and stored in secretory granules. In the presence of acid in the lumen of the stomach, the secreted **pepsinogen** is **converted to the active protease pepsin.**

Stimulation of acid secretion occurs when **receptors for acetylcholine (ACh), histamine, and gastrin** on the basolateral membranes of the **parietal cells** are stimulated. Occupation of the muscarinic ACh and the gastrin receptors results in an increase in intracellular free calcium; occupation of the histamine H$_2$ receptor results in an increase in cyclic adenosine monophosphate (cAMP). Calcium and cAMP act in a synergistic manner to bring about HCl secretion. ACh and gastrin also stimulate HCl secretion by acting on receptors on enterochromaffin-like cells (ECLs). These cells, which are adjacent to parietal cells, release histamine, which in turn acts in a paracrine manner to stimulate acid secretion. Antral G cells synthesize and store gastrin in secretory granules. Upon stimulation, gastrin is released into the bloodstream and circulates back to the stomach to act on parietal cells. Initially, the acid that is secreted is buffered by the ingested food. However, as more acid is secreted and the partially digested food empties into the duodenum, the pH falls. When antral pH falls to about 3 or below, somatostatin is released to inhibit gastrin secretion, thus decreasing further acid secretion. However, as in this case, gastrin also can be produced by tumors in areas that are not subject to this negative feedback. Thus, there is a continuous secretion of large amounts of acid. This can cause pain and damage, especially during times when there is no food in the stomach to buffer the acid.

In the pancreas, **acinar cells** synthesize and then store in secretory granules a large number of enzymes, such as **lipase and amylase,** and proenzymes such as **trypsinogen, chymotrypsinogen,** and the **prophospholipases.** These enzymes are required for the digestion of complex carbohydrates, proteins, and lipids. **Cells that line the pancreatic ducts,** in contrast, secrete a **fluid rich in bicarbonate** through a **secondary active transport system** that involves apical membrane chloride channels and chloride-bicarbonate exchangers. The **bicarbonate neutralizes the acid being emptied from the stomach** to bring the pH of the chyme closer to 7 to allow for optimal activity of the pancreatic enzymes. **Pancreatic acinar cells possess receptors mainly for ACh and cholecystokinin (CCK).** When occupied, both, but especially CCK receptors, result in enzyme secretion. Ductule cells, in contrast, possess receptors for secretin as well as for ACh and CCK. It is primarily occupation of the secretin receptor that results in stimulation of ductile secretion.

In the liver, **hepatocytes synthesize and secrete conjugated bile acids** (which at physiologic pH exist as bile salts), **phospholipids, and cholesterol** necessary for digestion and absorption of lipids. To these organic constituents is added an inorganic solution rich in bicarbonate that is secreted mainly by cells lining the biliary ducts. Only a small fraction of the bile acids that are secreted into the canaliculi at any given time are synthesized de novo. Most are resecreted as part of the **enterohepatic circulation.** This circulation is characterized by the secretion of bile acids into the duodenum. Once in the upper small intestine, the acids aid in the absorption of lipid-soluble materials. Most of the bile acids then are absorbed, mostly in the ileum, by a carrier-mediated process. They return to the liver in the portal blood and are extracted by the hepatocytes by another carrier-mediated process, pass through the cell, and are resecreted, thus completing the circulation. The small percentage lost during the circulation is replenished by hepatic synthesis. There seems to be little direct regulation of hepatocyte bile secretion by neurocrine, endocrine, or paracrine pathways; however, secretin does increase water and bicarbonate secretion by the bile ducts. The rate of hepatocyte bile secretion depends mostly on the rate of return of bile acids through the enterohepatic circulation and in part by the rate of de novo synthesis of bile acids.

During the **interdigestive state,** the **bile** that is secreted by the liver **enters the gallbladder** rather than the small intestine. There, the **organic components are concentrated as water and electrolytes are absorbed.** As the **bile acids, phospholipids, and cholesterol are concentrated,** they form **mixed micelles** that are water soluble and stay in solution. With the **ingestion of a meal, contraction of the gallbladder** and **relaxation of the sphincter of Oddi** accomplish the expulsion of bile into the duodenum, thus increasing the enterohepatic circulation. Gallbladder contraction is initiated during the cephalic phase of digestion through the release of **ACh** via extrinsic nerves, but most contraction occurs during the **intestinal phase of digestion** through the action of **CCK,** which appears to activate intrinsic nerves, which in turn cause contraction of gallbladder smooth muscle and relaxation of sphincter of Oddi smooth muscle.

COMPREHENSION QUESTIONS

[30.1]   A 25-year-old woman with inflammatory bowel disease has a large portion of her ileum removed. Bile acid metabolism in such a patient would be characterized by which of the following?

   A. Decreased loss of bile acids in the stool
   B. Increased de novo synthesis of bile acids
   C. Increased return of bile acids to the liver via the portal blood
   D. Increased secretion of bile acids by the liver

[30.2] A patient with duodenal ulcers has elevated serum gastrin levels that do not decrease upon acidification of the gastric antrum. In such a patient, which of the following is likely to be depressed?

A. Gastric acid secretion
B. Gastric pepsinogen secretion
C. Pancreatic bicarbonate secretion
D. Release of gastrin from antral G cells
E. Serum secretin levels

[30.3] A 32 year old alcoholic male with chronic pancreatitis in which more than 90% of pancreatic function is lost. Which of the following is most likely to be observed?

A. Decreased serum secretin levels
B. Depressed blood glucose levels
C. Enhanced bile acid micelle formation
D. Increased duodenal pH levels
E. Steatorrhea

Answers

[30.1] **B.** Removal of the ileum will interrupt the enterohepatic circulation of bile salts by removing the site of active reabsorption. This will result in a loss of bile acids in the feces and a decrease in the return of bile acids to the liver by the portal blood. The decreased flux of bile acids through hepatocytes will result in an upregulation of bile acid synthesis. Synthesis usually will not keep up with loss, and so the secretion of bile acids by the liver will be decreased.

[30.2] **D.** This patient probably has a tumor that is secreting gastrin in an unregulated manner. This will result in increased gastric acid secretion and very low gastric pH and duodenal pH. The low duodenal pH will lead to increased serum secretin levels and increased pancreatic bicarbonate secretion. The low gastric pH will lead to an increase in pepsinogen secretion but a decrease in the secretion of gastrin from antral G cells.

[30.3] **E.** This much destruction of the pancreas will lead to a deficiency in the secretion of bicarbonate, digestive enzymes, and islet cell hormones. Decreased bicarbonate will lead to decreased duodenal pH, which in turn leads to increased serum secretin levels and to a decreased solubility of bile acids in the intestinal lumen. The decreased secretion of lipase along with impaired micelle formation will lead to fat maldigestion and steatorrhea. The loss of adequate insulin secretion will result in elevated blood glucose levels (diabetes mellitus).

PHYSIOLOGY PEARLS

❖ Salivary secretion is hypotonic, rich in potassium, and produced in a large volume.

❖ Salivary secretion is stimulated when either or both of its sympathetic and parasympathetic nerves are stimulated.

❖ Acid secretion by gastric parietal cells is accomplished by primary active transport.

❖ Major stimulants of acid secretion are the neurocrine ACh, the hormone gastrin, and the paracrine histamine.

❖ Gastrin release is inhibited in a paracrine fashion by somatostatin, which is released when antral pH drops below approximately 3.

❖ Pancreatic enzymes are secreted by acinar cells, primarily in response to ACh and CCK. Pancreatic bicarbonate is secreted by duct cells, primarily in response to secretin. However, CCK potentiates the effect of secretin on bicarbonate secretion.

❖ Bile is formed in the liver and concentrated in the gallbladder. Bile is expelled by the gallbladder into the duodenum, primarily in response to CCK released from the small intestine.

❖ Bile salts secreted into the duodenum take part in the digestion and absorption of lipids and then are reabsorbed in the ileum to be returned to the liver in the portal blood.

REFERENCES

Johnson LR. Gastrointestinal physiology. In: Johnson LR, ed. *Essential Medical Physiology*. 3rd ed. San Diego, CA: Elsevier Academic Press; 2003:465-558.

Johnson LR. Salivary secretion, gastric secretion, pancreatic secretion. In: Johnson LR, ed, *Gastrointestinal Physiology*, 7th ed. Philadelphia, PA: Mosby; 2007:57-95.

Kutchai HC. Digestive system. In: Levy MN, Koeppen BM, and Stanton BA, eds. Berne & Levy, *Principles of Physiology*. 4th ed. Philadelphia, PA: Mosby; 2006:429-494.

Weisbrodt NW. Bile secretion and gallbladder function. In: Johnson LR, ed. *Gastrointestinal Physiology*. 7th ed. Philadelphia, PA: Mosby; 2007:97-106.

A 23-year-old male college student presents to his primary care physician with abdominal pain, bloating, flatulence, and diarrhea after eating ice cream. He denies fever, sick contacts, or recent travel. His father has a history of similar symptoms. The patient is diagnosed with lactose intolerance and is given medications to help him digest dairy products.

◆ **What products of carbohydrate digestion are absorbed in the small intestine?**

◆ **What products of protein digestion are absorbed in the small intestine?**

◆ **What products of lipid digestion are absorbed in the small intestine?**

ANSWERS TO CASE 31: GASTROINTESTINAL DIGESTION AND ABSORPTION

Summary: A 23-year-old man has a history of abdominal pain, bloating, flatulence, and diarrhea shortly after eating ice cream.

◆ **Carbohydrate digestion products absorbed:** Glucose, galactose, and fructose.

◆ **Protein digestion products absorbed:** Amino acids, dipeptides, and tripeptides.

◆ **Lipid digestion products absorbed:** Fatty acids, monoglycerides, cholesterol, and lysophospholipids.

CLINICAL CORRELATION

Lactose intolerance is a problem that results from an absence of lactase in the brush border of the small intestine. Lactase is responsible for breaking down lactose into glucose and galactose, which are absorbed. The undigested and unabsorbed lactose increases the osmotic gradient of the luminal contents, preventing the absorption of water. The increased retention of fluid results in the symptoms of diarrhea with its abdominal distention and cramping. The bacteria in the colon ferment the lactose into a variety of gases, leading to increased flatulence. This condition may be inherited (adult lactase deficiency) or secondary (temporary) after acute infectious gastroenteritis or mucosal damage from nonsteroidal anti-inflammatory drugs (NSAIDs) or other medications. Chronic small intestinal disorders also may cause lactase deficiency because of brush border mucosal damage. Patients with this condition are encouraged to study ingredient labels on foods and avoid products that contain milk, lactose, or dry milk solids. Lactase supplements may be taken 30 minutes before consumption of the lactose-containing products to prevent symptoms.

APPROACH TO GASTROINTESTINAL DIGESTION AND ABSORPTION

Objectives

1. Describe the digestion and absorption of carbohydrates.
2. Describe the digestion and absorption of proteins.
3. Describe the digestion and absorption of lipids.
4. Discuss the absorption of vitamins.

Definitions

α-dextrinase: An enzyme located on enterocyte brush border membranes that is involved in the digestion of starch.
Maltase-glucoamylase: An enzyme located on enterocyte brush border membranes that is involved in the digestion of starch and maltose.
Sucrase-isomaltase: An enzyme located on enterocyte brush border membranes that is involved in the digestion of starch and sucrose.
Lactase: An enzyme located on enterocyte brush border membranes that is involved in the digestion of lactose.

DISCUSSION

The **complex nutrients** ingested in a meal for the most part cannot be absorbed intact from the gastrointestinal tract. They **first must be broken down,** mostly by **enzymatic** processes, to **simpler molecules.** These molecules then are absorbed by a variety of passive and active mechanisms. The major nutrients involved are **carbohydrates, proteins, lipids, and vitamins.**

Carbohydrates

The **major carbohydrates** in the diet are **complex starches** (amylopectin and amylose) and the **disaccharides sucrose, maltose, lactose, and trehalose,** none of which can be absorbed as such. The digestion of starch begins in the mouth through the action of **salivary amylase.** This enzyme is active not only in the mouth as the food is chewed and swallowed but also in the orad stomach until it mixes with and becomes inactivated by gastric acid. No further carbohydrate digestion takes place after that until gastric contents are emptied into the duodenum. There, contents are mixed with **pancreatic amylase,** which continues the breakdown. The products of salivary and pancreatic amylase digestion are **maltose, maltotriose, and α-dextrins.** Ingested disaccharides undergo no breakdown until they reach the small intestine. In the intestine, the digestion of the **oligo- and disaccharides** continues through the actions of **enzymes** located on **enterocyte brush borders.** The **enzymes α-dextrinase, maltase-glucoamylase, and sucrase-isomaltase hydrolyze** the products of **starch** digestion by **amylase to yield glucose. Sucrase-isomaltase** also hydrolyzes **sucrose to glucose and fructose. Lactose** is hydrolyzed entirely by **lactase** to yield **glucose and galactose,** and **trehalose** is hydrolyzed entirely by **trehalase** to yield **glucose.**

The **glucose and galactose liberated during digestion** are **absorbed** across the **enterocyte apical membrane** by a shared **secondary active transport system (termed SGLT-1)** that is driven by the **coabsorption of sodium. Fructose,** in contrast, is **absorbed via facilitated diffusion** through the actions of the **carrier GLUT-5.** After entering the enterocyte, all three monosaccharides exit from the basolateral membrane by **facilitated diffusion,** using the **carrier GLUT-2.** Most of the enzymes involved in carbohydrate digestion are present in relatively high amounts throughout life. **Lactase, however, is high at birth and then in most people decreases in later life.** In many people, the enzyme decreases to such low levels by the third and fourth decades that lactose intolerance develops, as described in this case.

Proteins

Dietary protein and the protein contained in gastrointestinal secretions and from cells shed into the lumen of the gastrointestinal tract are acted on by several enzymes to yield amino acids and oligopeptides. The process of **protein digestion** begins in the **stomach** through the action of **pepsin,** which itself is an enzyme protein derived from the **precursor pepsinogen,** which is secreted by **chief cells of the stomach.** Once activated by acid, **pepsin acts as an endopeptidase to cleave interior peptide bonds.** The major digestion of protein, however, takes place in the small intestine. There, contents are mixed with the many proteases secreted by the pancreas as proenzymes. A key enzyme is **trypsin,** which is secreted as **trypsinogen.** The initial secreted trypsinogen is converted to trypsin through the action of the **brush border enzyme enterokinase.** This trypsin then not only attacks peptide bonds in the ingested proteins but also converts additional trypsinogen and the precursors chymotrypsinogen, proelastase, and the procarboxypeptidases to their active forms. Together, these endo- and exopeptidases liberate amino acids and peptides of varying length.

In addition to this luminal digestion, there are **peptidases** on the **brush border** that assist in the **breakdown of larger peptides to di- and tripeptides and amino acids.** Unlike the situation in carbohydrate absorption, where only monosaccharides are absorbed, **di- and tripeptides are absorbed readily across enterocyte apical membranes along with amino acids.** Several carrier-mediated transport systems are involved in peptide and amino acid absorption, including some that are secondary active systems that require sodium. Once in the cell, most dipeptides and tripeptides are hydrolyzed to amino acids, which then exit with the other amino acids through transporters on enterocyte basolateral membranes.

Lipids

Triglycerides, phospholipids, and cholesterol esters are the **major lipids** contained in the diet. Their digestion and absorption are rather complicated because of their **insolubility in water.** The breakdown of triglycerides begins in the mouth through the actions of **lingual lipase.** However, this activity, along with the activity of gastric lipase, accounts for only about 10% of triglyceride breakdown. Perhaps more important is the **mechanical dispersal**

and emulsification of lipids that take place in the **stomach** as a result of **gastric contractions.** This prepares the lipids for further emulsification and breakdown by chemical (bile) and enzymatic processes in the small intestine. Once in the **small intestine,** the lipid is acted on by **pancreatic lipase,** which is anchored to emulsified lipid droplets by **colipase,** which also is **secreted by the pancreas.** Colipase serves to anchor lipase to the fat droplet and to facilitate the passage of fat digestion (fatty acids and monoglycerides) to adjacent bile salt micelles.

Phospholipids present in the diet and in biliary secretions and sloughed cells are broken down by **pancreatic phospholipases, mainly phospholipase A_2, to fatty acids and lysophospholipids.** Cholesterol esters are broken down by pancreatic cholesterol ester hydrolase (nonspecific hydrolase). The **products of lipid digestion,** except for some of the medium-chain and short-chain fatty acids, are **taken up into micelles,** which deliver them to **enterocyte apical membranes.** There they diffuse from the micelles and are absorbed, along with the medium- and short-chain fatty acids, mostly by **simple diffusion.** Once inside the enterocyte, **triglycerides,** containing mostly **long-chain fatty acids** and **phospholipids** are **resynthesized and combined with cholesterol** to form, along with **apoproteins, chylomicrons.** These **relatively large lipoproteins** fuse with the enterocyte basolateral membrane and are secreted by **exocytosis** to be taken up in the **lymph.** The **medium- and short-chain fatty acids pass through the enterocytes unchanged** and are taken up into the bloodstream.

Vitamins

Vitamins are contained in the complex foods that humans ingest and are liberated and absorbed through some of the same processes discussed above. Many of the vitamins, such as **thiamine (B_1), riboflavin (B_2), C, biotin, folic acid, niacin, and pantothenic acid, are water soluble** and **enter across enterocyte apical membranes by secondary active transport coupled to sodium. Pyridoxine (B_6) is water soluble** and appears to be **absorbed by restricted diffusion.** The **cobalamin (B_{12})** that is released during digestion in the stomach is bound to and **protected by glycoproteins (R proteins)** secreted by salivary glands and gastric cells. The B_{12} released from this complex and from food during digestion in the upper small intestine is bound to **intrinsic factor,** another glycoprotein secreted by gastric parietal cells. This complex, which is protected from further digestion, is propelled to the **ileum,** where it is **taken up by a carrier-mediated transport** mechanism. Other vitamins, such as **A, D, E, and K, are fat soluble.** Once released from foods during digestion, mainly in the small intestine, they are taken up into micelles and delivered to enterocyte apical membranes, where they are absorbed mainly by **simple diffusion.**

COMPREHENSION QUESTIONS

[31.1]   Tests show that glucose is absorbed as expected by a patient if sucrose, lactose, or glucose is ingested, but not if complex starches are ingested. These data indicate a defect in which of the following?

A. Bile acid secretion
B. Brush border enzyme levels
C. Epithelial sodium-coupled glucose transport
D. Pancreatic enzyme secretion
E. Villus surface area

[31.2]   A patient is experiencing steatorrhea. Tests show that the enterohepatic circulation of bile salts is normal and that absorption of orally administered glucose is normal. A disorder in which of the following is most likely to be present?

A. Brush border enzyme levels
B. Gastric motility
C. Ileal motility
D. Pancreatic enzyme secretion
E. Villus surface area

[31.3]   A patient presents with signs of cystinuria. Tests indicate that when a solution of free amino acids is infused intraduodenally, absorption of arginine is impaired; however, if a solution of dipeptides is infused intraduodenally, arginine absorption is almost normal. These data indicate that the patient has a deficiency in which of the following?

A. All sodium-coupled secondary active transport pathways in intestinal epithelia
B. Basic amino acid transporters in intestinal epithelia
C. Bile acid synthesis
D. Epithelial cell peptidase activity
E. Pancreatic enzyme secretion

Answers

[31.1]   **D.** The fact that free glucose is absorbed readily indicates that villus surface area and sodium-coupled transport are normal. The fact that glucose is absorbed when disaccharides are ingested indicates that brush border enzymes are intact. Because complex starches must be broken down first by enzymes secreted by salivary glands (minor) and the pancreas, the impaired glucose absorption seen when starches are ingested, points toward a problem with pancreatic enzyme secretion.

[31.2]   **D.** Steatorrhea is the presence of fat in the stool. It can be because of defects in fat digestion and/or defects in the absorption of the products of fat digestion. Digestion requires lipase secreted mostly by the pancreas. Absorption requires an intact enterohepatic circulation of bile salts (stated as being normal) and an adequate intestinal surface area (indicated by the normal absorption of glucose). Brush border enzymes are not involved. Gastric contractions act to emulsify lipids, but because glucose must be emptied to be absorbed, gastric motility appears to be normal. Ileal motility is required for bile salt reabsorption from the ileum, and so it probably is normal in this patient.

[31.3]   **B.** Neither pancreatic enzymes nor bile salts are required for the absorption of free amino acids or dipeptides. What is required for the absorption of free amino acids is the presence of sodium-coupled amino acid transporters. Because glucose is absorbed readily, not all sodium-coupled transporters are affected, only those specific for basic amino acids. The fact that arginine absorption is almost normal when dipeptides are given indicates that epithelial cell peptidase activity is normal.

PHYSIOLOGY PEARLS

❖ Enzymes involved in carbohydrate digestion are secreted by salivary glands and the pancreas.

❖ Proteases, phospholipases, and colipase are secreted as proenzymes.

❖ Glucose and galactose are absorbed by sodium-coupled secondary active transport; fructose is absorbed by facilitated diffusion.

❖ Pancreatic secretions must be reduced by 80% or more for pancreatic enzyme deficiency to be manifested. Lipid absorption is affected more markedly than are carbohydrate absorption and protein absorption.

❖ Sugars must be hydrolyzed to monosaccharides for absorption, but protein digestion products can be absorbed as dipeptides and tripeptides as well as amino acids.

❖ Bile acids facilitate fatty acid and fat-soluble vitamin absorption from the jejunum and then are absorbed by sodium-coupled transport in the ileum.

❖ Ileal resection results in decreased bile acid absorption and bile acid secretion, but increased bile acid synthesis.

REFERENCES

Johnson LR. Digestion and absorption. In: Johnson LR, ed. *Essential Medical Physiology*. 3rd ed. San Diego, CA: Elsevier Academic Press; 2003:529-546.

Johnson LR. Digestion and absorption. In Johnson LR, ed, *Gastrointestinal Physiology*. 7th ed. Philadelphia, PA: Mosby; 2007:107-125.

Kutchai HC. Digestive system. In: Levy MN, Koeppen BM, and Stanton BA, eds. *Berne & Levy, Principles of Physiology*. 4th ed. Philadelphia, PA: Mosby; 2006:429-494.

A 17-year-old boy presents to his primary care physician with complaints of diarrhea for the last 2 days. The patient states that he just returned to the United States after visiting relatives in Mexico. The diarrhea began suddenly and is described as "water." He has noticed no abdominal pain or blood in his stool. On examination, he appears dehydrated, but otherwise his physical examination is normal. His stool is examined and appears like "rice water." The patient is diagnosed with an infectious form of diarrhea, most likely due to *Vibrio cholerae.*

◆ **What location in the gastrointestinal (GI) tract has tight, or impermeable, junctions between the epithelial cells?**

◆ **Why do patients with diarrhea often have hypokalemia?**

◆ **How does *V. cholerae* cause diarrhea?**

ANSWERS TO CASE 32: INTESTINAL WATER AND ELECTROLYTE TRANSPORT

Summary: A 17-year-old boy has profuse watery diarrhea from a *V. cholerae* infection.

◆ **Location of impermeable gap junctions:** Large intestine.

◆ **Hypokalemia with diarrhea:** Intestinal secretions are enriched in potassium, and so there is increased loss with diarrhea.

◆ *V. cholerae* **and diarrhea:** Toxin binds to receptors on apical membrane of crypt cells and activates adenylate cyclase, which increases intracellular cyclic adenosine monophosphate (cAMP) and secretion of chloride. Both sodium and water follow the chloride into the lumen and result in the secretory diarrhea.

CLINICAL CORRELATION

Diarrhea can be seen in a variety of conditions and disease processes. There are four basic mechanisms that result in diarrhea: **osmotic** (lactose intolerance), **exudative disorders** (inflammatory bowel disease), **secretory** (*V. cholerae*), and **motility** disturbance (hyperthyroidism). Diarrhea from cholera has a rapid onset and can lead to progressive dehydration and even death. The incubation period is about 24 to 48 hours, after which the patient will begin having painless watery diarrhea. The diarrhea is free from blood and appears like rice water. Patients often complain of muscle cramps that result from electrolyte abnormalities. Complications are a result of the fluid loss and electrolyte abnormalities. When patients are adequately hydrated and electrolytes are replaced, the process is self-limiting and resolves in a few days. The diagnosis can be confirmed by the identification of *V. cholerae* in stool.

APPROACH TO WATER ABSORPTION

Objectives

1. Discuss sodium and water absorption and secretion in the small intestine and colon.
2. Describe potassium, chloride, and bicarbonate absorption and secretion in the small intestine and colon.

DISCUSSION

Approximately 9 L of water and **30 g of sodium** are **absorbed from the small intestine and colon each day,** but **only about 2 L of water and 5 g of sodium are ingested.** The difference between absorbed and ingested values is because of salivary, gastric, pancreatic, biliary, and intestinal secretions, which then are reabsorbed. The vast **majority** of this fluid is **absorbed by the small intestine,** with **only about 1 to 2 L being absorbed from the colon.** Normally, only about 0.1 to 0.2 L is excreted in the feces.

Throughout the GI tract, **water permeates membranes passively** to **maintain isosmotic conditions** (except for salivary secretions, which are hypotonic, and colonic contents, which are hypertonic) as solutes are actively secreted and absorbed. Salivary glands, the stomach, the pancreas, and the liver are mainly secretory organs, as discussed in Case 30. The intestine, in contrast, has both secretory and absorptive functions. **Under normal conditions, absorption dominates,** but as in this case, that is not always the case. The mechanisms involved in small intestinal absorption of the products of digestion are covered in Case 31. This absorption, which is accompanied by significant amounts of sodium, chloride, and water, is accomplished by villus epithelial cells. Intestinal secretion, by contrast, is accomplished by crypt epithelial cells.

There are multiple pathways and mechanisms by which **sodium is absorbed by villus cells of the intestine.** The major ones are the sodium-coupled absorption of sugars and amino acids, sodium-chloride cotransport, sodium-hydrogen countertransport, and the entry of sodium by restricted diffusion. All these are secondary active processes that are **"powered" by the sodium-potassium ATPase** located on the basolateral borders of the villus cells. With this absorption comes the passive absorption of anions, mostly chloride, and water. Potassium is absorbed by both passive and active processes. In the small intestine, potassium is concentrated in the chyme as sodium and water are absorbed, but because the paracellular pathways are "leaky," potassium is absorbed passively down its electrochemical gradient. In the colon, which is less leaky, potassium is absorbed through a primary active process involving a potassium-hydrogen ATPase. Potassium also is secreted actively by colonic villus cells because of the restricted diffusion of potassium through apical membrane channels. Thus, as sodium is absorbed, potassium is lost. **The net result is that fecal fluid has a relatively high potassium concentration.** The situation with bicarbonate is also complicated. Most of the secreted bicarbonate acts to neutralize the acid secreted by the stomach. This results in no net loss or gain of bicarbonate because the secretion of acid involves the production of bicarbonate to balance that which is secreted by the pancreas and liver. In the distal small intestine and colon, bicarbonate is secreted in exchange for chloride through the action of a chloride-bicarbonate countertransporter on the apical membrane of villus cells. Thus, **fecal secretions tend to be alkaline.**

There normally is a **low level of secretion of sodium, chloride, and water by crypt epithelial cells of the small intestine** because of the **secondary active transport of chloride.** A **sodium-potassium-chloride cotransporter** is located on the **basolateral surface of these cells (see Figure 32-1).** Thus, the movement of sodium down its electrochemical gradient facilitates the uptake of chloride. This chloride then exits the apical membrane down its electrochemical gradient by restricted diffusion through a chloride channel. Sodium and

Lumen   Interstitium

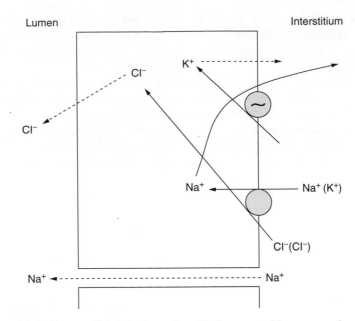

Figure 32-1. Crypt cells of the intestine. Cl⁻ is secreted by a secondary active process.

water follow passively through paracellular pathways. The fluid secreted by these cells helps maintain the liquidity of the intestinal contents and aids in digestion and absorption. The activity of the **chloride channel is regulated by both calcium and cAMP.** Elevations of either caused by actions of neuro-transmitters, or in this case toxins, increase flux through the channels and result in an increase in secretion. This secretion can exceed the ability of the villus cells to absorb, thus resulting in diarrhea rich in volume, potassium, and bicarbonate. Fortunately, the absorptive abilities of the villus cells are large and can be maximized by orally administering fluids that are rich in sodium and glucose. This is the basis for the oral rehydration (replacement) therapies that have been so successful in decreasing mortality from secretory diarrhea.

COMPREHENSION QUESTIONS

[32.1]   Oral rehydration formulas are noted to facilitate the absorption of sodium chloride and water. This observation is due in particular because of the inclusion of which of the following?

A. Bile salts
B. Other chloride salts
C. Carbohydrates
D. Fatty acids
E. Proteins

[32.2]   Which of the following is the rank order, from greatest to least, of areas of water absorption in the GI tract in a normal individual?

A. Colon, small intestine, stomach
B. Colon, stomach, small intestine
C. Small intestine, colon, stomach
D. Small intestine, stomach, colon
E. Stomach, small intestine, colon

[32.3]   Patients with cystic fibrosis have a defect in apical chloride channels in many epithelial cells. Such patients have a major defect in which of the following?

A. Colonic sodium chloride and water absorption
B. Gastric acid secretion
C. Ileal bile acid absorption
D. Jejunal glucose absorption
E. Small intestinal sodium chloride and water secretion

Answers

[32.1]   **C.** Owing to the presence of sodium-coupled glucose transporters in intestinal epithelial cells, sodium and water absorption are greatly enhanced by the inclusion of carbohydrates. Although amino acid and bile salt absorption also are sodium coupled, those transporters are not as abundant. Absorption of fatty acids is not sodium coupled.

[32.2]   **C.** By far, the greatest volume of intestinal contents is absorbed by the small intestine. The volume absorbed by the colon is significant and can increase when the functioning of the small intestine is impaired. However, the volume absorbed is much less than in the small intestine. The stomach absorbs little, if any, water. It mostly is a secretory organ.

[32.3]   **E.** Sodium, potassium, and chloride are transported actively into intestinal crypt cells across their basolateral borders. Chloride then exits the cells down its electrochemical gradient through apical chloride channels. These channels are defective in cystic fibrosis. HCl secretion by the gastric parietal cells does not involve these chloride channels. Also, the chloride that is absorbed along with sodium in the small intestine and large intestine does not pass through these channels. Bile acids are anions at the pH existing in the ileum and are not associated with chloride absorption.

PHYSIOLOGY PEARLS

❖ Water absorption and secretion in the intestine are passive and are driven by the absorption and secretion of solutes.

❖ Small intestinal villus epithelial cells absorb sodium and water; villus crypt cells secrete sodium and water.

❖ The majority of water absorption takes place in the proximal small intestine and is isosmotic.

❖ Sodium absorption in the ileum and colon is partially regulated by aldosterone.

❖ If bile salts are not absorbed in the ileum and pass into the colon, they increase secretion of electrolytes and water by the colon.

❖ Loss of gastric contents by vomiting results in alkalosis because of loss of hydrochloric acid. Diarrhea results in acidosis because of loss of bicarbonate.

REFERENCES

Johnson LR. Fluid and electrolyte absorption. In: Johnson LR, ed. *Gastrointestinal Physiology*. 7th ed. Philadelphia, PA: Mosby; 2007:127-135.

Johnson LR. Intestinal electrolyte and water transport. In: Johnson LR, ed. *Essential Medical Physiology*. 3rd ed. San Diego, CA: Elsevier Academic Press; 2003:547-555.

Kutchai HC. Digestive system. In: Levy MN, Koeppen BM, and Stanton BA, eds. *Berne & Levy, Principles of Physiology*. 4th ed. Philadelphia, PA: Mosby; 2006:429-494.

❖ **CASE 33**

A 44-year-old woman presents to her gynecologist with complaints of not having had a period for the last 8 months. She reports a negative pregnancy test at home. Upon further questioning, she reports a daily headache, changes in vision, and a milky discharge from the breast. She has no medical problems and is not taking any medications. On physical examination, she is noted to have galactorrhea and diminished peripheral vision bilaterally. The remainder of her examination is normal. A pregnancy test is repeated and is negative. A thyroid-stimulating hormone (TSH) level is drawn and is normal. Her serum prolactin level is elevated significantly. After a thorough workup is completed, she is found to have a prolactin-secreting pituitary adenoma.

◆ **How does hyperprolactinemia cause amenorrhea?**

◆ **Why would a physician need to check thyroid studies in patients with hyperprolactinemia?**

◆ **Where are the posterior pituitary hormones synthesized?**

ANSWERS TO CASE 33: PITUITARY ADENOMA

Summary: A 44-year-old woman has secondary amenorrhea, galactorrhea, headache and visual changes, and hyperprolactinemia. She is diagnosed as having a pituitary prolactinoma.

◆ **Elevated prolactin and amenorrhea:** Elevated prolactin levels inhibit pulsatile gonadotropin-releasing hormone (GnRH) secretion.

◆ **Thyroid disease and elevated prolactin:** Hypothyroidism is associated with an elevated thyrotropin-releasing hormone (TRH) level that increases the secretion of prolactin.

◆ **Synthesis of the posterior pituitary hormones:** Hypothalamic nuclei—hormones are synthesized in nerve cell bodies, packaged in secretory granules, and transported down the nerve axon to the posterior pituitary.

CLINICAL CORRELATION

An elevated prolactin level can be seen in numerous conditions. Patients should be screened initially with a pregnancy test and thyroid studies. Many different medications can cause an elevated prolactin level, including birth control pills, metoclopramide, and many antipsychotic medications. Patients present with amenorrhea secondary to inhibition of GnRH and/or galactorrhea. When adenomas are present, a patient may present with symptoms of headache or even changes in vision. The visual changes (bitemporal hemianopia) and headache usually are related to the prolactinoma compressing the optic chiasm. Normally, prolactin inhibits its own secretion by stimulating the release of dopamine from the hypothalamus. However, when pituitary adenomas are present, prolactin is secreted without inhibition from normal feedback mechanisms. Treatment of microadenomas that are not symptomatic is usually medical with bromocriptine (a dopamine agonist). However, when microadenomas are symptomatic or do not respond to medical management, surgical intervention is often necessary. Macroadenomas usually are treated surgically.

APPROACH TO THE PITUITARY GLAND

Objectives

1. Discuss the synthesis and secretion of the hormones of the anterior and posterior pituitary.
2. Describe the role of the hypothalamus in the synthesis and secretion of the hormones of the anterior and posterior pituitary.
3. Know the factors that increase and decrease prolactin secretion.

Definitions

Hypothalamohypophysial portal system: The vasculature that allows for peptides secreted by hypothalamic cells to travel to, and act on, cells in the pituitary.

Arcuate nucleus: The region of the hypothalamus whose cells secrete growth hormone-releasing hormone and gonadotropin-releasing hormone,

Paraventricular nucleus: The region of the hypothalamus whose cells secrete thyrotropin-releasing hormone and corticotropin-releasing hormone.

DISCUSSION

The **pituitary gland** is composed **of two lobes** that are derived embryonically from the **primitive gut** (anterior lobe) and the **brainstem** (posterior lobe). The pituitary secretes a large number of peptide hormones into the blood that affect the growth and secretions of other endocrine glands and/or the function of many end organs directly. Although it plays a major role in regulating many body functions, the **pituitary** itself is **regulated** in large part **by the hypothalamus** and/or by secretory products of other endocrine glands.

Concerning the **posterior pituitary, nerves extend from the supraoptic and paraventricular nuclei** of the **hypothalamus** to end in the posterior pituitary. **Cell bodies in the hypothalamus,** not in the posterior pituitary, **synthesize and package peptide hormones** in secretory granules that then undergo **axonal transport** to be stored in nerve endings in the posterior pituitary until they are released. The **major hormones released from the posterior pituitary** are **antidiuretic hormone (ADH),** also known as **vasopressin,** and **oxytocin.** These hormones are released from nerve endings in the pituitary when their nerve cells bodies in the hypothalamus receive stimulatory input. Input for the secretion of ADH comes from **hypothalamic osmoreceptors** responding to the **osmotic pressure of the blood** and from receptors located within the **cardiovascular system** (eg, the right atrium) responding to blood volume (pressure). Input for secretion of **oxytocin** comes from **receptors in the cervix** and in **mammary glands.** Stretching of the cervix during labor and delivery stimulates secretion of oxytocin, which stimulates uterine contractions that result in further stretching of the cervix. This is an example of a positive feedback loop. In nursing females, **oxytocin** also is released in **response to suckling** and often as a conditioned reflex in response to the thought of nursing. In this case, oxytocin stimulates milk ejection from the mammary gland. The release of ADH and oxytocin does not appear to be under direct negative feedback from circulating levels of the hormones.

The situation for the anterior pituitary differs. Peptide hormones of the **anterior pituitary** are **synthesized and stored in secretory cells** in the pituitary itself. Communication with the hypothalamus is via the **hypothalamohypophysial**

portal system, one of only two portal systems in the body. **Capillaries in the median eminence of the hypothalamus** and in the infundibular stem converge to form portal vessels that travel to the anterior lobe, where they branch into a second set of capillaries that supply the anterior pituitary. Thus, mediators released by cells in the hypothalamus can circulate to and affect pituitary secretory cells.

The major peptide hormones released from the **anterior pituitary** are **growth hormone (GH); thyroid-stimulating hormone (TSH), also known as thyrotropin; follicle-stimulating hormone (FSH); luteinizing hormone (LH); adrenocorticotropic hormone (ACTH); and prolactin (PRL).** The secretion of all these hormones is regulated in large part by mediators secreted into the hypothalamohypophysial portal system by cells in the hypothalamus. In addition, secretion of most of the anterior pituitary hormones is modulated by feedback inhibition from hormones released from the endocrine glands they influence.

Secretion of **GH** is stimulated by **growth hormone-releasing hormone (GHRH),** and perhaps by **ghrelin,** which is secreted by cells in the **arcuate nucleus.** GH secretion is modulated in a complex fashion. In peripheral tissues, GH stimulates the production of insulin-like growth factor-1 (IGF-1). IGF-1 in turn inhibits GH release at the level of the pituitary and the level of the hypothalamus by inhibiting the release of GHRH and stimulating the release of somatostatin, which in turn inhibits the release of GH from pituitary cells. Secretion of **TSH** is stimulated by the **tripeptide TRH** secreted by hypothalamic cells in the **paraventricular nucleus.** At the level of the **thyroid gland, TSH** stimulates growth of the thyroid and the synthesis and secretion of the thyroid hormones T_3 and T_4. As part of their actions, circulating T_3 and T_4 exert feedback inhibition primarily at the level of the pituitary and perhaps also at the hypothalamus. Secretion of **FSH and LH** is stimulated by the secretion of gonadotropin-releasing hormone **(GnRH)** from cells in the **arcuate nucleus.** Unlike the other hypothalamic hormones, to be effective, **GnRH** must be secreted in a **pulsatile** manner at a frequency of around **1 pulse per hour.** Frequencies much higher or lower than that are not effective at stimulating FSH and LH secretion. Also, GnRH, and hence FSH and LH, secretion is very low during childhood. Starting at puberty and continuing during reproductive life, pulsatile GnRH secretion occurs and FSH and LH are secreted from the pituitary to influence the maturation and function of the reproductive organs. In addition to the control exerted by GnRH, FSH and LH secretion are influenced by both positive and negative feedback.

In females, **estrogen** secreted by the developing **graafian follicle** suppresses FSH and LH secretion at the level of the pituitary. However, **before ovulation, estrogen levels** are reached that **trigger a surge in secretion of FSH and LH.** After ovulation, rising levels of **progesterone suppress FSH and LH secretion** through actions on both the pituitary and the hypothalamus. In **males, testosterone secreted from the testes suppresses LH secretion**

through actions on both the pituitary and the hypothalamus. FSH secretion is suppressed by inhibin, which also is secreted by the testes and acts at the level of the pituitary. Secretion of ACTH is stimulated by the peptide **corticotropin-releasing hormone (CRH),** which is secreted by cells in the paraventricular nucleus. At the level of the adrenal gland, **ACTH** stimulates growth of the adrenal cortex and the synthesis and secretion of **cortisol, corticosterone,** and small amounts of **adrenal androgens and estrogens.** ACTH secretion exhibits a diurnal rhythm that peaks early in the morning. The mechanisms controlling this rhythm are not understood completely. As part of their actions, circulating **cortisol** (mainly) and corticosterone exert feedback inhibition at the level of both the pituitary and the hypothalamus.

The regulation of **prolactin** secretion differs from that of the other pituitary hormones in that PRL secretion is under tonic inhibition from the hypothalamus. **If the hypothalamohypophysial portal system is disrupted, PRL secretion increases** rather than decreases as is the case for the other pituitary hormones. Most evidence points to **dopamine** rather than a peptide as being the **prolactin inhibitory hormone. In** addition to this **inhibitory pathway,** PRL secretion can be **stimulated by TRH.** The main target of PRL is the mammary gland, where it promotes the secretion of colostrum and milk. PRL levels rise during pregnancy. After parturition, basal levels fall, but there are spikes in PRL levels during and after periods of nursing. The spikes in PRL secretion are because of neural signals from the breast acting at the level of the hypothalamus to decrease dopamine release into the hypothalamohypophysial portal system. This reflex and the high levels of PRL suppress the hypothalamic secretion of GnRH, thus inhibiting the menstrual cycle.

COMPREHENSION QUESTIONS

[33.1] A 45-year-old woman is noted to have fatigue and cold intolerance and is diagnosed with hypothyroidism. Her physician suspects a pituitary etiology. Which of the following laboratory findings is most consistent with this condition?

    A. Low TSH, low free thyroxine

    B. Elevated TSH, low thyroxine

    C. Elevated TSH, elevated thyroxine

    D. Low TRH

[33.2]   A 35-year-old woman experiences anterior pituitary hemorrhagic
         necrosis (Sheehan syndrome) after a postpartum hemorrhage. She
         feels light-headed, dizzy, and weak. Which of the following hormones
         most likely is responsible for her symptoms?

         A. ACTH
         B. GnRH
         C. Prolactin
         D. TSH
         E. GH

[33.3]   A 25-year-old woman is undergoing ovulation induction for infertil-
         ity. She is given an injection of GnRH on Monday. Serum estradiol is
         low, and ovarian ultrasound reveals small follicles on Wednesday and
         Friday. What is the most likely explanation?

         A. Ovarian failure
         B. Pituitary failure
         C. Need for pulsatile hormone
         D. More time needed to see an effect

Answers

[33.1]   **A.** Usually, hypothyroidism is diagnosed by an elevated TSH,
         because the vast majority of cases of hypothyroidism involve a pri-
         mary gland (thyroid) failure. A much less common etiology is a pitu-
         itary etiology, which would be reflected by a low TSH. This would
         lead to a low free thyroxine but elevated hypothalamic secretion of
         TRH.

[33.2]   **A.** This female with anterior pituitary failure after postpartum hem-
         orrhage has symptoms of dizziness and light-headedness. This prob-
         ably is because of lack of ACTH and thus lack of mineralocorticoids
         such as aldosterone. The inability to retain sodium leads to hypov-
         olemia and the symptoms of hypotension.

[33.3]   **C.** Unlike the other pituitary hormones, GnRH needs to be secreted
         in a pulsatile fashion to effect gonadotropin (FSH and LH) secretion
         from the pituitary.

PHYSIOLOGY PEARLS

❖ The posterior pituitary secretes two hormones: antidiuretic hormone (also known as vasopressin) and oxytocin.

❖ The anterior pituitary secretes six hormones: GH, TSH, ACTH, FSH, LH, and PRL.

❖ Posterior pituitary hormones are released from endings of nerves that originate in the hypothalamus.

❖ The secretion of hormones by cells of the anterior hypothalamus is regulated by factors released from the hypothalamus into a portal venous system that runs from the hypothalamus to the anterior pituitary.

❖ The secretion of all the anterior pituitary hormones except prolactin requires stimulatory peptide factors to be released from the hypothalamus. Prolactin secretion is tonically inhibited by dopamine secreted by the hypothalamus.

❖ Peripheral neural and humoral inputs that regulate posterior pituitary hormone secretion act at the level of the hypothalamus.

❖ Peripheral neural and humoral inputs that regulate anterior pituitary hormone secretion act at the level of the hypothalamus and the pituitary.

REFERENCES

Genuth SM. Hypothalamus and pituitary gland. In: Levy MN, Koeppen BM, and Stanton BA, eds. *Berne & Levy, Principles of Physiology*. 4th ed. Philadelphia, PA: Mosby; 2006:647-662.

Goodman HM. Pituitary gland. In: Johnson LR, ed. *Essential Medical Physiology*. 3rd ed. San Diego, CA: Elsevier Academic Press; 2003:573-585.

❖ CASE 34

A 41-year-old woman presents to her primary care physician with weight and hair loss, diarrhea, nervousness, and eye pressure. She has no medical problems, but some of her family members have similar symptoms and require medication. On examination, she is noted to have exophthalmos, an enlarged nontender goiter, hyperreflexia, and a tremor when her arms are outstretched. The patient has a decreased thyroid-stimulating hormone (TSH) level and an increased free thyroxine (T_4) level and is diagnosed with Graves disease (hyperthyroidism).

 What is the mechanism by which high levels of iodine inhibit thyroid production?

 How does propylthiouracil (PTU) inhibit thyroid synthesis?

 What affect does pregnancy have on the free thyroid hormone level?

ANSWERS TO CASE 34: THYROID DISEASE

Summary: A 41-year-old woman has weight and hair loss, diarrhea, nervousness, eye pressure, nontender goiter, exophthalmos, and laboratory evidence of hyperthyroidism.

◆   **High levels of iodine:** Inhibit the iodine pump (Wolff-Chaikoff effect).

◆   **Mechanism of action of PTU:** Inhibits peroxidase enzyme activity in the follicular cell membrane, resulting in an inability to oxidize iodine.

◆   **Effect of pregnancy on free thyroid levels:** No change in free levels. The total level would be elevated because of an increase in thyroxine-binding globulin. Because the free levels remain the same, the patient is euthyroid.

CLINICAL CORRELATION

Patients with abnormalities of the thyroid may present with many different clinical symptoms. Patients with hyperthyroidism may present with weight loss, tremor, weakness, diarrhea, hair and nail changes, heat intolerance, goiters, exophthalmos, and/or tachycardia. The most common cause of hyperthyroidism is Graves disease. This disease results from stimulation of the thyroid gland by the binding of antibodies to the TSH receptor. The normal negative feedback mechanism does not stop the thyroid because antibody levels, unlike TSH levels, are not modulated by T_3 and T_4 levels. Laboratory findings suggestive of hyperthyroidism include a decreased TSH and an elevated T_4 or T_3 count. Treatment is often with PTU (blocks peroxidase activity), iodine (inhibits the iodine pump), radioactive iodine (ablates the thyroid), or surgery (thyroidectomy). Beta-blocker medications often are used when tachycardia is present.

APPROACH TO THYROID PHYSIOLOGY

Objectives

1.   Describe the synthesis of thyroid hormones.
2.   Understand the regulation of thyroid synthesis and secretion.
3.   Describe the various actions of thyroid hormones.

Definitions

Colloid: The material that fills the lumen of the thyroid follicles. It is comprised mostly of thyroglobulin, the storage form of thyroid hormone.
Thyroxin-binding globulin: The plasma protein to which most of the thyroid hormone in the circulation is bound.

DISCUSSION

The **thyroid gland** is composed of **many follicles** that consist of **epithelial (follicular) cells surrounding a lumen where thyroglobulin,** the precursor of the thyroid hormones T_3 and T_4, is synthesized and stored. Thus, **thyroglobulin** is stored outside the apical membranes of the follicular cells and away from the capillaries perfusing those cells' basolateral membranes. **Thyroglobulin is a glycoprotein** that is synthesized in the **endoplasmic reticulum** of the **follicular cells** and **secreted across their apical membranes into the lumen** by the Golgi apparatus. The other hormone component, **iodide, is taken up from the blood on the cells' basolateral membranes** by a **sodium-coupled active transport process** that can concentrate iodide 30 to 200 times. The iodide then passes through the cell to be **oxidized** on the apical surface by H_2O_2 through the action of the **enzyme thyroperoxidase.** The oxidized iodide then reacts with a small number of the **tyrosines of thyroglobulin** to form **mono- and diiodotyrosine.** Synthesis is completed by the coupling of two diiodotyrosines to form T_4, the major product, and by the coupling of monoiodotyrosines with diiodotyrosines to form T_3, the minor product. This coupling takes place while the tyrosines are still part of the thyroglobulin molecule and is catalyzed by thyroperoxidase. Normally, this storage form of thyroid hormone is sufficient to provide the body with adequate amounts of hormone for 1 to 3 months.

   Secretion of thyroid hormones begins with the **uptake of thyroglobulin** by the apical membrane of follicular cells by **endocytosis.** Lysosomal vesicles then fuse with the endocytotic vesicles, and lysosomal enzymes hydrolyze the thyroglobulin to form T_4, T_3, mono- and diiodotyrosine, free amino acids, and peptides. The T_4 **and** T_3 **diffuse across the follicular cell basolateral membrane** to enter the circulation. The **mono- and diiodotyrosines are deiodinated, and the iodide is recycled.**

   Synthesis and secretion of T_3 and T_4 will take place at low levels without any stimulus. However, normally, thyroid function is enhanced to various levels by the pituitary hormone **TSH. TSH binds to receptors** on the **basolateral surface** of follicular cells and through a **G protein-linked pathway increases cyclic adenosine monophosphate (cAMP) levels in the cell.** This leads to stimulation of hormone synthesis and secretion, and, if TSH levels are high enough for a long enough time, to an increase in size and number of follicular cells. In certain conditions, as in this case, antibodies to the TSH receptor can bind to and activate the receptor. This leads to a marked increase in the synthesis and secretion of thyroid hormone and to growth of the thyroid gland. Circulating thyroid hormones exert a negative feedback at the level of the pituitary, thus decreasing the release of TSH (see Case 33).

   Once secreted, T_3 **and** T_4 **are tightly bound to plasma proteins,** primarily thyroxin-binding globulin with lesser amounts bound to thyroxin-binding prealbumin and albumin. **Less than 1% of these hormones is in free solution** and thus in equilibrium with the interstitial fluid. Because of the tight binding to plasma proteins and the rather slow uptake of hormone by cells of the body, circulating T_3 and T_4 have plasma half-lives of around 1 and 6 days, respectively. Much of the T_3 circulating in the blood arises not from secretion from the thyroid but instead from the deiodination of T_4 by deiodinases primarily in the liver and kidney. Also, many cell types have deiodinases that convert T_4 to T_3 upon the uptake of T_4 into the cell. This is important because T_3 seems to be the most active hormone at the level of cellular receptors. T_4 also can be degraded to an inactive T_3, called rT_3 (reverse T_3), by the removal of an iodide from the internal ring of T_4 by deiodinase. The regulation and importance of this reaction are not clear.

The **effects of thyroid hormones** have a **slow onset** and a **long duration** and do not bring about moment-to-moment regulation. T_3 and T_4 enter cells by simple diffusion. Most of the T_4 is converted to T_3, which then binds with **nuclear receptors** to **modulate the transcription of a number of proteins** involved in cellular metabolism. By upregulating the synthesis of these proteins, **thyroid hormones increase the oxygen consumption and adenosine triphosphate (ATP) production** of all tissues in the adult body except brain, testis, and spleen. Much of the ATP produced is consumed to produce **body heat.** To support the increased metabolism, there is an increase in carbohydrate absorption from the intestine and in hepatic glycogenolysis and gluconeogenesis.

The effects of thyroid hormones on lipid and protein metabolism are somewhat complex. A certain hormone level is needed to provide the carbohydrate for lipogenesis to take place. However, thyroid hormone also is needed for fatty acid mobilization, and as hormone levels increase, mobilization predominates. Thyroid hormones affect protein metabolism in much the same way as they affect lipid metabolism. Optimal synthesis and degradation of protein require a certain low level of hormone. At high levels, although both synthesis and degradation are increased, degradation predominates.

In general, thyroid hormone stimulates the metabolic activity of most cells in the body. Because overall metabolism is enhanced by thyroid hormone, cardiac output and respiration are positively correlated with hormone levels.

More specifically, thyroid hormones are required for normal brain development during the perinatal period. In adults, the effects of thyroid hormone on the central nervous system (CNS) are complex and are not completely understood. **Hypothyroidism** is accompanied by **slow thought processes and somnolence. Hyperthyroidism** is characterized by **nervousness, anxiety, paranoia, and difficulty sleeping.** Fine muscle **tremor** also is prominent in hyperthyroidism.

In many tissues innervated by the autonomic nervous system, especially the sympathetic branch, thyroid hormones increase the number of adrenergic receptors, particularly β-adrenergic receptors, and/or the concentration of intracellular signaling mediators coupled to the receptors. Thus, **heart rate and myocardial contractility** are **increased in hyperthyroidism. Gastrointestinal secretions and motility** also are **stimulated by thyroid hormone.** This may be due to an action on the enteric nervous system. T_3 and T_4 **play little role in fetal growth** but are essential for growth to adulthood. Thyroid hormones appear to have few direct actions on skeletal growth by themselves; however, they are essential for growth hormone and other growth factors to be effective.

COMPREHENSION QUESTIONS

[34.1] A 33-year-old woman is noted by her physician to have some fatigue and some coarse skin. Her only medication is an oral contraceptive agent. The following laboratories have been returned:

TSH	1.0 mU/L (0.35-6.0 mU/L)
Free thyroxine	1.0 ng/dL (0.8-2.7 ng/dL)
Total thyroxine	13.0 µg/dL (4.5-12.0 µg/dL)
Thyroid-binding globulin (TBG)	55 ng/mL (15-34 mg/L)

Which of the following is the most likely diagnosis?

A. Hyperthyroidism
B. Hypothyroidism
C. Normal thyroid status
D. Transient hyperthyroidism

[34.2] A 33-year-old chemist takes L-thyroxine (Synthroid) 1 µg orally each day. He asks how the thyroxine works on a cellular level. Which of the following is the best explanation?

A. It binds onto membrane surface receptor and activates protein synthesis.
B. It binds onto membrane surface receptor and activates a secondary messenger.
C. It binds onto a cytoplasmic receptor, and the hormone–receptor complex diffuses to the nucleus to affect transcription.
D. It has a direct effect on the hypothalamic nuclei affecting metabolism.

[34.3] A 15-year-old adolescent is suspected of having anorexia nervosa. Thyroid function tests are also drawn. Her TSH is in the normal range, but the rT_3 level is elevated. Which of the following is the most accurate statement regarding her status?

A. Reverse T_3 has little biological effect.
B. This patient probably has T_3 thyroiditis.
C. The free rT_3 would be the next step to assess possible hyperthyroidism.
D. This patient probably has hypothyroidism.

Answers

[34.1] **C.** This patient has an elevated total thyroxine level because of increased TBG. However, the free (active) thyroxine is normal, and the TSH is in the normal range, both of which indicate a normal euthyroid state. Women who are pregnant or on an oral contraceptive agent may develop an increased TBG; hence, free T_4 or TSH levels are better tests to assess thyroid status.

[34.2]   **C.** Thyroxine behaves similarly to steroid hormones in that it binds
          onto cytoplasmic receptors, and the hormone–receptor complex then
          diffuses to the nucleus to affect the transcription of DNA and ulti-
          mately protein synthesis. Most protein hormones bind to surface
          membrane receptors; thyroid hormone is an exception.

[34.3]   **A.** Reverse T_3 has no biological effect. Individuals with anorexia ner-
          vosa often have an increased rT_3 level and a lower T_3 level, reflecting
          a lower metabolism rate as compensation for the markedly decreased
          caloric intake. The fact that her TSH is in the normal range makes it
          difficult to make a diagnosis of hypothyroidism.

PHYSIOLOGY PEARLS

❖ Iodide necessary for the synthesis of thyroid hormone is taken up by
   thyroid follicular cells against an electrochemical gradient by
   sodium-coupled secondary active transport.

❖ The oxidative reaction steps linking iodide to tyrosine residues of
   thyroglobulin take place extracellularly in the colloid stored
   within thyroid follicles.

❖ Thyroid hormone secretion requires the pinocytotic uptake and
   breakdown of colloid by follicular cells.

❖ TSH, which is secreted by the pituitary in response to thyrotropin-
   releasing hormone from the hypothalamus, simultaneously stimulates thyroid hormone synthesis and thyroid hormone secretion.

❖ Thyroid hormone exists in two forms: triiodothyronine (T_3) and
   tetraiodothyronine (T_4). Both circulate in the blood bound to
   plasma proteins, but at the cellular level, T_4 is converted to T_3,
   which then binds to thyroid hormone receptors.

❖ Thyroid hormone is essential for normal brain development in the
   perinatal period.

❖ Thyroid hormone stimulates oxidative metabolism in all tissues
   except brain, spleen, and testis. ATP utilization and heat production are increased.

❖ Thyroid hormone binds to nuclear receptors to regulate the transcription of genes involved in metabolic events.

REFERENCES

Genuth SM. Thyroid gland. In: Levy MN, Koeppen BM, and Stanton BA, eds. *Berne
   & Levy, Principles of Physiology*. 4th ed. Philadelphia, PA: Mosby; 2006:663-675.
Goodman HM. Thyroid gland. In: Johnson LR, ed. *Essential Medical Physiology*.
   3rd ed. San Diego, CA: Elsevier Academic Press; 2003:587-605.

A 36-year-old woman presents to her gynecologist with complaints of amenorrhea and hirsutism. She has also noticed an increase in her weight (especially in the trunk region) and easy fatigability. She denies any medical problems. Her periods were always normal until 6 months ago, and her hirsutism has been gradual in onset. On examination, she has a very rounded hirsute face with centripetal obesity. Her blood pressure is elevated, as is her weight compared with previous visits. On abdominal examination, she is noted to have striae and a male-like distribution of hair on the lower abdomen. The patient then undergoes studies that demonstrate increased cortisol production and failure to suppress cortisol secretion normally when dexamethasone is administered. She is diagnosed with Cushing syndrome.

◆ **Where in the adrenal cortex is cortisol produced?**

◆ **How do glucocorticoids inhibit prostaglandin production?**

◆ **Why is hyperpigmentation not found in patients with secondary adrenocortical insufficiency?**

ANSWERS TO CASE 35: ADRENAL GLAND

Summary: A 36-year-old woman with amenorrhea, hirsutism, elevated blood pressure, weight gain, insuppressible cortisol, and abdominal striae is diagnosed with Cushing syndrome.

◆ **Cortisol production:** Zona fasciculata.

◆ **Glucocorticoids and prostaglandins:** Inhibit cyclooxygenase and phospholipase A_2, which are needed for prostaglandin formation.

◆ **Secondary adrenocortical insufficiency and hyperpigmentation:** There is a low level of adrenocorticotropic hormone (ACTH) with secondary adrenocortical insufficiency. ACTH contains the MSH fragment, and when it is elevated (primary adrenocortical insufficiency), hyperpigmentation may occur.

CLINICAL CORRELATION

Cushing syndrome is a condition caused by increased cortisol production. This increase may be the result of overproduction of ACTH (Cushing disease) or excess production of cortisol by the adrenal gland (adrenal hyperplasia). A patient's symptoms may include truncal obesity, a round "moon" face, a "buffalo hump," hypertension, fatigability and weakness, amenorrhea, hirsutism, abdominal striae, osteoporosis, and hyperglycemia. The diagnosis is presumed when there is increased cortisol production and failure to suppress cortisol secretion with dexamethasone. The level of ACTH will help differentiate whether the problem is from overproduction of ACTH or from increased adrenal cortisol production. Treatment depends on the etiology. Overproduction from an ACTH-secreting tumor usually requires surgical intervention. Medical management of adrenal hyperplasia may include the use of ketoconazole or other medications that inhibit steroidogenesis.

APPROACH TO ADRENAL PHYSIOLOGY

Objectives

1. Understand the structure of the adrenal cortex and medulla.
2. Know about regulation of adrenocortical hormones.
3. Understand the actions of adrenocortical hormones.

Definitions

1. **Glucocorticoids:** Steroid hormones, primarily cortisol, secreted by the adrenal cortex that promote the synthesis of enzymes involved in energy balance and fuel utilization. They have potent immunosuppressant and

anti-inflammatory activities and their secretion is increased in response to stress.

2. **Mineralocorticoids:** Steroid hormones, primarily aldosterone, that are secreted by the adrenal cortex and are essential for the maintenance of salt and water balance by the kidney.

3. **ACTH:** Adrenocorticotrophic hormone is secreted by the anterior pituitary gland and directly controls the rate of production of the glucocorticoids and androgens by the adrenal cortex.

DISCUSSION

The **suprarenal,** or **adrenal, glands** are a **pair of structures just above the kidneys.** The adrenals form a complex structure consisting of functionally and morphologically distinct regions: an outer region, the adrenal cortex, and the inner medulla. The **adrenal cortex** is the site of **synthesis and secretion of steroid hormones** known as the **mineralocorticoids,** the **glucocorticoids,** and the **androgens.** The bulk of the adrenal gland is the cortex, which is composed of morphologically and functionally distinct segments. Descending into the gland just below the capsule is the **zona glomerulosa,** clusters of cells that secrete the **mineralocorticoid** aldosterone. The **zona fasciculata** penetrates deeply into the cortex and overlays the **zona reticularis.** These two regions produce the glucocorticoids and the **adrenal androgens.** The innermost region is the medulla. The adrenal **medulla** is heavily innervated and is a source of the circulating sympathetic hormones **epinephrine and norepinephrine.**

Regulation of Adrenal Cortical Hormone Secretion

The rate of secretion of the adrenal cortical hormones is dependent on their rate of production. Unlike the peptide hormones, for example, the steroid hormones are permeable to the plasma membranes of cells, and their concentration in the cell is the determinant of the rate at which they leave the cell and enter the plasma. In the plasma, they bind to and are transported by globular proteins such as corticosteroid-binding protein and albumin. The adrenal cortical hormones act on target tissues by diffusing into the cell and forming a complex with a specific intracellular receptor. Complex formation exposes a DNA-binding site and is translocated into the nucleus. In the nucleus, the hormone–receptor complex binds to a specific site on the DNA target molecule, the hormone responsive element, and enhances or inhibits gene transcription.

The production of **glucocorticoids** and **androgens** is directly controlled by **ACTH.** ACTH binds to a receptor on the cell surface which mediates the activation of the enzymes involved in the synthesis of pregnenolone, the precursor molecule of adrenocortical hormones produced in the zona fasciculata and the zona reticularis. ACTH actions result in the direct activation of enzymatic activities and a slower increase in the synthesis of these enzymes. Cortisol secretion normally follows that of ACTH, with a diurnal pattern of secretion peaking in the early morning hours. **ACTH** is produced in the **anterior lobe of the pituitary gland** in response to hypothalamic release of **corticotropin-releasing hormone (CRH)** from the paraventricular nuclei. The circulating level of cortisol is regulated by a negative feedback control of ACTH secretion. Cortisol inhibits ACTH secretion by acting directly on the ACTH-producing cells and indirectly by inhibition of the hypothalamic neuronal release of CRH. The mechanism of cortisol inhibition involves cortisol binding to corticosteroid receptors in these tissues and inhibition of specific gene transcription.

Cushing syndrome is often the result of increased pituitary secretion of ACTH because of a pituitary adenoma. There are however other types of tumors (outside the pituitary) that secrete ACTH and stimulate cortisol production. To help identify the cause of the elevated cortisol a test is conducted with the administration of dexamethasone, a synthetic analog of cortisol, to inhibit ACTH release and thus cortisol production. The failure to lower cortisol production indicates a nonpituitary source of the problem.

Physiology of Glucocorticoids

Cortisol has a permissive effect on a number of enzymes that mediate the breakdown of fats and protein and hepatic glucose production and is essential for the maintenance of energy balance and fuel utilization in the body. **Cortisol** also has potent **anti-inflammatory** and **immunosuppressant** activities that make it an extremely important therapeutic agent. The glucocorticoids, primarily cortisol and to a lesser extent corticosterone, play a central role in the physiologic response to stress, and their secretion is increased during **stress.** Factors such as **surgery, hypoglycemia, and pain** stimulate ACTH secretion and consequently stimulate cortisol production and secretion. Severely stressful conditions will override both diurnal ACTH production and the feedback inhibition of cortisol on ACTH secretion, resulting in a sustained ACTH level and maximal levels of cortisol production.

The **physiology of the glucocorticoids** is complex and can influence and alter the function of every system in the body. The dominant and most crucial functions involve energy metabolism through the control of the expression of proteins that are essential for the maintenance of energy balance during periods of food deprivation. During periods of fasting, the body rapidly exhausts its carbohydrate supplies and depends on other sources of fuel for metabolic energy. In the liver, cortisol increases the synthesis of enzymes in the gluconeogenic pathway, as well as enzymes in muscle tissue for the breakdown of proteins to provide glucogenic precursors for glucose synthesis. **Glucocorticoid-dependent enzymes** catalyze the breakdown of fats through **lipolysis** to **generate free fatty acids and keto acids** for energy production. The combined effect of these actions is to decrease glucose utilization by providing alternate fuels and to maintain plasma glucose levels for tissues that have an absolute requirement for glucose as oxidizable substrate.

Corticosteroids have potent anti-inflammatory activity. Tissue injury or other stimuli lead to an increased production of the arachidonic acid derivatives, prostaglandins and leukotrienes. The injury activates a phospholipase (PLA_2) that releases arachidonic acid from phospholipids. The newly formed arachidonic acid then is converted to the prostaglandin structure by a cyclooxygenase. Physiologically, prostaglandins have localized effects of dilating the vessels in the area of the injury and sensitizing the nerve endings and increasing the sensation of pain.

Glucocorticoids are also negative regulators of cytokine production, particularly interleukin-1 (IL-1) and tumor necrosis factor-α (TNF-α) and numerous other mediators. These cytokines are produced primarily in macrophages after stimulation by immune complexes and arachidonic acid metabolites and after injury. In addition to inhibiting their production, the steps outlined above identify loci where glucocorticoids interfere with the signaling pathways and the actions of their products. IL-1 production by macrophages plays a central role in the immune response; thus, glucocorticoids are immunosuppressive. The glucocorticoids are effective immunosuppressive agents and are an important therapeutic tool. Proliferation of β-lymphocytes requires cytokines released from helper T cells. Glucocorticoids inhibit macrophage and T-cell cytokine production, which reduces B-cell proliferation. T-cell proliferation is induced by IL-2 after exposure to an antigen. Glucocorticoids inhibit IL-2 production, thereby reducing T-cell proliferation. By these mechanisms, glucocorticoids are able to suppress both humoral and cellular immune responses.

The Physiology of Mineralocorticoids

The mineralocorticoids, primarily aldosterone, are essential for the maintenance of salt and water balance by the kidney by regulating sodium reabsorption and potassium secretion. Aldosterone is produced in the zona glomerulosa from the common pregnenolone precursor. Regulation of aldosterone secretion is dependent on several factors. ACTH-dependent pregnenolone synthesis is required for maximal aldosterone production, but secretion is controlled directly by angiotensin II and the extracellular ($[K^+]$) potassium concentration. Increasing plasma $[K^+]$ stimulates aldosterone secretion. Atrial natriuretic factor has a negative modulatory effect on aldosterone secretion. As with the other adrenal cortical hormones, aldosterone binds to and is carried in the blood by corticosteroid-binding globulin (CBG).

The physiologic role of aldosterone is the maintenance of fluid and electrolyte balance, and its secretion is tightly coupled to the vascular volume. A decrease in vascular volume initiates a cascade response with an increase in renal renin secretion from smooth muscle cells of the afferent glomerular arteriole. Renin catalyzes the conversion of angiotensinogen to angiotensin I. Angiotensin-converting enzyme (ACE) converts angiotensin I to angiotensin II. The target of angiotensin II is the zona glomerulosa, which responds by increasing the production and secretion of aldosterone.

COMPREHENSION QUESTIONS

[35.1] Dexamethasone is a synthetic analogue of cortisol. Therapeutically, it can be used to block the effects of conditions with excessive cortisol secretion. Which of the following is the best description of the mechanism of action of dexamethasone?

A. Binds to cortisol
B. Binds to the adrenal gland
C. Competes for cortisol-binding sites
D. Inhibits ACTH secretion

[35.2] Mineralocorticoids play a critical role in fluid and electrolyte balance in the body. A normal response to aldosterone is to increase acid secretion in the kidney. The hyperaldosteronism that occurs with some adrenal tumors has interesting and profound effects on acid–base balance as a result of increased renal H^+ secretion. Which of the following would be the most likely result of hyperaldosteronism?

A. Excretion of excess bicarbonate
B. Generation of metabolic alkalosis
C. Hyperkalemia caused by renal K^+ resorption
D. Increased H^+ resorption by renal tubular cells
E. Movement of K^+ out of cells in exchange for H^+

[35.3] Adrenalectomized animals are unable to survive even brief periods of food deprivation. Cortisol replacement restores the ability to survive a fast. Which of the following is the best explanation for this observation?

A. Cortisol can act synergistically with insulin.
B. Cortisol can act antagonistically to the action of growth hormone.
C. Cortisol has a permissive effect on enzymes involved in the mobilization of various fuels.
D. Cortisol increases glucose utilization and decreases glycogen storage.

Answers

[35.1] **D.** Cortisol production and secretion are controlled by ACTH, which is secreted from the anterior lobe of the pituitary gland. A feedback inhibition loop allows cortisol to inhibit ACTH secretion. The synthetic glucocorticoid dexamethasone effectively and abruptly blocks ACTH secretion, thereby suppressing cortisol secretion.

[35.2] **B.** Hyperaldosteronism leads to a loss of potassium and hypokalemia. The hypokalemia leads to a loss of potassium from cells largely in exchange for H^+. This causes a metabolic alkalosis and an intracellular acidosis. Renal tubular cells respond with an increase in the rate of H^+ secretion. Paradoxically, despite the metabolic alkalosis, there is an increased rate of H⁺ secretion and bicarbonate reabsorption with the addition of bicarbonate to the blood. There are increased reabsorption of bicarbonate and maintenance of the metabolic alkalosis.

[35.3]   **C.** Cortisol is essential for the expression of numerous enzymes involved in the maintenance of fuel supplies in preparation for and during a fast. At each stage of metabolism, enzymes have been identified as cortisol-dependent, beginning with the generation of glucogenic precursors. Muscle protein catabolism is an essential source of carbohydrate precursors. Cortisol increases proteolysis and induces the transaminases necessary to convert pyruvate into alanine for transport to the liver for gluconeogenesis. Key enzymes in the gluconeogenic pathway ranging from pyruvate to glycogen, and those involved in the release of glucose from the liver are all known to be inducible by cortisol. Thus, one of its main functions is the continued production of glucose for metabolism by glucose-dependent tissues during a fast. Glucose utilization by tissues that can utilize alternative fuels is reduced by cortisol, which antagonizes insulin-dependent processes. To provide the energy necessary for gluconeogenesis, cortisol enhances triglyceride breakdown and free fatty acid mobilization from fat stores. In addition, cortisol acts synergistically with glucagon to enhance hepatic gluconeogenesis.

PHYSIOLOGY PEARLS

❖ Adrenal glands have an outer cortical region that produces the mineralocorticoids (aldosterone), glucocorticoids (cortisol), and androgenic hormones.

❖ The inner, medullary region of the adrenal gland is highly innervated and produces the circulating sympathetic hormones epinephrine and norepinephrine.

❖ The adrenocortical hormones are steroid hormones. The steroid hormones are permeable to the cell membrane; thus, their rate of secretion is dependent on their rate of production.

❖ Cortisol production is dependent on ACTH and in part is controlled by a negative feedback loop with cortisol-inhibiting ACTH production. In the present case, there is an increase in ACTH secretion that causes an overproduction of cortisol (Cushing syndrome). Adrenal hyperplasia also can cause overproduction of cortisol.

❖ Understanding the mechanisms of action of the adrenocortical hormones has produced a number of novel therapies for the control of hypertension (ACE inhibitors), anti-inflammatories (COX 2 inhibitors), and immunosuppression (cortisol).

REFERENCES

Genuth SM. The adrenal glands. In: Berne RM, Levy MN, eds. *Physiology*. 4th ed. St. Louis, MO: Mosby; 1998:930-964.

Goodman HM. Adrenal glands. In: Johnson LR, ed. *Essential Medical Physiology*. 3rd ed. San Diego, CA: Elsevier Academic Press; 2004:607-635.

❖ CASE 36

A 12-year-old boy presents to the emergency department with complaints of weight loss, fatigue, polydipsia (excess thirst), polyphagia (excess hunger), and polyuria (excess urination). The patient has no medical problems but there are many family members with diabetes and hypertension. On examination, the patient is a thin ill-appearing male in no acute distress with normal vital signs. His examination is unremarkable. A urinalysis reveals glucosuria and a markedly elevated serum fasting blood sugar. The patient is diagnosed with type I diabetes mellitus (insulin-dependent), and is advised by the physician to start insulin therapy. The patient's parents ask whether oral agents such as sulfonylurea tablets can be used instead of insulin.

 What is the major factor that regulates insulin secretion?

 What hormones do the delta cells of the pancreas produce?

 How do sulfonylurea drugs increase insulin secretion?

ANSWERS TO CASE 36: PANCREATIC ISLET CELLS

Summary: A 12-year-old boy with weight loss, fatigue, polydipsia, polyphagia, polyuria, and elevated fasting blood sugar is diagnosed with type I diabetes mellitus.

◆   **Major regulating factor:** Serum sugar levels.

◆   **Delta cells produce:** Somatostatin and gastrin.

◆   **Sulfonylurea medications:** Close the K_{ATP} potassium channels in the beta cells allowing activation of voltage dependent Ca^{2+} channels resulting in insulin secretion.

CLINICAL CORRELATION

Type I diabetes (juvenile) is caused by destruction of pancreatic islet cells, leading to insulin deficiency. The destruction of the pancreatic islet cells may have multifactorial causes, such as genetic predisposition, viral, or autoimmune. Patients usually present in childhood or early adulthood and account for about 10% of all cases of diabetes. These patients' symptoms include polydipsia, polyphagia, weight loss, and recurrent infections. Severe derangements may induce diabetic ketoacidosis, characterized by markedly elevated blood sugar levels, elevated serum ketone levels, metabolic anion gap acidosis, and a variety of metabolic derangements such as hypokalemia. A fasting blood sugar will help make the diagnosis of diabetes. Because the primary deficit is lack of insulin, patients will need insulin replacement to improve their symptoms. Oral agents usually cannot be used as primary therapy in type I diabetes because of the basic defect caused by insulin deficiency. Type II diabetes occurs because of peripheral tissue resistance to insulin.

APPROACH TO PANCREATIC PHYSIOLOGY

Objectives

1. Understand glucagon secretion, action, and regulation.
2. Understand insulin secretion, action, and regulation.
3. Understand somatostatin secretion, action, and regulation.

Definitions

Islets of Langerhans: Highly vascularized and innervated structures in the pancreas containing three major cell types that secrete insulin (beta cells), glucagon (alpha cells) and somatostatin (delta cells).

Insulin: A small polypeptide anabolic hormone that promotes the sequestration of carbohydrate, fat and protein mainly in liver, adipose tissue and skeletal muscle. In the absence of insulin these substances are mobilized from tissues to meet the fuel demands of the body.

Glucagon: A small polypeptide hormone that targets mainly the liver to promote glucose production through gluconeogenesis and glycogenolysis, and fatty acid oxidation with the production and release of keto acids to meet the energy demands of the body during periods of fasting.

Sulfonyl ureas: A class of small therapeutic molecules that are potent stimulants of insulin secretion by pancreatic beta cells.

DISCUSSION

The **cells of the islets of Langerhans** in the **endocrine pancreas** are the site of **synthesis and secretion** of the **peptide hormones glucagon, insulin, and somatostatin.** The **islets are highly vascularized,** with a blood flow pattern that **drains directly into the portal vein,** delivering the hormones directly to the liver. The islets are innervated in the areas of the secretory cells with both **sympathetic** (middle splanchnic nerve) and **parasympathetic** (vagus nerve) input.

Mechanism of Secretion

A general model applies to the mechanism of secretion for each of the three hormones, but the specific stimuli vary. The **hormones are synthesized on the rough endoplasmic reticulum (ER) as propeptide hormones.** They are processed in the ER and transported to the Golgi apparatus for sorting and packaging into secretory vesicles. **Secretory vesicles bud off of the trans-Golgi network** and are directed toward the plasma membrane. The vesicles containing the prohormone and the hormone-converting enzyme accumulate in proximity to and just below the plasma membrane. After the appropriate stimulus, the vesicles are recruited to the cell surface, where they fuse with the plasma membrane, and their contents are ejected from the cell. During this process of degranulation, there is a conversion to the hormone by specific enzymatic cleavage of the prohormone.

The specifics of the activation of the secretory process are more fully characterized for insulin than for the other hormones. The mechanism is clinically relevant because it is the site of therapeutic intervention to increase insulin secretion from the beta cells. **Insulin secretion is dependent on a rise in the intracellular calcium concentration** according to the following sequence of events:

1. The main stimulus is an **increase in the plasma glucose** concentration that causes an **increase in intracellular glucose.**
2. Increased glucose in the cell promotes an **increase in adenosine triphosphate (ATP) levels.**
3. **ATP inhibits a potassium channel** in the plasma membrane, with a resultant **depolarization of the membrane potential.**
4. Depolarization of the membrane activates a **voltage-dependent calcium channel, permitting calcium influx** and **the initiation of secretory vesicle fusion.**

The importance of this sequence of events is underscored by the finding that the **potassium channel is blocked by sulfonylureas.** Thus, therapeutic use of these agents can enhance insulin secretion in patients with an insulin-deficient or resistant disease.

Regulation of Secretion

There is a **complex physiologic interaction between insulin and glucagon** that is reflected in their regulation and mechanism of action. Generally, factors that result from stresses to the individual, such as **starvation and low plasma glucose** and **elevated** levels of **epinephrine, norepinephrine, cortisol, or growth hormone** all stimulate **glucagon** secretion and **suppress insulin** secretion. During unstressful periods with adequate food, metabolic factors such as carbohydrates, fatty acids, and amino acids stimulate insulin secretion.

Insulin

Insulin is an anabolic hormone that **promotes the utilization and storage of glucose, fatty acids, and amino acids.** Insulin is **secreted by the beta cells of the islet** in response to numerous stimuli, including metabolites, hormones, and neural mediators. The most important regulator of insulin secretion is the **plasma glucose concentration.** Increasing plasma glucose causes a stimulation of insulin secretion, whereas a fall in glucose is accompanied by a decline in insulin secretion. Regulation of insulin secretion by other factors such as amino acids, fatty acids, and ketone bodies for the most part is a complex interaction and is dependent on the circulating level of glucose and not relevant to the present case.

Insulin secretion is stimulated by several hormones. There is a class of hormones called **incretins** that are **mainly enteric hormones** that **stimulate insulin secretion.** Interestingly, these hormones are secreted in response to the ingestion and absorption of carbohydrate, protein, or lipid and are secreted in advance of an increase in the circulating levels of the metabolites. The insulin response is thus anticipatory of the increase. The ultimate effect is to enhance insulin secretion by the beta cells. In the experimental setting, there are several hormones that exhibit this response; however, the physiologically relevant agents are **glucose-dependent insulinotropic peptide (GIP) and glucagon-like peptide-1 (GLP-1).** A paracrine effect of **glucagon** is to **stimulate insulin secretion,** presumably to potentiate the effect of glucagon on the elevation of plasma glucose levels. **Secretion of insulin** also is **enhanced by cortisol and growth hormone. Somatostatin inhibits insulin secretion** through a paracrine effect.

The **islets** are **innervated with both sympathetic and parasympathetic** neurons. **The beta cells** are stimulated by the **parasympathetic release of acetylcholine or vasoactive intestinal peptide (VIP).** The **sympathetic hormones, epinephrine and norepinephrine,** are **potent inhibitors** of **insulin secretion.** A strong sympathetic response can shut down insulin secretion completely, thereby minimizing glucose utilization as part of the flight or fight response.

The role of **insulin** is to **promote the storage of metabolic fuels** in the form of **glycogen, triglyceride, and protein.** The main targets of insulin action are the **liver, muscle, and adipose tissue.** The mechanism of action of insulin is complex, eliciting both rapid responses and longer term effects on cell metabolism. Insulin action is mediated by a **plasma membrane insulin receptor** that is one of the **tyrosine kinase receptors** that can activate multiple intracellular signaling pathways (see Case 2). In the short term, the **effects of insulin on the cell are increased glucose transport (adipose and muscle), glycogen synthesis, and fatty acid synthesis.** In the long term, a parallel pathway involving MAP kinase activation leads to the activation of transcription factors that regulate specific protein synthesis.

Glucagon

Glucagon is produced and secreted by the alpha **cells of the islets,** although the regulation and mechanism of secretion are not clearly understood (see above). As is the case with insulin secretion, the **most important determinant** in the **secretion of glucagon** is the **blood glucose concentration.** However, the **rate of glucagon secretion decreases with increasing blood glucose. Glucagon secretion is maximal** at plasma glucose concentrations **less than 50 mg/dL** and completely blocked at concentrations above 200 mg/dL. A comparison of several effectors on glucagon secretion by the alpha cell shows that the response is the opposite of the effect on beta-cell secretion of insulin. In addition to glucose, ketone bodies and free fatty acids inhibit glucagon secretion. The enteric hormones GIP and GLP-1 that stimulate insulin secretion inhibit glucagon secretion. Finally, insulin itself and somatostatin inhibit glucagon secretion.

Alpha cells also **secrete glucagon** in response to **neural stimulation** from both **sympathetic and parasympathetic** neurons. In contrast to the beta cell, epinephrine and norepinephrine are potent stimuli for glucagon secretion, as are acetylcholine and VIP from parasympathetic neurons.

The **major target tissue for glucagon** is the **liver,** and in most regards glucagon is counterregulatory to insulin action. The mechanism of glucagon action is very well defined and well described. Although glucagon receptors are found on other tissues, the concentration of the hormone necessary to elicit a response is well above the physiologic range. The **hepatic glucagon receptor** is a **G protein–coupled receptor.** Binding of glucagon leads to **activation of adenyl cyclase** and **synthesis of cyclic adenosine monophosphate (cAMP).** Elevated cAMP activates **protein kinase A,** resulting in the **phosphorylation** of a number of key **regulatory enzymes.** The result is a stimulation of glycogen breakdown and gluconeogenesis with a net production and release of glucose into the blood. During periods of fasting (low circulating levels of insulin) glucagon will also limit fatty acid synthesis and promote its breakdown and production of ketone bodies.

Control of the Plasma Glucose Concentration

The opposing actions of insulin and glucagon on hepatic function are the basis of a simple but elegant feedback mechanism to control net glucose production. The key regulator of pancreatic secretion of insulin and glucagon is the plasma glucose concentration, which is controlled by the action of these two hormones on the liver. As plasma glucose concentrations approach fasting levels below 90 mg/dL, glucagon secretion increases and insulin secretion decreases. These changes promote the production of glucose in the liver and its release into the blood.

Somatostatin

Pancreatic somatostatin is secreted by the **delta cells of the islets.** The role of pancreatic somatostatin is poorly understood. From a number of experimental studies, somatostatin has been shown to **inhibit both alpha-cell and beta-cell secretion of glucagon and insulin,** respectively, suggesting a possible paracrine role for the hormone.

COMPREHENSION QUESTIONS

[36.1] Insulin secretion is inhibited by which of the following?

  A. Glucagon
  B. Epinephrine
  C. Amino acids
  D. Glucose

[36.2] An experimental animal is instrumented to monitor plasma glucose and insulin levels. After a control fasting period to establish a steady state, a test substance is administered to the animal. Shortly after the administration of the substance, there is an increase in the plasma insulin concentration and a fall in the plasma glucose concentration. The substance is most likely which of the following?

  A. Glucagon
  B. Epinephrine
  C. A sulfonylurea compound
  D. Somatostatin
  E. Glucose

[36.3] In a normal individual, the liver is the main regulator of the plasma glucose concentration. When there is an increase in the plasma glucose concentration, the liver extracts glucose from the blood and converts it into glycogen and, to a lesser extent, triglycerides. When the plasma glucose concentration falls, the liver will begin to produce glucose and release it into the blood to maintain its concentration. In an untreated type I diabetic patient, the liver fails to extract glucose and continues to produce glucose regardless of its plasma concentration. Which of the following most likely contributes to this failure?

A. Increased glucokinase activity
B. Decreased phosphorylase activity
C. Increased gluconeogenesis
D. Diminished muscle protein catabolism
E. Insulin-dependent glucose transport in the liver

Answers

[36.1]   **B.** Insulin secretion is stimulated by amino acids and glucose and inhibited by somatostatin and epinephrine and sympathetic stimulation. Epinephrine is a potent blocker of insulin secretion and stimulates glucagon secretion. This is the so-called flight or fight response to provide a burst of glucose for rapid and immediate utilization.

[36.2]   **C.** The correct answer is a sulfonylurea compound. These compounds block the ATP-inhabitable K^+ channel in the beta cells, which causes a depolarization and activation of a Ca^{2+} channel. The influx of Ca^{2+} stimulates insulin secretion. As insulin levels rise, there is increased glucose utilization by liver, muscle, and adipose tissues, causing a fall in the plasma glucose concentration. Glucagon or glucose would stimulate insulin secretion; however, there would be a transient increase in the plasma glucose concentration. Epinephrine and somatostatin would inhibit insulin secretion.

[36.3]   **C.** The liver has no insulin-dependent glucose transport system. Glucose transport is insulin-independent, and glucose rapidly equilibrates across the hepatocyte membrane. One of the most important factors in the failure of the liver to extract glucose in a chronically insulin-deficient state is reduced glucokinase activity. Glucokinase is liver-specific and has several important features that distinguish it from the analogous hexokinase in other cell types. It also has a higher Km and is not feedback-inhibited by its product glucose-6-phosphate. Therefore, even at high glucose concentrations, glucokinase does not saturate and continues to produce glucose-6-phosphate, which can accumulate in the cell. Insulin has a permissive effect on glucokinase, and in its absence, glucokinase levels can fall to very low levels. As a consequence, glucose entry into the glycolytic or glycogen synthetic pathway is limited. The lack of insulin also reduces the activities of key regulatory enzymes (eg, glycogen synthase, phosphofructokinase, and pyruvate kinase) involved in directing glucose toward glycogen synthesis or glycolysis, further limiting glucose utilization. Insulin also promotes protein synthesis in muscle tissue, and in its absence, there is an increased protein catabolism with a release of glucogenic precursors into the blood. These precursors are taken up by the liver and used to produce glucose through the gluconeogenic pathway.

PHYSIOLOGY PEARLS

❖ The major hormones regulating energy metabolism are glucagon and insulin. They are produced and secreted by the alpha and beta cells of the pancreatic islets of Langerhans.

❖ Insulin is an anabolic hormone that targets the liver, adipose tissue, and muscle tissue and promotes glycogen synthesis, fatty acid synthesis and triglyceride formation, and protein synthesis.

❖ Glucagon targets the liver and is counterregulatory to insulin, promoting glycogenolysis, fatty acid oxidation, and gluconeogenesis.

❖ Glucagon action is mediated by G protein–coupled plasma membrane receptor activation of adenyl cyclase and protein kinase A activation.

❖ Insulin targets mainly the liver, muscle, and adipose tissues, and its action is mediated by a plasma membrane tyrosine kinase receptor and has short-term and long-term effects on the target cell. The immediate effects are the activation of protein kinase B and phosphoprotein phosphatase-1, which antagonize cAMP-dependent reactions and promote glycogen synthesis, fatty acid synthesis, and triglyceride formation.

❖ Longer term insulin effects are mediated by the MAP kinase signaling pathway, with activation of specific transcription factors that leads to increased protein synthesis.

❖ During starvation, there is a dramatic fall in insulin levels, leading to a decrease in insulin-dependent processes and allowing glucagon-dependent processes to prevail. The fall in plasma glucose stimulates glucagon secretion, which promotes hepatic fatty acid oxidation, glycogen breakdown, and gluconeogenesis. The lack of insulin allows protein breakdown to occur, with a release of glucogenic precursors from muscle into the circulation. Glucagon-dependent gluconeogenesis from these precursors in the liver is driven by energy derived from fatty acid oxidation.

REFERENCE

Goodman HM. The pancreatic islets. In: Johnson LR, ed. *Essential Medical Physiology*. 3rd ed. San Diego, CA: Elsevier Academic Press; 2003:259-276.

A 46-year-old man presents to his primary care physician with complaints of confusion, headache, disorientation, and visual difficulties in the morning upon awakening. He also has episodes of heart palpitations, sweating, and tremor in the morning. All the symptoms usually resolve after he eats break-fast and do not recur unless he skips a meal. His physical examination is completely normal. A complete blood count is normal, and a basic metabolic panel reveals a fasting blood sugar < 50 mg/dL. The patient denies any alcohol or drug use. The patient subsequently is diagnosed with an insulinoma that is causing hypoglycemia. The physician explains to the patient that the insulin secreting tumor causes a low blood sugar, and the body increases the hormones epinephrine and cortisol to try to elevate the blood sugar.

◆ **What effect does epinephrine have on pancreatic islet cells?**

◆ **What effect does prolonged fasting have on cortisol secretion?**

◆ **How many calories per gram does glucose provide?**

ANSWERS TO CASE 37: HORMONAL REGULATION OF FUEL METABOLISM

Summary: A 46-year-old man has symptoms of hypoglycemia in the morning and when meals are skipped secondary to an insulin-secreting insulinoma.

 Effect of epinephrine on pancreatic islet cells: Stimulate glucagon secretion and inhibit insulin secretion.

 Cortisol and prolonged fasting: Follow the normal basal diurnal rhythmic pattern.

◆ **Calories provided in glucose:** About 4 calories per gram.

CLINICAL CORRELATION

The etiology of hypoglycemia can be broken down into two categories. The first category is postprandial hypoglycemia, in which symptoms occur 2 to 4 hours after eating, resulting in diaphoresis, anxiety, irritability, palpitations, and tremor. Epinephrine release is thought to be the cause of these symptoms. The second category is fasting hypoglycemia. These patients generally have symptoms of headache, confusion, mental dullness, fatigue, visual changes, seizures, and, rarely, loss of consciousness. Etiologies for this type of hypoglycemia include excess insulin (self-administered medications, insulinoma), alcohol abuse and liver disease (decreased gluconeogenesis), and pituitary or adrenal insufficiency. Insulinomas are endocrine tumors of the pancreas derived from beta cells that autonomously secrete insulin without normal regulatory control. The diagnosis can be confirmed by finding elevating serum insulin levels at the time of hypoglycemia. The levels of insulin and glucose also should be checked during a period of prolonged fasting.

APPROACH TO HORMONAL REGULATION OF FUEL METABOLISM

Objectives

1. Know the basic body fuels: glucose, glycogen, fat, protein.
2. Understand the regulation of blood glucose.
3. Describe the regulation of metabolism during fasting and after eating.
4. Know the effects of exercise on glucose metabolism.

Definitions

Body fuel reserves: The body stores metabolic fuels in the form of carbohydrates, fat and protein mainly in the liver, skeletal muscle, and adipose tissue.

Plasma glucose balance: The primary regulator of insulin and glucagon secretion is glucose. Elevation of circulating glucose levels stimulates insulin secretion and inhibits glucagon secretion, in turn stimulating hepatic glucose uptake and inhibiting glucose production. A fall in circulating glucose has the opposite effect resulting in hepatic glucose production and release into the blood. Thus the circulating levels of glucose provide a feedback mechanism to control the relative rate of glucose uptake and glucose production by the liver.

DISCUSSION

The **body has three fuel reserves** that may be drawn on during a fasting state: **carbohydrate, fat, and protein.** In terms of pure energy yield, **fat is the most economical,** yielding about **9.4 kcal/g** compared with about **4.2 kcal/g for protein and carbohydrate.** An examination of the distribution of fuel reserves reveals that about 76% of the caloric content is fat, 23% is protein, and 1% is carbohydrate, principally as glycogen. The **glycogen reserves are stored in liver and muscle. Fats** are stored in **adipose tissue and the liver.** The protein reserves are distributed throughout the body, but are drawn mainly from the muscle mass of the body. An **average adult ingests and expends about 2500 kcal/day.** Excess caloric intake provides nutrients for storage in the fuel reserves of the body. During periods of fasting the body draws on those reserves. The **glycogen stores** are the smallest and most rapidly depleted, **lasting about a day or two,** depending on the level of activity. Despite this rapid depletion, the plasma glucose concentration remains at a constant level of 80 to 90 mg/dL for the duration of the fast. The body must maintain this fasting level of glucose to provide a fuel source for tissues that have an **absolute requirement for glucose as an oxidative substrate.**

Shortly after the **initiation of the fast,** there is an **increase in lipolysis** in adipose tissue with **a release of free fatty acids (FFA) into the circulation.** The liver oxidizes FFA through β-oxidation, resulting in the production of ketoacids. The ketoacids are transported into the blood and used as an oxidizable substrate to minimize the demand for glucose. Because the main carbohydrate stores are depleted rapidly, the body draws on the protein mass to provide glucogenic precursors. The problem that the body faces is that **fat can be used only to provide oxidative energy** and **cannot serve as a glucogenic precursor.** Protein catabolism releases **amino acids** that can serve as **glucogenic precursors.** Drawing on the protein reserves is problematic in that it necessitates a loss of muscle mass and connective tissue. Return to a normal feeding cycle permits restoration of the fuel reserves.

Control of Plasma Glucose Concentration

Maintaining the plasma glucose concentration and managing the fuel reserves include a highly choreographed series of events that are directed mainly by **two hormones: insulin and glucagon.** In a general sense, insulin may be viewed as an anabolic hormone and glucagon as a catabolic hormone.

The Role of the Liver in Fuel Metabolism

The major site of action is the liver, which is a target tissue for both hormones; depending on their relative concentrations, the liver either extracts glucose from the blood (high insulin/glucagon ratio) or produces and adds glucose to the blood (low insulin/glucagon ratio). The responses can be divided into short-term ones such as the changes occurring during a normal daily cycle of feeding and long-term adaptive responses to prolonged fasting.

In the **short term,** the effects of **insulin and glucagon** on several key regulatory reactions in intermediary metabolism are **directly opposed to each other.** These key points of regulation have been described as **futile cycles** because there is always some basal activity. For example, **glycogen synthesis and glycogenolysis occur simultaneously** at a very low rate, with a **continuing cycling of glucose between glucose-1-phosphate and glycogen.** Net production or breakdown of glycogen is dependent on the relative rates of the two reactions. Regulation of the process is exerted by activating one reaction and inhibiting the counterreaction. Often these reactions are controlled by phosphorylation-dephosphorylation cycles, and in large part these effects can be attributed to **one common factor: cyclic adenosine monophosphate (cAMP). Glucagon activates adenyl cyclase, causing an increase in cellular cAMP levels** and **protein kinase A (PKA)** activity. This stimulates glycogenolysis and glucose production. In contrast, insulin binding to its receptor, a **tyrosine kinase,** activates a signaling pathway that activates **protein kinase B (PKB) and protein phosphatase-**1 which inhibits glycogenolysis and activates glycogen synthesis.

Thus, after the ingestion of a carbohydrate-containing meal, the rise in plasma insulin levels will cause an activation of glycogen synthase and an inhibition of phosphorylase. A fall in the plasma glucose concentration reduces pancreatic insulin secretion and stimulates glucagon secretion. The hepatocyte responds to these changes by initiating a decrease in protein phosphatase activity (as a result of decreased insulin levels) and an increase in PKA activity (as a result of elevated glucagon levels). The overall effect is an increase in glycogenolysis with the production of glucose. Similar mechanisms in the glycolytic pathway control the relative rates of glycolysis and gluconeogenesis. With elevated plasma insulin, there is an activation of glycolysis. Glucagon inhibits the glycolytic pathway and activates gluconeogenesis.

Insulin also **promotes hepatic glucose uptake and utilization** through activation of **lipogenesis.** Insulin activates pyruvate oxidation by the mitochondria, increasing production of acetyl-CoA. The acetyl-CoA is directed into the lipogenic pathway for fatty acid synthesis. Therefore, in the presence of insulin, glucose also enters into the glycolytic pathway, providing substrates for increased fatty acid production. In the absence of insulin, these pathways are reversed, that is, reduced glycolysis and reduced fatty acid synthesis but there is an increase in fatty acid oxidation and an increase in the gluconeogenic enzymes favoring the production of glucose.

The Role of Adipose Tissue in Fuel Metabolism

Adipose tissue is another major site of insulin action. Adipocytes have an insulin-dependent glucose permeability that is similar to that of muscle cells; however, its main function is to provide the substrate **α-glycerophosphate** for triglyceride formation. The key step in the regulation of triglyceride synthesis and breakdown is highly regulated. There is a continuous low rate of lipolysis catalyzed by hormone-sensitive lipase (HSL) in adipose tissue with the production of FFA. The FFA produced by this reaction is reesterified to triglyceride in the presence of insulin and sufficient glucose to supply the α-glycerophosphate backbone. In the absence of insulin, the FFA produced by this reaction is released into the blood. This is an important control mechanism because it couples FFA production to plasma glucose and insulin levels. Other counterregulatory hormones (eg, cortisol, growth hormone, catecholamines) stimulate HSL, accelerating lipolysis and the release of FFA. In diabetes mellitus, the failure of insulin-dependent regulation of this reaction permits the massive production of FFA and leads to diabetic ketoacidosis.

After the ingestion of a carbohydrate-containing meal, plasma insulin rises as a consequence of elevated plasma glucose levels. Increased insulin stimulates glucose utilization by the liver through synthesis of glycogen and, with sufficient glucose levels, FFA. Muscle glucose uptake increases, and glycogen synthesis is stimulated. The glucose permeability of adipose tissue increases, providing a substrate for triglyceride formation and storage. The **combined effect is net glucose utilization and storage as glycogen and fats.** The increase in glucose utilization results in a fall in the plasma glucose concentration and a parallel fall in insulin secretion. The fall in insulin is accompanied by a fall in glucose tissue utilization. As the **glucose concentration approaches fasting levels, glucagon secretion increases.** The increase in plasma glucagon stimulates hepatic glycogenolysis and gluconeogenesis, and the liver converts from a glucose-utilizing to a glucose-producing organ. In this case, the patient is suffering from an increased and uncontrolled level of insulin. As a consequence, glucose utilization is not limited by factors such as permeability and reduced enzyme activities; instead, this is because of the availability of glucose itself. This results in the severe hypoglycemia that accompanies this disorder.

The Role of Muscle in Fuel Metabolism

Insulin acts on other tissues to promote glucose utilization. Muscle stores glucose in the form of glycogen. The glucose is taken up from the plasma and converted to glycogen in a series of regulated reactions that are analogous to hepatic glycogen synthesis. **Muscle lacks the enzyme glucose-6-phosphatase;** thus, glucose generated by glycogen breakdown cannot be released into the blood and is destined for oxidation by the muscle. An important difference between muscle and hepatic glucose utilization is that glucose uptake by resting muscle is insulin dependent. A specific **insulin-dependent** glucose transporter, **GLUT-4, is required for glucose uptake by the muscle cell.** Therefore, **insulin** promotes muscle glucose utilization by **activating glycogen synthesis** and **glucose uptake.** In the absence of insulin, the glucose permeability of the resting muscle cell is low. In **exercising muscle,** there is an **insulin-independent** increase in **glucose permeability** that is dependent on the level of exercise.

Muscle utilizes FFA as oxidizable substrate preferentially over glucose. During prolonged exercise, for example, the body's supply of glycogen can be exhausted. As described above, there is an increase in fatty acid mobilization from adipose tissue which is delivered to the muscle tissue on albumin. Muscle oxidizes FFA as its primary source of energy limiting further glucose utilization.

Adaptive Mechanisms to Stress and Prolonged Food Deprivation

The **central nervous system** responds to **severe hypoglycemia** with an increase in **sympathetic output to the pancreas and the adrenal medulla.** Catecholamine release at the nerve endings directly stimulates alpha **cells to secrete glucagon** and **inhibits beta-cell secretion of insulin.** Catecholamines released by the adrenals stimulate muscle glycogenolysis and adipose lipolysis and act in synergy with glucagon to stimulate hepatic glucose production. The central nervous system (CNS) also stimulates hypothalamic ACTH and growth hormone secretion. Their effects are somewhat delayed, with the major effect resulting from cortisol secretion. Cortisol alone has a minimal effect, but in combination with glucagon and epinephrine, it evokes a very pronounced increase in hepatic glucose production.

The **glucocorticoids** play a **major role in the maintenance of fuel supplies** and the **mobilization of fats and protein breakdown. Cortisol has a permissive effect** on a number of enzymes that are involved in fuel metabolism. In the experimental setting, fasting adrenalectomized animals fail to generate glucogenic precursors and die shortly after depletion of their carbohydrate stores. The major deficit is the failure to initiate muscle protein breakdown to provide the carbohydrate backbone for gluconeogenesis. In the normal animal, these enzymes are always present because of the secretion of cortisol. During a prolonged fast, there is a gradual small increase in glucocorticoid secretion throughout the fast.

During periods of **prolonged food deprivation,** a series of adaptive responses result from the **lack of insulin.** Glucagon secretion is increased to maintain a fasting level of plasma glucose, however, the body reacts by mobilizing alternative fuel supplies (FFA and ketone bodies) and glucogenic precursor molecules (amino acids derived from protein breakdown). These changes result from a lack of insulin caused by decreased insulin secretion during starvation, the failure of the pancreas to produce and secrete insulin, or insulin resistance. All the short-term changes in enzymatic activities described above occur, but there are several longer term responses to insulin. For example, **glucokinase** is a liver-specific enzyme that is required for glucose phosphorylation to glucose-6-phosphate. The **synthesis of glucokinase is insulin dependent.** The actual turnover of the protein is such that during a normal cycle of food intake, there is not a significant enough change in the enzyme level to interfere with glucose utilization. However, during prolonged food deprivation, the levels of glucokinase fall to near-zero levels. This is an appropriate adaptive response to starvation because it limits glucose utilization by the liver. A number of enzymes involved in glucose metabolism and the regulation of energy metabolism in general are insulin dependent in this fashion. For example, lipoprotein lipase is the committed step in triglyceride accretion and storage in the adipocyte and is synthesized in an insulin-dependent fashion. This minimizes glucose utilization by the adipocyte by preventing the uptake and storage of triglycerides during fasting. Finally, insulin has a general effect of increasing protein synthesis.

More than 150 genes have been shown to be insulin dependent. In the absence of insulin, there is an **increase in protein catabolism** with an **increase in the rate of amino acid release into the blood.** Under normal conditions, with the onset of a fast there is a fall in plasma insulin levels and an increase in the glucagon concentration. The fall in insulin reduces glucose utilization and, if continued, results in a decrease of several enzymes involved in glucose utilization. As a consequence, there will be **increased mobilization of FFA from adipose tissue.** FFA is transported to the liver, which in the absence of insulin is in a ketogenic state. **FFA β-oxidation results in the production** of **ketoacids** and their release into the blood. **FFA and ketoacids are the preferred oxidative substrates of a number of tissues,** further minimizing glucose utilization and conserving the carbohydrate backbone. Muscle protein catabolism results in a release of amino acids. Glucogenic amino acids are transported to the liver to serve as a substrate for gluconeogenesis.

Exercise markedly increases the demand for fuels. The glucose stores are sufficient for short-duration exercise, and these needs are met by the **glycogen stores, creatine phosphate, and adenosine triphosphate (ATP) reserves in the muscle.** Exercise of longer duration results in significant alterations of insulin and the counterregulatory hormones, resulting in the breakdown of hepatic glycogen and the mobilization of FFA from adipose tissue. There is a **fall in insulin secretion and an increase in catecholamines, glucagon, growth hormone, and cortisol.** These factors combined result in

an overall increase in hepatic glucose production as a consequence of catecholamines and glucagon, and a decrease in glucose utilization by the liver as
a result of the fall in insulin. Decreased insulin levels also minimize glucose
uptake in the adipocyte, resulting in an increase in FFA production. The
increased levels of the counterregulatory hormones will activate hormone-
sensitive lipase (HSL) in the adipocyte to increase the production of FFA to
serve as an alternative source of oxidizable substrate. **During prolonged exercise (> 3 hours), glycogen stores are depleted nearly completely** and there
is an **increased demand for FFA for oxidizable substrates.**

COMPREHENSION QUESTIONS

[37.1]   A 36-year-old female biochemist reflects on the action of insulin as
         she is eating toast at breakfast. Insulin action on target cells results in
         which of the following?

         A. Activation of a tyrosine kinase
         B. Activation of adenyl cyclase
         C. Increased glucagon secretion
         D. Increased gluconeogenesis

[37.2]   Glucagon action on the liver is mediated by which of the following?

         A. A cell surface receptor tyrosine kinase receptor
         B. A specific G protein–coupled receptor and activation of adenyl
            cyclase
         C. Binding to an intracellular receptor
         D. Ligand binding to specific enzymes

[37.3]   An 8-year-old child is diagnosed with type I diabetes. Insulin defi-
         ciency results in which of the following?

         A. Decreased glycogenolysis
         B. Decreased lipolysis
         C. Increased protein synthesis
         D. Ketogenesis

Answers

[37.1]   **A.** Insulin does not activate adenyl cyclase. It does bind to a receptor
         tyrosine kinase that autophosphorylates upon insulin binding. The
         phosphorylation activates the tyrosine kinase to phosphorylate spe-
         cific insulin receptor substrate molecules. These substrate molecules
         then lead to the activation of short- and long-term signaling pathways.
         Short-term pathways involve phosphorylation of protein phosphatase-1
         by PKB. Protein phosphatase-1 catalyzes the dephosphorylation of
         phosphoproteins such as glycogen synthase, leading to their activation.
         Although details of the short-term pathway have not been elucidated

completely, the result is enhanced glucose utilization through glycogen synthesis and glycolysis, increased glucose permeability in muscle and adipose tissue, and increased synthesis of triglycerides in adipose and hepatic tissue. The long-term response is mediated by activation of the MAP kinase pathway and the activation of specific transcription factors for the synthesis of key regulatory enzymes in anabolic pathways and protein synthesis in muscle cells.

[37.2]　**B.** Glucagon is a peptide hormone that binds to a specific plasma membrane receptor that is coupled by G proteins to adenyl cyclase. Activation of the cyclase results in elevated levels of cAMP and activation of PKA. PKA specifically targets enzymes in the hepatocyte that promote glycogenolysis, gluconeogenesis, and the oxidation of FFA. The net effect is to increase glucose production and release from the liver. Secondarily, there is an increase in ketogenesis with their release into the blood.

[37.3]　**D.** Insulin deficiency promotes a series of reactions in the body that are similar to adaptation to food deprivation or starvation. The initial response is to maintain the plasma glucose concentration through increased glycogenolysis and hepatic gluconeogenesis. Without the insulin-dependent control, there will be a decrease in the rate of glucose utilization as a result of decreased permeability in insulin-dependent tissues such as muscle and adipose tissue. Limiting glucose permeability to adipose tissue will inhibit triglyceride formation, resulting in increased release of FFA into the circulation. Hepatic oxidation of FFA will produce ketone bodies that will enter the circulation, providing alternative energy sources for tissues, and reduce glucose utilization further. Insulin promotes muscle protein synthesis, and in its absence protein catabolism will prevail, with a release of glucogenic precursors into the circulation for hepatic gluconeogenesis.

PHYSIOLOGY PEARLS

❖ Management of the body's fuel supplies is dependent on multiple hormonal interactions and the coordinated activities of several key organ systems. Both short-term and long-term hormonal responses are due primarily to changes in the plasma glucose concentration.

❖ Immediate changes occur in the phosphorylation state and the activities of rate-limiting enzymes in the pathways of carbohydrate, fat, and protein metabolism. Long-term effects are because of changes in the rate of protein synthesis and breakdown that alter the expression of key rate-limiting enzymes in anabolic and catabolic pathways.

❖ The liver can be viewed as a "glucostat" that controls plasma glucose. The liver can either extract glucose from the blood or produce and release glucose into the blood, depending on the circulating levels of glucagon and insulin. A feedback control mechanism is built into the system in that the plasma glucose level controls the rates of insulin and glucagon secretion.

❖ Insulin and glucagon have relatively short half-lives in the circulation. Their circulating levels are dependent on their rates of secretion, which are controlled primarily by the plasma glucose concentration. Thus, there is a very tight coupling between the hepatic glucose metabolism and its plasma concentration.

❖ Cortisol has a permissive effect on enzymes that are in the pathways of protein breakdown for the production of glucogenic precursors and lipolytic pathways that produce FFA. In its absence, fasting animals fail to maintain plasma glucose levels and soon die.

REFERENCES

Goodman HM. Hormonal regulation of fuel metabolism. In: Johnson LR, ed. *Essential Medical Physiology*. 3rd ed. San Diego, CA: Elsevier Academic Press; 2003:259-276.

Goodman HM. The pancreatic islets. In: Johnson LR, ed. *Essential Medical Physiology*. 3rd ed. San Diego, CA: Elsevier Academic Press; 2003:259-276.

A 70-year-old woman is brought to the emergency department with right flank pain, nausea, vomiting, and blood in her urine. She has no fever or urinary tract symptoms. She has recurrent kidney stones, vague abdominal pain, muscle weakness, and atrophy. On examination, she is in moderate distress secondary to her flank pain. She appears thin and fragile. Other than right back pain, her physical examination is normal. Urinalysis reveals large amounts of blood but no signs of infection. An intravenous pyelogram (IVP) is performed and reveals numerous kidney stones. A metabolic panel shows an extremely elevated calcium level. Further workup demonstrates that the patient has hyperparathyroidism from a parathyroid adenoma.

◆ **How does parathyroid hormone (PTH) increase intestinal calcium absorption?**

◆ **What effect do elevated levels of PTH have on renal phosphate reabsorption?**

◆ **What are three factors that increase the activity of 1 α-hydroxylase in the kidney?**

ANSWERS TO CASE 38: CALCIUM METABOLISM

Summary: A 70-year-old woman who presents to the emergency department with kidney stones, abdominal pain, and muscle weakness is found to have hyperparathyroidism.

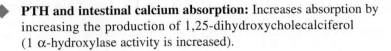 **PTH and intestinal calcium absorption:** Increases absorption by increasing the production of 1,25-dihydroxycholecalciferol (1 α-hydroxylase activity is increased).

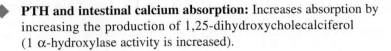 **Elevated levels of PTH and effect on phosphate:** Inhibits renal phosphate reabsorption in proximal tubule, resulting in phosphate excretion.

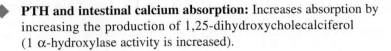 **Three factors that increase 1 α-hydroxylase activity:** Increased PTH, decreased serum calcium and phosphate levels.

CLINICAL CORRELATION

Hypercalcemia can be caused by a variety of conditions, including those which increase calcium absorption (milk-alkali syndrome), decrease calcium excretion (thiazide use), increase mobilization of the bone (hyperparathyroidism), and involve metastatic cancer (breast, prostate, etc.). A patient's symptoms depend on the level of hypercalcemia. With a mild elevation, a patient may be asymptomatic. With increasing levels, patients may have constipation, anorexia, nausea, vomiting, abdominal pain, nephrolithiasis, renal failure, emotional lability, confusion, psychosis, or coma.

Objectives

1. Understand the synthesis, regulation, and secretion of PTH.
2. Understand the synthesis, regulation, and secretion of calcitonin.
3. Know about the role of vitamin D in calcium metabolism.

Definitions

PTH: A hormone that plays a critical role in controlling calcium and phosphate balance.
1,25-dihydroxyvitamin D (calcitriol, 1,25-dihydroxycholecalciferol): The most active form of vitamin D.
25-hydroxyvitamin D (calcidiol, 25-hydroxycholecalciferol): An inactive form of vitamin D.
1α-hydroxylase: The enzyme that converts the inactive form of vitamin D, 25-hydroxyvitamin D, to the active form, 1,25-dihydroxyvitamin D.

DISCUSSION

Calcium plays an essential role in many cellular processes, including **muscle contraction, hormone secretion, cell proliferation, and gene expression.** Hence, calcium balance is critical for the maintenance of normal body functions. **Calcium balance** is a **dynamic process** that reflects a balance among calcium **absorption by the intestinal tract,** calcium **excretion by the kidney,** and **release and uptake of calcium by bone** during bone formation and resorption (see the references at the end of this case). **Most body calcium is stored in bone** (~1000 g), which is a very dynamic site as bone is remodeled continuously, with only approximately 0.1% in the extracellular fluid (~1 g). Although only a small fraction of total body calcium (and phosphate) is located in the plasma, it is the plasma concentration of **ionized calcium (and phosphate) that is tightly regulated,** primarily under the control of **PTH and vitamin D.** Both of these hormones regulate calcium absorption by the intestine, bone formation and resorption, and urinary calcium excretion. **Calcitonin** and, to a smaller extent, **estrogens** also regulate calcium and phosphate homeostasis, although the mechanisms are not fully understood.

PTH, a **peptide** hormone, is synthesized and secreted by the **chief cells of the parathyroid glands.** In contrast to most secretory processes, **low levels of extracellular calcium** (ionized plasma calcium) **induce secretion of PTH,** whereas **high levels inhibit secretion of PTH.** The ionized calcium levels are sensed by a **calcium-sensing receptor, CaSR,** in the plasma membrane; this is a **G protein–coupled receptor.** Upon binding of calcium during periods of high calcium levels, phospholipase C (PLC) is activated, generating 1,4,5-triphosphate (IP_3) and diacylglycerol (DAG) and, in turn, inducing release of calcium from internal storage sites and activation of protein kinase C (PKC), respectively. Both the elevation of intracellular calcium levels and the activation of PKC inhibit the secretion (and synthesis) of PTH. In contrast, in the presence of low plasma calcium levels, less calcium is bound to the CaSR, leading to enhanced PTH secretion (and synthesis).

PTH is a potent regulator of plasma-ionized calcium levels, **acting at three sites** to increase plasma levels. First, PTH **enhances intestinal calcium** (and **phosphate**) absorption in the presence of permissive amounts of vitamin D (see below). Second, PTH **stimulates bone resorption,** resulting in the release of calcium phosphate. Third, PTH stimulates the **active reabsorption of calcium from the kidney** (see Case 26). The effects of PTH at the three sites lead to an elevation in ionized plasma calcium levels. In the presence of **low PTH levels, these effects are reversed,** resulting in a lowering of plasma calcium levels (see Figure 38-1).

Vitamin D is a **steroid hormone** that is intimately involved in the regulation of plasma calcium levels. Its role in calcium metabolism first was recognized in the childhood disease **rickets,** which is associated with a deficiency of a fat-soluble vitamin and is characterized by a hypocalcemia with various skeletal abnormalities. The disease is corrected by dietary vitamin

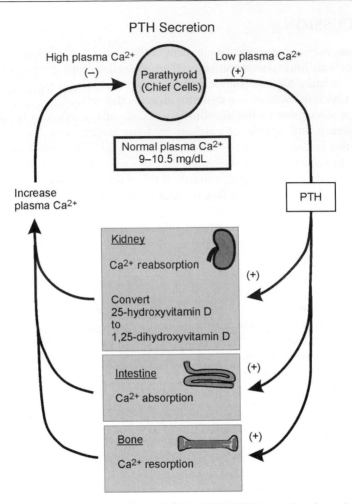

Figure 38-1. Regulation of plasma Ca^{2+} by PTH. PTH secretion from the chief cells of the parathyroid gland is regulated by plasma Ca^{2+} levels. High plasma Ca^{2+} levels are sensed by the chief cell calcium-sensing receptor to inhibit PTH synthesis and secretion, while low plasma Ca^{2+} levels have the opposite effect, stimulating PTH synthesis and secretion. In the presence of low plasma Ca^{2+}, PTH secretion works to increase plasma Ca^{2+} at three sites: the kidney, where PTH promotes Ca^{2+} reabsorption from the late distal tubule and connecting tubule and promotes conversion of 25-hydroxyvitamin D to its active form, 1,25-dihydroxyvitamin D, in the proximal tubule; the intestine, where the elevated levels of 1,25-dihydroxyvitamin D (because of elevated PTH) stimulate calcium absorption; and bone, where PTH promotes net bone resorption. All three sites lead to an increase in plasma Ca^{2+} levels back toward normal values (see text for more details).

D replacement therapy. Vitamin D is present in the diet and can be **synthesized in the skin** from 7-dehydrocholesterol in the presence of **ultraviolet light.** As this molecule passes through the liver, it is **hydroxylated to 25-hydroxyvitamin D** (25-hydroxycholecalciferol), the **inactive** form of vitamin D. 25-Hydroxyvitamin D travels by the circulation to the **kidney,** where proximal tubule cells contain the enzyme **1 α-hydroxylase,** which converts the molecule to **1,25-dihydroxyvitamin D, the most active form of vitamin D.** The activity of the 1 α-hydroxylase is tightly controlled by PTH and plasma phosphate levels. **PTH and hypophosphatemia stimulate** 1 α-hydroxylase **activity,** resulting in elevated vitamin D levels and the maintenance of calcium (and phosphate) balance (see below). In contrast, **low PTH levels and hyperphosphatemia inhibit the enzyme,** reducing the production of vitamin D.

Although **vitamin D** has numerous actions, its **two dominant actions** appear to be to **enhance the availability of calcium and phosphate for new bone formation** and to **prevent an abnormal rise or fall in plasma calcium and phosphate levels** such as symptomatic hypocalcemia and hypophosphatemia. It does this by acting on all three primary sites of regulation of calcium balance. First, **vitamin D increases the production of several intestinal proteins,** including a **luminal membrane calcium channel** and a **high-affinity cytosolic calcium-binding protein (calbindin),** that enhance transcellular absorption of calcium. PTH also is thought to stimulate intestinal calcium absorption, but this may be an indirect effect in which the PTH-induced increase in vitamin D formation in the kidney leads to enhanced intestinal calcium absorption. Second, in the kidney, vitamin D appears to act in a **synergistic fashion with PTH** to **induce active calcium reabsorption in the distal convoluted tubule** and **connecting tubule** (see Case 26) by increasing the synthesis of a distinct luminal membrane calcium channel and a cytosolic calcium-binding protein (calbindin). Third, vitamin D **induces resorption of bone,** mobilization of calcium, and bone mineralization after an elevation of plasma calcium levels. Hence, the actions of vitamin D on calcium metabolism are complex, but all point to control of the prevention of alterations in plasma calcium levels.

Calcitonin is a third hormone that is thought to underlie control of calcium balance, although its role in humans is not well defined. Calcitonin is **synthesized and secreted by C cells in the thyroid gland.** It is stored in secretory vesicles within the C cells and **released after an elevation in extracellular calcium levels above normal.** The role of calcitonin in calcium homeostasis, however, is questioned. With complete removal of calcitonin in thyroidectomized individuals or with overproduction of calcitonin in individuals with rare C-cell tumors, plasma calcium, vitamin D, and PTH levels are normal. Nonetheless, calcitonin may play a secondary role in calcium homeostasis in tissue that expresses a calcitonin receptor. The **osteoclast bone cells** appear to be a particular target of calcitonin; high levels of calcitonin are sensed and lead to inhibition of bone resorption, thereby **slowing bone turnover** and **potentially**

contributing to the generation of hypocalcemia. In the **kidney,** calcitonin causes **mild natriuresis and calciuresis,** which may contribute to the hypocalcemic (and hypophosphatemic) actions of calcitonin. Hence, a central role of calcitonin in regulating calcium metabolism in humans is not evident.

COMPREHENSION QUESTIONS

[38.1] Parathyroid hormone plays a critical role in regulating plasma calcium levels, as is evident in individuals with hyperparathyroidism, in which persistent hypercalcemia is evident. Under normal conditions, low plasma calcium stimulates PTH secretion, which in turn activates and/or inhibits calcium-handling processes at a number of different sites. High PTH levels stimulate and/or inhibit which of the following processes to return plasma calcium levels toward normal?

A. Inhibit calcium secretion by the gastrointestinal tract
B. Reduce the expression of plasma calcium-binding proteins
C. Stimulate bone resorption, leading to the release of calcium into the plasma
D. Stimulate calcium reabsorption by the renal proximal tubule
E. Stimulate the release of calcium from muscle cells

[38.2] A 50-year-old individual is admitted to the emergency room with a fractured tibia. The fracture occurred while this person was lifting light boxes. Bone scans of the spine and hip reveal low bone density. Laboratory tests show low plasma calcium, elevated PTH levels, and low vitamin D levels. The patient indicates that she is on a balanced diet with sufficient fruits and vegetables. However, the patient's plasma creatinine and blood urea nitrogen (BUN) levels are elevated markedly. Which of the following is the most likely reason for the hypocalcemia and reduced bone mass?

A. Excessive urinary excretion of calcium
B. Impaired secretion of calcitonin
C. Low dietary calcium
D. A parathyroid gland tumor generating excessive amounts of PTH
E. Reduced renal activity of 1 α-hydroxylase activity (which converts the inactive form of vitamin D to the active form)

[38.3] A 35-year-old woman undergoes a thyroidectomy for papillary serous thyroid cancer. The surgeon suspects that the parathyroid glands have been removed. Which of the following findings is most likely to be seen in the patient 1 week postoperatively?

A. Coma
B. Constipation
C. Esophagitis
D. Muscle spasms and tetany

Answers

[38.1]   **C.** One of the major actions of PTH is on bone. Binding of PTH to receptors on bone cells stimulates bone resorption, particularly in the presence of permissive amounts of vitamin D. This leads to the release of calcium phosphate and the elevation of plasma levels of both calcium and phosphate. Separately, PTH can act on the gastrointestinal tract to stimulate calcium absorption and on the renal thick ascending limb and distal convoluted tubule to stimulate calcium reabsorption. Hence, PTH plays a major role in regulating plasma calcium levels through its actions on calcium handling by several organ systems.

[38.2]   **E.** The key observation is that the patient has renal insufficiency or is in the early stages of chronic renal failure. This reduces the levels of 1 α-hydroxylase in the proximal tubule cells, thereby reducing the conversion of 25-hydroxyvitamin D, the inactive form of vitamin D, to 1,25-dihydroxyvitamin D, the most active form.

[38.3]   **D.** Removal of the parathyroid glands may lead to hypocalcemia. Symptoms include nerve paresthesias, muscle spasms, and tetany. A physical sign is the Trousseau sign, the development of carpal spasm when the blood pressure cuff is inflated for about 2 to 3 minutes. The Chvostek sign is twitching of facial muscle when the facial nerve is percussed lightly anterior to the ear. Severe hypocalcemia can lead to seizures, laryngospasm, and lethargy. The other answers refer to symptoms or signs of hypercalcemia.

PHYSIOLOGY PEARLS

❖   The dominant site of calcium storage in the body is bone, which contains nearly 99.9% of body calcium.

❖   Calcium balance is regulated by three dominant processes: intestinal calcium absorption, bone mineral absorption and resorption, and kidney calcium reabsorption.

❖   Plasma calcium regulates the synthesis and secretion of PTH by the parathyroid glands. In contrast to most secretory processes, low calcium levels stimulate PTH secretion and high calcium levels inhibit PTH secretion.

❖   The active form of vitamin D, 1,25-dihydroxyvitamin D, is converted from the inactive form, 25-hydroxyvitamin D, by 1α-hydroxylase in the kidney.

REFERENCES

Barrett EJ, Barrett P. The parathyroid glands and vitamin D. In: Boron WF, Boulpaep EL, eds. *Medical Physiology: A Cellular and Molecular Approach.* New York: W. B. Saunders; 2003:Chap 51.

Goodman HM. Hormonal regulation of calcium metabolism. In: Johnson LR, ed. *Essential Medical Physiology.* 3rd ed. San Diego, CA: Elsevier Academic Press; 2003:Chap 43.

A 13-year-old boy is brought to the pediatrician by his mother because of concerns about his growth. The patient is considerably taller than all his classmates, has coarse facial features, and has a prominent jaw. Both parents are short in stature, and his growth is very abnormal for other family members. On examination, the patient is noted to be extremely tall for his age with frontal bossing, increased hand and foot size, and coarse facial features with a prominent jaw and an enlarged tongue. His skin is noted to be oily with numerous skin tags. After further workup is performed, the patient is diagnosed with gigantism.

◆ **With what other pituitary hormone is growth hormone homologous?**

❖ **How does somatostatin inhibit growth hormone?**

ANSWERS TO CASE 39: GROWTH HORMONE

Summary: A 13-year-old boy has abnormal growth and a diagnosis of gigantism.

 Hormone homologous with growth hormone: Prolactin.

 Inhibition of growth hormone: Somatomedins stimulate the production of somatostatin and act directly on the anterior pituitary.

CLINICAL CORRELATION

Growth hormone production is critical for normal adult growth. If overproduction occurs in childhood, gigantism will result. Overproduction during adolescence (after puberty) will result in acromegaly. Once a child's growth plates have fused, responsive osteoblastic progenitor cells are stimulated in the periosteum. This results in thickening of the cranium (frontal bossing), the mandible, and the bones of the hands and feet. These patients also have thickening of the skin (increased growth of skin tags) and other soft tissue structures. Growth hormone excess can be treated with somatostatin analogues. Failure of growth hormone secretion in childhood results in pituitary dwarfism. These children have normal growth during early infancy but have abnormal growth thereafter.

APPROACH TO GROWTH HORMONE PHYSIOLOGY

Objectives

1. Know about growth hormone (GH), including synthesis, secretion, and mode of action.
2. Understand the physiologic effects of GH.
3. Describe the regulation of GH secretion.

Definitions

Growth hormone: Small peptide hormone secreted by the anterior pituitary gland that binds to a plasma membrane receptor in target tissues having both direct and indirect actions to promote growth of the organism. Direct actions result in increased gluconeogenesis, and amino acid uptake in liver and muscle and lipolysis in adipose tissues. Indirect actions involve activation of specific transcription factors that generate growth factors to stimulate bone elongation.

Growth hormone binding protein: A circulating protein derived from the proteolytic breakdown of the GH receptor complex that binds to and stabilizes circulating GH.

IGF-1 and IGF-2: Insulin-like growth factors are peptide hormones that are produced and secreted mainly by the liver in GH dependent fashion that mediate indirect GH actions on growth of the organism.

DISCUSSION

Growth hormone, also known as **somatotropin,** is a **191-amino acid peptide** hormone with a mass of approximately **22,000 Da.** It is **synthesized in the anterior pituitary gland** in cells that are called **somatotrophs** and stored in dense granules in secretory vesicles. After stimulation of the cell, the secretory vesicles are translocated to the plasma membrane and undergo fusion, with release of granule content into the circulation. Although labile when free in the blood, GH is stabilized by binding to a specific binding protein. A **novel aspect of the GH-binding protein** was the finding that it is **homologous** to the **extracellular domain of the GH receptor.** The receptor is the source of the binding protein after proteolytic scission of its extracellular domain. The **mode of action of GH is complex,** with both **direct and indirect actions** on target cells and tissues. The **GH receptor** is a **member of a superfamily of plasma membrane receptors known as tyrosine kinase–associated receptors** that includes the **prolactin receptor and several cytokine receptors.** Characteristically, these receptors have an **extracellular domain and a single membrane-spanning domain**. Hormone binding induces the dimerization of two receptor molecules. Dimer formation forms an intracellular domain that binds to and activates the tyrosine kinase Janus kinase 2 (JAK-2). JAK-2 activation phosphorylates tyrosine residues on the receptor molecule which then serve as docking sites for other receptor-binding proteins that themselves are activated with subsequent activation of the STAT and mitogen activated protein (MAP) kinase signaling pathways. These pathways lead to the activation of specific transcription factors.

Among the gene products are a family of **peptide hormone intermediates** that are required for some GH-dependent processes: the **somatomedins** or **insulin-like growth factors (IGF-1 and IGF-2).** The IGFs are **structurally related to insulin,** and IGF-1 has about 50% homology with the A and B chains of proinsulin. There are specific receptors for IGFs in many cell types that are structurally related to the insulin receptor and exhibit tyrosine kinase activity. IGF-1 also binds to the insulin receptor. Their mechanism of action appears to be similar to that of the insulin receptor. IGF-1 seems to be the physiologically more relevant molecule. It is synthesized and released from multiple GH target tissues and in some studies appears to have an autocrine or paracrine role in regulation. However, the IGFs do enter the circulation with an extended half-life as a result of binding with six specific insulin-like growth factor–binding proteins (IGFBP$_{1-6}$). The primary site of synthesis is the liver, which seems to maintain the circulating level of IGFs. Many GH-dependent actions are mediated by these hormones. In the absence of GH, the hormones are not present in the circulation.

The **role of GH** is to **regulate growth of the organism.** The physiologic actions of GH are **primarily anabolic,** characterized by an **increase in RNA and protein synthesis.** GH tends to **favor lipolysis in adipose tissue** but **promote gluconeogenesis, amino acid uptake, protein synthesis in the liver and muscle,** and **IGFs and IGFBPs in the liver** and target tissues. Most of the effects on other tissues (eg, bone, heart, lung) are indirect and are mediated by IGFs produced in the liver or the target tissue. Administration of GH to GH-deficient individuals causes an immediate nitrogen retention and decrease in urinary urea and phosphate excretion, signaling an increase in protein synthesis and structural remodeling.

GH stimulates skeletal elongation and growth through its **action on the bone epiphyseal plates.** GH **targets chondrocytes,** which are a major cell type populating the epiphyseal growth plate. Chondrocytes are cartilage-forming cells that generate a cartilage matrix that subsequently becomes calcified. Osteoblasts migrate into the calcified matrix, resulting in bone formation. Thus, **bone elongation** occurs by **continual generation** of **chondrocytes** in the epiphyseal growth plate and production of the cartilage matrix. GH stimulates amino acid uptake, protein synthesis, collagen synthesis, chondroitin sulfate production, and cartilage formation. There is an increase in cell number and cell size with a continual elongation of columns of chondrocytes. In the absence of GH, the epiphyseal growth plate atrophies and chondrocyte growth diminishes.

GH is **secreted in a pulsatile fashion** with an irregular frequency. Characteristically, GH secretion follows a pattern of frequent bursts of secretory activity throughout the day, with a maximal prolonged burst in the early morning hours. **GH secretion** occurs throughout life but is **maximal during the years with the highest growth rate,** peaking during **early puberty and adolescence.** Secretion is controlled by the hypothalamus through the two neuropeptides **growth hormone–releasing hormone** (GHRH) and **somatostatin.** The regulated release of these two hormones acts in concert to control the secretion of GH. GHRH stimulates the synthesis and secretion of GH, and somatostatin interferes with the pituitary response to GHRH. A third control is exerted through a negative feedback by IGF-1 to inhibit GH secretion. For each of these controls, there are specific receptors on the GH-secreting cells.

COMPREHENSION QUESTIONS

[39.1]   The actions of GH are mediated in part by which of the following?

    A. Insulin
    B. Somatomedins
    C. Thyroid hormone
    D. Estrogen

[39.2]   A 45-year-old woman has a cerebrovascular accident that causes necrosis of the posterior pituitary. Which of the following effects is most likely to be seen?

    A. Inability to lactate
    B. Hypothyroidism
    C. Hypoglycemia
    D. Hypernatremia

[39.3] GH acts on which of the following cells to cause long bone growth?

    A. Chrondrocytes

    B. Osteocytes

    C. Intracellular matrix

    D. Lymphocytes

Answers

[39.1] **B.** Somatomedins, also known as IGFs, are produced in response to GH by the liver and locally by GH target cells. Those produced by the liver enter the circulation and act in an endocrine fashion, whereas those produced locally act in a paracrine or autocrine fashion by binding to specific IGF receptors. Many GH actions are mediated by IGFs.

[39.2] **D.** The anterior pituitary secretes thyroid-stimulating hormone, GH, adrenocorticotropic hormone, prolactin, follicle-stimulating hormone, and luteinizing hormone, whereas the posterior pituitary secretes oxytocin and antidiuretic hormone (ADH). Lack of ADH would lead to the inability to resorb free water, leading to hypernatremia.

[39.3] **A.** Chondrocytes are the primary target for GH in the epiphyseal plate.

PHYSIOLOGY PEARLS

❖ GH is secreted in a pulsatile fashion and follows a circadian pattern. The two main regulators are GHRH and somatostatin, with bursts of GH secretion occurring when somatostatin secretion is lowest.

❖ GH actions are mediated by IGFs produced by the liver and locally by the target tissues. There are specific receptors on target cells for the IGFs, which can act in an endocrine, paracrine, or autocrine fashion.

❖ GH stimulates the growth of long bones, and its absence during early puberty and adolescence prevents development into full adult stature.

❖ GH stimulates bone growth through the production of IGF-1, which stimulates chondrocyte growth and cartilage synthesis in the epiphyseal plates.

❖ GH acts on other tissues involved in energy metabolism and promotes lipolysis by adipose tissue and fatty acid utilization to reduce body fat. At the same time, GH promotes protein synthesis and muscle development. The combined effects result in an increase in the lean body mass with increased GH secretion.

❖ At puberty, there is an increase in the frequency and amplitude of the GH secretory pulses that are dependent on increased levels of gonadal hormones, driving the growth spurt through puberty and into adolescence.

REFERENCE

Goodman HM. Hormone control of growth. In: Johnson LR, ed. *Essential Medical Physiology*. 3rd ed. San Diego, CA: Elsevier Academic Press; 2003:701-718.

❖ CASE 40

A 17-year-old girl presents to her pediatrician because she has not had a menstrual period yet. She reports breast development but scant axillary and pubic hair. On examination, she is noted to have a blind vaginal pouch with no evidence of a uterus or cervix. A karyotype is performed and reveals that she is 46,XY. The patient is diagnosed with testicular feminization.

 What is the mechanism of this disorder?

 Why would this phenotypic female not have a uterus, a cervix, or fallopian tubes?

 What enzyme is responsible for the conversion of testosterone in the male to its active form?

ANSWERS TO CASE 40: REPRODUCTION IN THE MALE

Summary: A 17-year-old phenotypic female with XY chromosomes and absent müllerian structures is diagnosed as having androgen insensitivity.

 Pathophysiology of disorder: Defective androgen receptors that result in atrophy of wolffian ducts.

 Absent müllerian structures: Testes secrete antimüllerian hormone that causes atrophy of the müllerian ducts.

 Conversion of testosterone to active form: 5 α-Reductase.

CLINICAL CORRELATION

Patients with androgen insensitivity are often diagnosed after a workup for primary amenorrhea. The disorder is caused by defective or absent androgen receptors and is inherited in a maternal X-linked recessive pattern. Testosterone and estrogen levels measured in a patient's blood are similar to male levels. However, because of defective receptors, the target tissues do not recognize the testosterone that is present. With end-organ insensitivity to the testosterone, the primordial tissues develop in a female pattern and the patient is a phenotypical female. Because the patient still has testes (abdominal), antimüllerian hormone is present and prevents the development of internal female structures such as the uterus, cervix, upper vagina, and fallopian tubes. Clinically, patients appear as a female, with normal breast development but scant axillary and pubic hair and a blind vaginal pouch with absent uterus and cervix. Breast tissue develops as a result of peripheral conversion of testosterone to estrogen. Because there is an increased risk of gonadal tumors with intraabdominal testicular location, the testes are removed surgically after puberty.

APPROACH TO MALE REPRODUCTIVE PHYSIOLOGY

Objectives

1. Understand testes anatomy.
2. Know about the secretion of testosterone by the testes.
3. Describe the regulation of the testes.
4. Understand the changes associated with puberty.
5. Describe the actions of testosterone.

Definitions

Spermatogenesis: The process describing the mitotic division of spermatogonia (the stem cells) and their development into mature sperm.
5 α-reductase: The enzyme present in many cells that converts testosterone to dihydrotestosterone.

DISCUSSION

The **major portion of the testes,** which is involved in the **production of sperm** and **testicular hormones,** is composed of **seminiferous tubules** embedded in loose connective tissue. The **highly convoluted seminiferous tubules** are the site where **Sertoli cells and the germ cells that produce sperm precursors** are located. The **connective tissue** is the site where the **Leydig cells** are located. Within the seminiferous tubules, the developing sperm cells are enveloped by Sertoli cells, which effectively isolate them from the interstitial fluid. Secretions from Sertoli cells thus regulate the environment in which sperm develop through many of their stages. Sertoli cells also produce a watery fluid that facilitates the transport of developing sperm through the seminiferous tubules and into the epididymis. There they complete development into mature sperm and are stored until ejaculation.

Testosterone is **secreted by the testes and the adrenal gland,** with **more than 95% coming from the testes.** It is the primary sex steroid secreted by the testes, although small amounts of another androgen, androstenedione, and estrogen also are secreted. These hormones are **synthesized and secreted by the Leydig cells.** Cholesterol taken up from the circulation and synthesized de novo by the Leydig cells is the precursor for the **rate-limiting step** that leads to the **conversion of cholesterol to pregnenolone.** Pregnenolone then is processed to testosterone through a number of steps. Once secreted by the Leydig cell, testosterone diffuses to adjacent seminiferous tubules to act in a paracrine manner. Some also enters the bloodstream to act on distant structures in an endocrine manner. In the blood, testosterone circulates largely bound to plasma proteins. Less than 5% is free, with about 50% bound to albumin and 45% bound to sex hormone–binding protein.

Spermatogenesis is regulated by a complex, incompletely understood process. **Gonadotropin-releasing hormone (GnRH)** is **secreted by the hypothalamus in a pulsatile manner** similar to that seen during the luteal phase of the menstrual cycle in females. In response to GnRH, **both follicle-stimulating hormone (FSH) and luteinizing hormone (LH) are secreted by the pituitary.** Although **both FSH and LH are necessary to stimulate spermatogenesis,** it appears that neither acts directly on cells in the germinal epithelium. **LH binds to receptors located predominantly on Leydig cells,** where it **stimulates the production of testosterone.** As was stated above, much of the **testosterone then diffuses to adjacent tubules, where it binds to receptors on Sertoli cells.** FSH also binds to receptors located predominantly on Sertoli cells. Testosterone and FSH act together to stimulate the production of androgen-binding protein and several growth factors by the Sertoli cells. It is these products, perhaps along with a direct action of testosterone, that stimulate spermatogenesis. Once initiated, FSH does not seem to be required for spermatogenesis to continue as long as adequate testosterone is present. However, in the absence of FSH, the rate of spermatogenesis is reduced. The secretion of GnRH, LH, and FSH is regulated by negative feedback (see Figure 40-1).

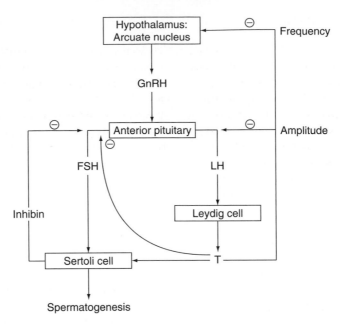

Figure 40-1. Neuroendocrine control of testicular function. GnRH = gonadotropin-releasing hormone; FSH = follicle-stimulating hormone; LH = luteinizing hormone; T = testosterone.

Testosterone (T) secreted primarily in response to LH acts within the hypothalamus to **decrease the pulse frequency** and hence the **amount of GnRH secreted.** The reduced GnRH in turn results in decreased LH secretion by the pituitary. In addition, testosterone may have a minor inhibitory effect directly on the pituitary. **Secretion of FSH is mainly under feedback inhibition by inhibin. Inhibin is a protein secreted by Sertoli cells** upon stimulation by FSH.

Testicular function and its regulation are present during embryonic development, and **relatively high levels of GnRH, LH, and FSH** are secreted in a pulsatile manner in the **perinatal period.** Then **levels fall until puberty.** During **early puberty,** mainly at **night,** the **amplitude of GnRH, LH, and FSH pulsatile secretion increases,** causing an increase in nocturnal testosterone secretion. This then develops into the adult pattern, in which secretion is relatively high all day. The mechanism controlling both the shutting down of the system shortly after birth and its turning back on at puberty is not known.

In addition to regulating its own secretion and its role in spermatogenesis, testosterone has many other actions. In many cells, **testosterone is converted to dihydrotestosterone (DHT), which is the predominant agonist.** The main actions of these androgen agonists are to bring about **expression of the**

male phenotype. Androgens promote development of the **male secondary sex organs** (which are absent in this patient). They also **stimulate growth of pubic, chest, axillary, and facial hair.** Androgens, especially DHT, are responsible for the **loss of scalp hair** that occurs in **male pattern baldness** and for stimulation of **sebaceous glands.** Androgens stimulate the **growth of skeletal muscle and help maintain muscle mass.** They stimulate **growth of the larynx and vocal cords,** thus causing the **vocal changes** associated with puberty. Androgens play a major role in the **growth spurt of the spine, long bones, and shoulder girdle** and in the **epiphyseal closure** that occurs during and shortly after puberty. Finally, androgens increase **libido.**

COMPREHENSION QUESTIONS

[40.1]   In a young boy diagnosed with precocious puberty, puberty is best delayed by the administration of a long-lasting preparation of which of the following?

A. Estrogen receptor antagonist
B. FSH receptor antagonist
C. GnRH receptor agonist
D. Growth hormone receptor antagonist
E. Testosterone receptor agonist

[40.2]   In experiments designed to accomplish male contraception, immunization to produce antibodies capable of both binding and neutralizing the bioactivity of human FSH is being investigated. Men immunized in this manner would be expected to exhibit which of the following?

A. Depressed hypothalamic GnRH secretion
B. Depressed serum inhibin levels
C. Depressed serum testosterone levels
D. Elevated serum LH
E. Enhanced secretion of growth factors by Sertoli cells

[40.3]   A 24-year-old male has been lacking the production of testosterone since early childhood and has not been treated. He will likely exhibit which of the following signs?

A. Be somewhat taller than average
B. Have a deep voice
C. Have abundant chest hair
D. Have no pubic or axillary hair
E. Undergo premature baldness

Answers

[40.1] **C.** Secretion of LH and FSH, which in turn stimulate testicular development and testosterone secretion, requires the pulsatile secretion of GnRH by the hypothalamus acting on the pituitary. Continuous stimulation of the pituitary by a GnRH agonist downregulates LH and FSH secretion. A testosterone receptor agonist would hasten puberty. FSH has minimal effects on testosterone secretion, which is required for many of the signs of puberty. Interfering with the actions of estrogens and growth hormone would not alter the events associated with puberty that are caused by testosterone.

[40.2] **B.** FSH stimulates the development and function of Sertoli cells. These cells secrete inhibin and growth factors that influence sperm maturation, and so serum inhibin levels would be decreased, as would growth factor secretion, by Sertoli cells. Inhibin acts mainly at the level of the pituitary to inhibit FSH secretion, and so GnRH secretion and LH secretion are affected minimally. Leydig cells would respond to LH by secreting normal levels of testosterone.

[40.3] **A.** Because testosterone plays a major role in causing epiphyseal closure, growth continues past the normal age of puberty. Although body hair is less abundant, pubic and axillary hair is present as a result of adrenocortical androgen secretion. In contrast, male pattern baldness, which is attributed to the actions of androgens, will not occur. Because androgens are required for growth of the larynx and vocal cords, the voice deepening associated with puberty will not take place.

PHYSIOLOGY PEARLS

❖ FSH and LH are secreted by the pituitary in response to the pulsatile secretion of GnRH by the hypothalamus.

❖ FSH acts on Sertoli cell receptors to promote the secretion of products that promote sperm development. LH acts on Leydig cell receptors to stimulate testosterone secretion.

❖ Testosterone secreted from the testes suppresses LH secretion through actions on both the pituitary and the hypothalamus.

❖ Inhibin, a peptide secreted by Sertoli cells, acts at the level of the pituitary to suppress FSH secretion.

❖ Testosterone acts in a paracrine manner to stimulate spermatogenesis through its action on Sertoli cells and in an endocrine manner to influence other tissues.

❖ Testosterone is converted to DHT in many tissues, such as the scalp and sebaceous glands. There DHT rather than testosterone is the active androgen.

❖ Sertoli cells have FSH receptors, and Leydig cells have LH receptors.

❖ In the absence of the production and secretion of testicular hormones, a genetic male will present with a female phenotype.

REFERENCES

Genuth SM. Male reproduction. In: Levy MN. Koeppen BM, and Stanton BA, eds. *Berne & Levy, Principles of Physiology*, 4th ed. Philadelphia, PA: Mosby; 2006:712-723.

Goodman HM. Hormonal control of reproduction in the male. In: Johnson LR, ed. *Essential Medical Physiology*. 3rd ed. San Diego, CA: Elsevier Academic Press; 2003:719-735.

A 19-year-old woman presents to her gynecologist with complaints of not having had a period for 6 months. She reports having normal periods since menarche at age 12. She denies sexual activity, thyroid symptoms, or a milky breast discharge. She has no medical problems and is not taking any medications. On examination, she is thin but otherwise normally developed. The patient makes several comments about the fact that she thinks she is fat and is not satisfied with her body image. In comparison to other patients of her age, she is extremely underweight. She reports exercising excessively to "lose weight." The remainder of the examination is normal except for a slow heart rate and dry skin with lanugo. A pregnancy test is negative, and thyroid function tests are normal. The patient is diagnosed with anorexia nervosa and referred for treatment and counseling.

◆ **What is the pathophysiologic cause of her amenorrhea?**

◆ **Which cells in the ovary secrete estrogen?**

◆ **What is the major hormone produced by the corpus luteum?**

ANSWERS TO CASE 41: REPRODUCTION IN THE FEMALE

Summary: A 19-year-old woman presents with secondary amenorrhea and anorexia nervosa.

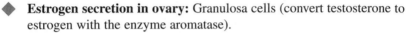 **Pathophysiology of amenorrhea:** Hypothalamic state caused by the patient's anorexia nervosa, resulting in decreased gonadotropin-releasing hormone (GnRH) secretion from the hypothalamus and, as a result, decreased luteinizing hormone (LH) and follicle-stimulating hormone (FSH) production and secretion.

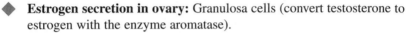 **Estrogen secretion in ovary:** Granulosa cells (convert testosterone to estrogen with the enzyme aromatase).

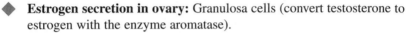 **Major hormone produced by the corpus luteum:** Progesterone.

CLINICAL CORRELATION

Many conditions may result in secondary amenorrhea. It is often helpful to remember the various levels where normal function may be lost. If there is a history of cervical surgery, cervical stenosis may be present, resulting in an anatomic obstruction of menses. Ovarian problems also result in amenorrhea and menstrual irregularities. Possible causes of ovarian dysfunction include premature ovarian failure, a history of chemotherapy and/or radiation causing destruction of ovarian tissue, and polycystic ovarian syndrome. Finally, if there is a problem with the hypothalamic axis, FSH and LH may not be secreted, and therefore the ovary will not be stimulated to produce estrogen/progesterone. Patients with hypothyroidism, hyperprolactinemia, anorexia, excessive stress, and excessive exercise all may have hypothalamic dysfunction that affects stimulation of their ovaries. A primary ovarian problem can be differentiated from a primary hypothalamic problem by checking the FSH level. If the FSH level is high, the ovary is where the problem is, and if the FSH is low, the hypothalamus is likely to be the source of the problem. If an FSH level were drawn on this patient with anorexia, it probably would be low. Her amenorrhea can be corrected by hormonal medications or by treating her anorexia.

APPROACH TO FEMALE REPRODUCTIVE PHYSIOLOGY

Objectives

1. Know the ovarian anatomy and hormones.
2. Understand the control of ovarian function.

3. Know the regulation of menstrual cycle.
4. Be able to chart the normal hormone levels throughout the menstrual cycle.

Definitions

Amenorrhea: Cessation of menses for 6 months or three times the normal menstrual interval.

Primary amenorrhea: Condition where a female has never had menses and has not had menses by the age of 16 years, regardless of secondary sexual development.

Secondary amenorrhea: Condition where a female has had menses previously and now has absence of menses as defined in amenorrhea.

Hypothalamic Dysfunction: Alterations of gonadotropin releasing hormone pulsatile secretion that may be due to a variety of disorders such as hyperprolactinemia, hypothyroidism, anorexia nervosa, or excessive exercise.

DISCUSSION

Ovarian Anatomy and Hormones

Human ovaries are paired ellipsoid pelvic structures that are attached to the uterus by the utero-ovarian ligament and the pelvic side wall by the infundibulopelvic ligament. They **produce the oocytes** and the hormones responsible for the events that lead to fertilization and the establishment of pregnancy. Ovaries are composed of two areas: a **central zone, or medulla,** and a **peripheral zone, or cortex.** The medulla contains the ovarian support structures, including the blood, lymph vessels, and nerve fibers. The **cortex contains the two functional ovarian structures, follicles and corpora lutea,** in varying states of development or regression. **Most follicles** exist in a **nondeveloping pool** and are called **primordial follicles.** A number of primordial follicles begin development, but usually only one develops into the ovulatory (graafian) follicle. Follicles that fail to continue to develop undergo self-destruction and are referred to as atretic. **Developing follicles** may be classified as **primary, secondary, tertiary,** and **graafian** as they mature. Tertiary (those which contain a fluid-filled cavity) and larger follicles have two primary cell types separated by a basement membrane. Granulosa cells surround the maturing oocyte and the fluid-filled cavity of the follicle. The basement membrane surrounds the granulosa cells and separates them from several outer layers of cells called thecal cells. Both **granulosa and thecal cells contribute to the synthesis of estradiol. Androgens are synthesized by the thecal cells,** cross the membrane and are **converted to estradiol by the granulosa cells.** After ovulation, the granulosa cells are transformed in a process called luteinization into the luteal cells of the corpus luteum, which is responsible for the synthesis of progesterone. If fertilization fails to occur, the corpus luteum undergoes self-destruction in a process called luteolysis. Corpora luteal structures in their early stages of development and late stages of regression are referred to as **corpus hemorrhagicum and corpus albicans,** respectively.

Control of Ovarian Function

Ovarian function is regulated primarily by **FSH** and **LH** secreted by the anterior pituitary. Their secretion is regulated by the **GnRH** produced by the hypothalamic area of the brain. The hypothalamus integrates numerous positive and negative signals that affect reproductive function. The integrated message is a **pulsatile secretion of GnRH** at a pulse frequency to facilitate the secretion of FSH and/or LH. GnRH pulses occur at hourly to less frequent intervals. Peripheral levels of estrogen and progesterone act (feedback) at the level of the hypothalamus and/or pituitary to influence FSH and LH (pulse frequency) secretion positively and/or negatively.

Follicular development is regulated by the peripheral levels of FSH and LH and/or LH pulse frequencies, depending on the state of follicle development. **Transformation** of **primordial follicles** into a cohort of developing primary follicles is **independent of FSH and LH support.** Several of the primary follicles continue to develop into tertiary follicles and then are recruited for further development by elevated levels of FSH during the first week of the menstrual cycle. A follicle at this state then is selected as the **dominant follicle** for further development and ovulation. The exact nature of dominant follicle selection is unknown, but hourly pulses of LH are important for further development of the dominant follicle. Elevated peripheral levels of estradiol from the developing dominant follicle suppress peripheral FSH (negative feedback) levels and ultimately stimulate (positive feedback) the preovulatory surge of LH to ovulate the mature graafian follicle.

Luteinization of the granulosa cells of the ovulated follicle to **form the corpus luteum** is dependent on the **preovulatory surge of LH. LH also is required for maintenance of the corpus luteum** with the resulting **progesterone** and a low-level estrogen secretion during the luteal phase of the cycle. The resulting elevated peripheral progesterone levels reduce the frequency of LH pulses from hourly to once every 3 to 4 hours (negative feedback). In the absence of implantation of a fertilized oocyte, the **corpus luteum has an inherent life span of 14 days.** Mechanisms involved in luteolysis of the human corpus luteum are not fully understood, but may involve intraovarian prostaglandin F_{2a}.

Menstrual Cycle Regulation

Most of the ovarian activities described above occur over a period of 28 days (Figure 41-1). This period in humans is called the menstrual cycle because it involves vaginal shedding of the uterine mucosa: menstruation. The first day

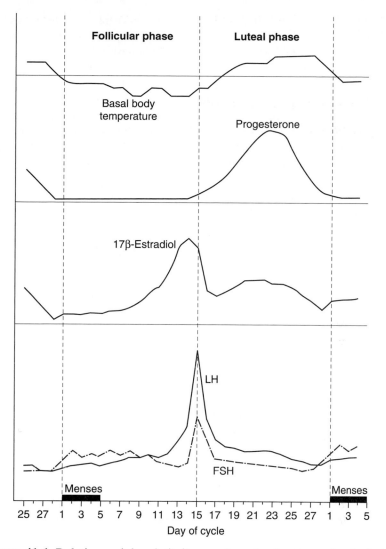

Figure 41-1. Relative peripheral pituitary and ovarian hormones levels during the menstrual cycle. The preovulatory surge of luteinizing hormone (LH) occurs on day 15. LH pulses are not shown. LH pulses occur hourly during the late follicular phase of the cycle and every 3 to 4 hours during the luteal phase.

of menstruation is designated as day 1 of the menstrual cycle. **Ovulation of the graafian follicle occurs around midcycle after the preovulatory LH peak.** The 14 days preceding ovulation are characterized by increasing peripheral levels of estradiol from follicular development and are called the follicular phase. The 14 days after ovulation are characterized by a transitory increase in peripheral progesterone and to a lesser extent estrogen levels from the corpus luteum and are called the luteal phase. There is greater variability in the duration of the follicular phase than the luteal phase, accounting for the considerable variation in the length of the menstrual cycle in humans. Undoubtedly, factors affecting follicular development contribute to the variation in length of the follicular phase. At the uterine level, the **follicular phase** is referred to as the **proliferative phase.** During this period of estradiol influence, the uterine endometrium increases in thickness and the uterine glands lengthen. During the **luteal phase,** when **progesterone levels are elevated,** the **uterine glands are coiled and secretory.** The phase with respect to the endometrium is called **secretory.** When the corpus luteum regresses and progesterone levels decline, the endometrial mucosa thins and is shed. This thinning is accompanied by necrosis of endometrial blood vessels, leading to spotty hemorrhages and contributing to the menstrual flow.

COMPREHENSION QUESTIONS

[41.1]   A patient with a 29-day menstrual cycle probably ovulated on which of the following days?

   A. Day 13
   B. Day 14
   C. Day 15
   D. Day 16

[41.2]   How does a basal body temperature chart reflect ovulation?

   A. Increased basal body temperature with LH surge
   B. Decreased basal body temperature with LH surge
   C. Increased basal body temperature with decreased progesterone level
   D. Increased basal body temperature with elevated progesterone level
   E. Increased basal body temperature with increased peripheral estradiol levels

[41.3]   How does progesterone affect the pulsatile release of GnRH from the hypothalamus?

   A. No change
   B. Increases
   C. Decreases
   D. Stops release altogether

[41.4]   Withdrawal of which of the following hormones results in menstruation?

   A. Estradiol
   B. FSH
   C. Progesterone
   D. LH

Answers

[41.1] **C.** The corpus luteum has an inherit life span of 14 days, resulting in a 14-day luteal phase. Ovulation occurs just before the luteal phase. Subtracting 14 days from the patient's menstrual duration (29 days) gives an approximate day of ovulation (day 15).

[41.2] **D.** The elevated progesterone level during the luteal phase causes an increase in the patient's basal body temperature by increasing the body's thermoregulatory set point in the hypothalamus. A basal body temperature chart can be helpful to infertility patients by documenting the presence or absence of ovulation during a menstrual cycle.

[41.3] **C.** Progesterone causes a decrease in pulsatile release of GnRH.

[41.4] **C.** Withdrawal of the hormone progesterone results in sloughing of the endometrium (menstruation). If pregnancy occurs, the corpus luteum is "rescued" and production of progesterone continues (no menstruation).

PHYSIOLOGY PEARLS

❖ The central zone of the ovary (medulla) contains support structures for the ovary, and the peripheral zone (cortex) contains the follicles and corpora lutea in various stages of development.

❖ The follicular phase of the menstrual cycle varies in length among different individuals, whereas the luteal phase is relatively constant (14 days).

❖ The predominant hormones in the follicular and luteal phases are estradiol and progesterone, respectively.

❖ Elevated peripheral levels of estradiol result in the LH surge by positive feedback on the anterior pituitary.

❖ Ovulation is dependent on the preovulatory LH surge.

REFERENCES

Adashi EY, Rock JA, Rosenwaks Z, eds. *Reproductive Endocrinology, Surgery, and Technology.* Vols. 1 and 2. Philadelphia, PA: Lippincott-Raven; 1995.

Becker KL, Belezikian JP, eds. *Principles and Practice of Endocrinology and Metabolism.* 3rd ed. Philadelphia, PA: Lippincott Williams & Wilkins; 2001.

❖ CASE 42

A 23-year-old woman presents to the emergency department with complaints of severe abdominal pain. She is known to be 7-weeks pregnant and did not have any problems with previous pregnancies. She denies any vaginal bleeding. On examination, the patient is in moderate distress and is slightly hypotensive with a normal pulse. Her abdomen is distended and tender on the right side with rebound and guarding. Her cervix is closed, and her uterus is consistent with 7 weeks of pregnancy. A beta-human chorionic gonadotropin (β-hCG) is drawn and is positive. A stat blood count is drawn and demonstrates a drop in hemoglobin from blood work done 3 days earlier. An ultrasound is performed and demonstrates a viable singleton pregnancy in the uterus. There is also a large amount of free fluid in her abdomen, and a right adnexal mass is noted. The patient is taken to the operating room to investigate the right adnexal mass, pain, and free fluid. A ruptured corpus luteum is identified intraoperatively, along with a large amount of blood in the abdomen. After the bleeding corpus luteum is removed, the surgery is completed and patient is taken to the recovery room.

◆ **What is the function of the corpus luteum during the first trimester of a pregnancy?**

◆ **Why does lactation not occur during pregnancy despite an increasing prolactin level?**

ANSWERS TO CASE 42: PREGNANCY

Summary: A 23-year-old woman at 7 weeks' gestation presents with acute abdominal pain from a ruptured corpus luteal cyst.

◆ **Function of corpus luteum in the first trimester:** Produces progesterone.

◆ **Lactation during pregnancy:** Estrogen and progesterone inhibit prolactin action on the breast.

CLINICAL CORRELATION

The formation of a corpus luteum cyst is a normal finding during pregnancy. At times, the corpus luteum may be large and even rupture. Rupture of the corpus luteum results in an intraabdominal hemorrhage and severe abdominal pain, usually requiring surgery. The corpus luteum secretes progesterone which is needed to maintain the pregnancy. After the first trimester, the corpus luteum will regress. In this case, the corpus luteum ruptured and was removed at 7 weeks (before the placenta can produce the hormone independently). Supplemental progesterone will be needed for this patient until after the first trimester to maintain the pregnancy. The risk of an ectopic pregnancy would be much higher if a viable pregnancy had not been seen in the uterus on ultrasound. The hormone hCG has two subunits, alpha and beta, and is produced early in the pregnancy by the placenta. The hCG rescues and maintains the corpus luteum's production of progesterone. The alpha subunit is similar to follicle-stimulating hormone (FSH), luteinizing hormone (LH), and thyroid-stimulating hormone (TSH). The beta subunit is unique to each hormone, and this is why the β-hCG level is measured to verify a pregnancy.

APPROACH TO EARLY PREGNANCY PHYSIOLOGY

Objectives

1. Be able to describe normal fertilization and implantation.
2. Be able to describe the role of the placenta and hormones (hCG, progesterone).
3. Know about lactation.

Definitions

Corpus luteum: A physiologic cyst of the ovary which forms after the oocyte is released; its major hormone secreted is progesterone.

Hemoperitoneum: An abnormal collection of blood in the peritoneal cavity, which can cause abdominal pain, hypotension, and tachycardia.

Threatened abortion: Vaginal bleeding occurring with a pregnancy in the first 20 weeks of gestation. This may signify a miscarriage, an ectopic pregnancy, or a normal gestation.

DISCUSSION

Fertilization and Implantation

Fertilization occurs when a **sperm penetrates the investments** (cumulus cell matrix and zona pellucida) surrounding an ovum and subsequently **activates the ovum to initiate embryo development.** In **humans,** fertilization occurs in the **ampulla region of the oviduct.** Ova reach the oviduct soon after ovulation, which occurs **12 hours after the preovulatory LH peak. Ova remain fertile in the oviduct for about 12 to 24 hours after ovulation.** Sperm remain fertile in the female genital tract for up to 48 hours. Before a sperm can fertilize an ovum, it must reside for a period of time in the uterus and/or oviduct to undergo **capacitation.** Capacitation—the capacity to fertilize— occurs by removal of epididymal-seminal plasma proteins from and/or alteration of the glycoproteins on the sperm plasma membrane. Capacitation results in sperm hypermotility to facilitate sperm passage through the cumulus matrix with the aid of a sperm membrane protein with hyaluronidase activity. Noncapacitated sperm fail to penetrate the cumulus matrix. Once the sperm has passed through the cumulus matrix, species-specific proteins on the sperm plasma membrane bind to specific receptor proteins on the zona pellucida. This is followed by the **acrosome reaction,** which involves release of a trypsin-like **protease** called **acrosin** from the sperm acrosome to **facilitate sperm penetration of the zona.** On penetrating the zona, the plasma membranes of the sperm and ovum fuse, resulting in ovum activation and the initiation of embryo development. Activation of the ovum also blocks penetration of the zona and membrane fusion by additional sperm to prevent polyspermy.

In humans, the embryo reaches the uterus in the **early blastocyst stage,** around **6 days after ovulation.** At this stage, the embryo consists of 50 to 150 cells (blastomeres) with a fluid-filled cavity (blastocoele). The blastomeres have differentiated into the trophectoderm and the inner cell mass. The trophectoderm is a thin layer of cells that forms the outer surface of the embryo and subsequently forms the fetal component of the placenta. The inner cell mass is a cluster of cells at a specific point on the inner surface of the trophectoderm. It forms the body of the embryo after implantation. Before implantation can occur, the zona pellucida surrounding the blastocyst must be removed by a process called hatching.

Implantation in humans occurs around day 7, when the blastocyst makes physical and subsequently physiologic contact with the endometrium in the fundal region of the uterus. Implantation can be divided into **three stages: apposition, adhesion, and penetration.** During the **apposition stage,** movement of the blastocyst is limited to enable microvilli of the trophoblast cells to interdigitate with those of the lumen epithelial cells. This stage provides sufficient stability to allow development of the **adhesion stage,** which involves firm molecular adhesion of the trophoblast cells to the surface of the epithelial cells. During the apposition stage, the blastocyst can be dislodged by gentle perfusion; however, with the beginning of the adhesion stage such dislocation is resisted. In humans, the **penetration phase** begins several hours after the initiation of implantation and involves aggressive movement of the blastocyst through the basement membrane of the uterine epithelium into the stroma of the endometrium. Implantation does not rely on the presence of the endometrium and is driven largely by the trophoblastic cells.

The highly invasive nature of the human blastocyst enables the pregnancy to implant in various locations outside the normal endometrial cavity, resulting in an **ectopic pregnancy.** In response to hormonal signals from the developing pregnancy, the endometrial stromal cells undergo an inflammatory-type response called **decidualization** to form the maternal component of the placenta. Decidualization involves the proliferation and differentiation of the endometrial stromal cells. Decidualization occurs even in the presence of an ectopic pregnancy, resulting in an enlarged uterus that may be mistaken for a normal intrauterine pregnancy. To form the fetal component of the placenta, the trophectodermal cells of the blastocyst fuse, forming a syncytium of cells consisting of two layers. The **inner layer,** the **cytotrophoblasts,** consists of mitotically active mononuclear cells and is prominent early during pregnancy. The **outer layer,** the **syncytiotrophoblasts,** consists of fused, primarily non-dividing multinuclear cells that become prominent later in pregnancy. The syncytiotrophoblasts appear to facilitate movement of the developing embryo into the decidual mass. The cytotrophoblasts and syncytiotrophoblasts contribute to the secretion of the placental hormones.

Estrogen (estradiol, estriol, and estrone) levels in the maternal circulation increase dramatically during pregnancy (Figure 42-1). The corpus luteum is the principal source of estrogens during the first several weeks, but subsequently nearly all estrogens are secreted by the syncytiotrophoblasts of the placenta. The **syncytiotrophoblasts** convert **dehydroepiandrosterone (DHEA) of adrenal origin to estrogens.** The role of the high estrogen levels in pregnancy is not well understood. However, the estrogens contribute to the stimulation of blood flow, uterine growth, development of the mammary gland, and the events leading to parturition.

Maternal levels of progesterone also increase throughout the pregnancy. The primary source of progesterone during pregnancy is the **syncytiotrophoblasts** of the placenta; however, until 6 to 8 weeks of pregnancy the **corpus luteum** is the major source. Removal of the corpus luteum before 8 to 10 weeks of pregnancy often leads to abortion unless the patient is given exogenous progesterone. **Maternal cholesterol is converted to progesterone by the placenta.** During the first week of pregnancy, progesterone stimulates the glands in the oviduct and uterus to secrete nutrients for the embryo. At this time, progesterone also prepares the uterine endometrium for implantation (the decidual response). Subsequently, progesterone inhibits uterine smooth muscle contractility, leading to myometrial quiescence. Progesterone may have a role in

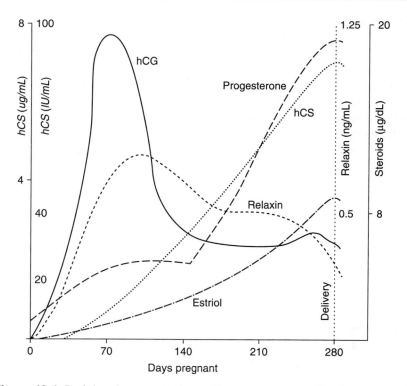

Figure 42-1. Peripheral concentrations of hormones secreted by the ovary and placenta throughout pregnancy. hCG = human chorionic gonadotropin; hCS = human chorionic somatomammotropin.

preventing immunologic rejection of the conceptus by the mother by inhibiting T lymphocyte–mediated activity.

In addition to the steroid hormones described above, the **placenta** is an important source of protein hormones that also contribute to the pregnancy. These hormones are **hCG; human chorionic somatomammotropin (hCS), also called human placental lactogen (hPL); relaxin;** and numerous other hormones and factors. The placental protein hormones are secreted by the **syncytiotrophoblasts.** The hCG plays a vital role in the establishment and maintenance of pregnancy. Secretion of hCG by the early embryo extends the life span of the corpus luteum, which otherwise would regress at the end of the menstrual cycle. hCG can be detected in the maternal circulation around 10 days after the midcycle LH surge and peaks around the tenth week of pregnancy. The presence of hCG in the blood and urine is the basis for the human pregnancy test and has been used for varying diagnostic purposes by clinicians. First trimester "morning sickness" often correlates with the hCG level and peaks at around 10-weeks gestation.

Lactation

Mammary gland function is controlled by many of the same hormones that regulate reproduction. After puberty, **estrogen causes proliferation of the mammary ducts, whereas progesterone in association with estrogen controls development of the lobules** containing the alveoli that are responsible for milk synthesis. **Prolactin, growth hormone, and the glucocorticoids enhance mammary gland development** in response to estrogen and progesterone. The stromal and fat tissue surrounding the mammary ducts and alveoli also proliferate at this time. Full proliferation of mammary alveoli and breast development occur during later stages of pregnancy, when levels of estrogen, progesterone, and prolactin are elevated.

Milk synthesis by the developed mammary gland is dependent on **high levels** of **prolactin in association with cortisol and insulin.** Although the milk secretory system is fully developed during the final stages of pregnancy, lactation does not begin until after parturition. **High levels of estrogen actually inhibit the stimulatory action of prolactin on milk synthesis.** The abrupt decline in estrogen at the time of parturition removes this inhibitory influence of estrogen, and lactation begins. In women it may take from 1 to 3 days or longer for full milk secretion or lactation to occur.

Continued lactation is dependent on the **removal of milk at regular intervals** by suckling in addition to the presence of the hormones described above. Failure to empty the alveoli will cause lactation to cease in about 1 week. This is accompanied by involution of the lobuloalveolar structures.

The **suckling stimulus** causes a **surge in prolactin secretion** and the **"milk letdown" reflex.** Prolactin enhances the production of milk, as was described above. The milk letdown reflex involves the rapid secretion of oxytocin by the posterior pituitary to stimulate contraction of the myoepithelial cells that surround each alveolus to express milk into the duct system of the mammary gland, causing milk letdown. It is well known that in humans resumption of menstrual cycles after parturition is delayed by the suckling stimulus. The high concentrations of the hormones resulting from suckling, especially prolactin, are associated with a suppression of LH secretion. High prolactin concentrations may act at the hypothalamus to decrease the frequency of the pulsatile LH secretions necessary for dominant follicle development. However, support for this inhibitory effect of prolactin on LH secretion is not beyond question.

COMPREHENSION QUESTIONS

[42.1]   Where does fertilization most often occur?

        A. Cervix

        B. Ovary

        C. Oviduct

        D. Uterus

[42.2]   Maintenance of the corpus luteum during the first 8 weeks of pregnancy is dependent on which of the following hormones?

A. Estrogen
B. hCG
C. Progesterone
D. DHEA-S

[42.3]   Implantation of the blastocyst into the endometrium usually occurs on which days after fertilization?

A. 2-3 days
B. 4-5 days
C. 6-7 days
D. 8-9 days

[42.4]   What important lactation hormone enhances contraception and inhibits ovulation?

A. Estrogen
B. Oxytocin
C. Progesterone
D. Prolactin

Answers

[42.1]   **C.** Fertilization and sperm capacitation usually occur in the fallopian tube (most often in the ampulla region).

[42.2]   **B.** Maintenance of the corpus luteum and its secretion of progesterone are dependent on the hormone hCG. Trophoblastic tissue (syncytiotrophoblasts) produces hCG, with peak levels around 10 weeks of gestation. Pregnancy tests (serum or urine) detect the presence of hCG (specifically the beta subunit). hCG has two subunits: alpha and beta. The alpha subunit is similar in structure to TSH, LH, and FSH.

[42.3]   **C.** The blastocyst typically enters the endometrial cavity 6 days after fertilization, and implantation occurs near the seventh day. During implantation, patients may have a "bloody vaginal discharge" or a brief episode of vaginal spotting that may be mistaken for a "light" period.

[42.4]   **D.** Elevated levels of prolactin during lactation (and other conditions with elevated prolactin, such as prolactinomas, medications, and hypothyroidism) inhibit hypothalamic GnRH secretion, which subsequently inhibits FSH and LH secretion, resulting in anovulation.

PHYSIOLOGY PEARLS

❖ Fertilization occurs in the fallopian tube.

❖ The ova remain fertile in the fallopian tube for 12 to 24 hours.

❖ Sperm undergo capacitation in the oviduct and remain fertile for up to 48 hours.

❖ The blastocyst enters the endometrial cavity on the sixth day, with implantation occurring on the seventh day.

❖ Trophoblastic tissue is the driving force for implantation; the presence of the endometrium is not required.

❖ The corpus luteum is "rescued" from regression by hCG secreted by the syncytiotrophoblasts. The corpus luteum produces progesterone until about 8 to 10 weeks, when the developing placenta can maintain progesterone production.

❖ Early secretion of progesterone by the corpus luteum is important in the maintenance of early pregnancy.

❖ Prolactin is necessary for milk production, which is maintained after delivery by the infant's suckling. Oxytocin is necessary for milk ejection.

REFERENCES

Adashi EY, Rock JA, Rosenwaks Z, eds. *Reproductive Endocrinology, Surgery, and Technology*. Vols. 1 and 2. Philadelphia, PA: Lippincott-Raven; 1995.

Becker KL, Belezikian JP, eds. *Principles and Practice of Endocrinology and Metabolism*. 3rd ed. Philadelphia, PA: Lippincott Williams & Wilkins; 2001.

❖ CASE 43

A 65-year-old man presents to his primary care doctor complaining of difficulties with his vision, particularly at night. The blurred vision is primarily in the right and left peripheral fields. He has myopia and wears corrective lenses. The physical examination reveals visual acuity of 20/100 bilaterally with visual field deficits on the right and left periphery.

◆ **Where is the cranial lesion that results in bitemporal hemianopia?**

◆ **What type of lens is necessary to correct myopia?**

◆ **Why does a deficiency of vitamin A result in night blindness?**

ANSWERS TO CASE 43: VISUAL SYSTEM

Summary: A 65-year-old man having difficulty with night vision presents with bitemporal hemianopia.

 Location of lesion causing bitemporal hemianopia: Optic chiasm.

 Lens needed for myopia: Biconcave lens.

 Vitamin A and night blindness: Regeneration of 11-*cis*-retinal in photoreceptors is dependent on vitamin A. 11-*cis*-retinal is necessary for photoisomerization.

CLINICAL CORRELATION

An often neglected but important part of a physical examination is the eye examination. A thorough eye examination can identify and localize many disease processes. Tumors or ischemic events may affect various nerve tracts, including the optic nerve tract. Depending on the location of the lesion, a predictable visual change can be recognized on the basis of knowledge of the optic tract. Lesions that affect the optic chiasm affect both of the peripheral visual fields, sparing the midline visual fields. An example of this type of lesion would be a pituitary tumor that compresses the optic chiasm. A lesion in an optic nerve will result in blindness in the ipsilateral eye, and a lesion in an optic tract will result in homonymous hemianopia. Pupil size and retinal changes also can reflect underlying medical conditions.

APPROACH TO VISION PHYSIOLOGY

Objectives

1. Understand the peripheral processing of visual information.
2. Know about the central processing of visual information.
3. Describe the oculomotor system.

Definitions

Fovea: Region of the retina, in line with the visual axis, which has become specialized for high-acuity vision by the radial displacement of blood vessels and all cell layers that can interfere with light reaching the outer segments of the cone photoreceptors that are concentrated there.

Rods: Low-acuity, achromatic photoreceptors having long outer segments that are specialized for high sensitivity in dim light.

Cones: High-acuity, chromatic photoreceptors having short outer segments that are specialized for high temporal, spatial, and chromatic resolution in bright light.

Saccades: Quick, preprogrammed, ballistic eye movements used in searching for visual targets (contrasted with smooth pursuit movements that track already engaged targets).

DISCUSSION

Light enters the **pupil** and passes through the **lens,** the **vitreous humor,** and the **inner layers of the retina** before encountering **photopigment molecules in the outer segments of cone or rod photoreceptors.** In each case the **chromophore is 11-*cis* retinal** (derived from **vitamin A**), which **absorbs a photon to isomerize to all-*trans*-retinal.** In rods the chromophore is attached to the protein **opsin** (forming rhodopsin), and in cones the same chromophore is attached to one of three different cone opsins that alter the absorbance spectrum of the chromophore so that it is most sensitive to short (blue-violet), medium (green-yellow), or long (yellow-red) wavelengths. Transition to the all-*trans* form of retinal causes a conformational change in the opsin (this semi-stable conformation is called metarhodopsin II in rods) that activates the G protein transducin, which then activates a phosphodiesterase that hydrolyzes cyclic guanosine monophosphate (cGMP).

Sensory transduction in the retina is unusual because the effective stimulus, light, does not excite photoreceptors; instead it hyperpolarizes them. In the **dark, cGMP is synthesized continuously** by a **constitutively active guanylyl cyclase,** and the resulting cGMP binds to and opens cGMP-activated cation channels, causing an influx of Na^+ that maintains the photoreceptor at a depolarized potential (~ -40 mV). The **tonic depolarization** causes a **continuous release of glutamate** from the photoreceptor's terminals onto bipolar cells. **During illumination,** the **decrease in cGMP** reduces the opening of cGMP-activated cation channels, causing the **photoreceptor** to **hyperpolarize** and reducing tonic release of glutamate onto bipolar cells. Bipolar cells in the "off" channel have ionotropic glutamate receptors that depolarize the cell in the presence of glutamate and hyperpolarize the cell when glutamate release from the photoreceptors decreases in response to light. Bipolar cells in the "on" channel have metabotropic glutamate receptors that hyperpolarize the cell in the presence of glutamate; therefore, light causes a depolarizing response in these cells, inverting the signal from inhibitory to excitatory. These *on* and *off* responses are maintained through much of the subsequent visual pathway.

The **bipolar cells excite ganglion cells in the retina,** and the ganglion cells send long axons through the optic nerve, optic chiasm, and optic tract to excite neurons in the **lateral geniculate body;** those axons then project to the **primary visual cortex.** At each level from the retina to the visual cortex, the visual information is sharpened by **center versus surround inhibition** mediated by local inhibitory interneurons such as the horizontal cells in the retina.

In the **optic chiasm,** ganglion cell axons from the nasal half of each retina cross and merge with uncrossed axons from the temporal retina of the contralateral eye so that **each optic tract carries information exclusively from the contralateral visual field.**

Lesions at different locations along the visual pathway produce characteristic visual deficits. For example, **section of one optic nerve** produces **complete ipsilateral anopia.** A section through the **optic chiasm** produces **heteronymous hemianopia,** with loss of vision from the **temporal half of each retina.** Section of **one optic tract** produces **homonymous hemianopia,** with loss of vision from the **temporal half of one retina and the nasal half of the other.** In the visual cortex, visual images are reconstructed in a series of steps that go through different areas of the primary visual cortex and into other regions in the parietal lobe. Processing depends on highly ordered representation of different components of visual information in specific, sometimes overlapping neuronal populations (eg, ocular dominance layers, orientation-specific columns, color-specific blobs).

Highest-acuity vision occurs when light strikes photoreceptors in the **fovea,** a specialized area of the retina **in line with the visual axis through the center of the lens.** The oculomotor system is designed both for rapid visual exploratory movements and to keep a selected image focused on the fovea. Eye movements in three axes are produced by coordinated activity in three pairs of extraocular muscles: the medial and lateral rectus muscles, which rotate the eye in the horizontal plane; the superior and inferior rectus muscles; and the superior and inferior oblique muscles, which cause vertical and torsional movements. **Eye movements** are composed of **saccades** (extremely rapid ballistic movements) that have an exploratory function and **slower smooth pursuit** movements that keep a target on the fovea and are subject to continuous modification. These movements are programmed and controlled by groups of interneurons in the brainstem (saccades) and cerebral cortex, cerebellum, and pons (smooth pursuit movements). Eye movements are coordinated with head movements and vestibular input and are influenced by visual attention and experience.

Intrinsic muscles of the eye are innervated by the **autonomic nervous system. Parasympathetic fibers excite ciliary muscles** that control the shape of the lens and mediate the **accommodation reflex.** Contraction of ciliary muscle relieves tension on the lens, which becomes more spherical and brings near objects into focus. **Parasympathetic** fibers also innervate **pupillary constrictor muscles,** which mediate the pupillary reflex to bright light. Pupillary dilator muscles, which oppose constriction, are tonically excited by **sympathetic fibers.** During states of increased sympathetic activity (eg, certain emotions, fight or flight situations), the pupils dilate noticeably.

COMPREHENSION QUESTIONS

[43.1] Isomerization to all-*trans*-retinal after absorption of light is associated with which of the following features?

A. A conformational change that inactivates guanylyl cyclase
B. A series of conformational changes that activate transducin
C. Occurrence in rods but not cones
D. Direct binding of retinal to a cGMP phosphodiesterase
E. Opening of cGMP-activated cation channels

[43.2] Retinal ganglion cells in the *on* and *off* pathways show opposite responses to a narrowly focused beam of light because of which of the following reasons?

A. *On* bipolar cells are hyperpolarized by glutamate released from photoreceptors, whereas *off* bipolar cells are depolarized.
B. *On* bipolar cells excite horizontal cells, whereas *off* bipolar cells inhibit horizontal cells.
C. *On* bipolar cells excite retinal ganglion cells, whereas *off* bipolar cells inhibit retinal ganglion cells.
D. *On* photoreceptors are hyperpolarized by light, whereas *off* photoreceptors are depolarized by light.
E. *On* retinal ganglion cells are depolarized by glutamate release from bipolar cells, whereas *off* bipolar cells are hyperpolarized by glutamate release.

[43.3] A saccade has which of the following properties?

A. It can be modified continuously during its execution.
B. It causes the lens to become more spherical.
C. It functions primarily to protect the fovea from extreme illumination.
D. It is evoked by the release of acetylcholine (ACh) from parasympathetic postganglionic fibers.
E. It is a ballistic movement designed for rapid visual exploration.

Answers

[43.1] **B.** Isomerization to all-*trans*-retinal leads to the activation of the G protein transducin, which then activates a phosphodiesterase that hydrolyzes cGMP. This sequence occurs in both rods and cones and results in the closing of cGMP-activated cation channels.

[43.2] **A.** Light reduces tonic glutamate release from all ocular photoreceptors, and this will depolarize *on* bipolar cells (which in the absence of
light are tonically hyperpolarized by glutamate release) and hyperpolarize *off* bipolar cells (which in the absence of light are tonically
depolarized by glutamate release). Both the *on* and the *off* bipolar
cells excite retinal ganglion cells, which then excite neurons in the
lateral geniculate body that in turn excite neurons in primary visual
cortex, maintaining distinct *on* and *off* channels.

[43.3] **E.** A saccade is a ballistic movement that cannot be modified during
its execution. It is mediated by somatic motor neurons, and its function is to enhance rapid visual exploration of the environment.

PHYSIOLOGY PEARLS

❖ Photopigments in rods and cones utilize the same chromophore, 11-*cis*-
retinal, to absorb light, but the chromophore is attached to different
opsins, which confer different spectral absorption properties to each
photopigment.

❖ Depolarization of a photoreceptor in the dark is maintained by a
continuous synthesis of cGMP, which opens cGMP-activated
cation channels, permitting a steady influx of Na^+. The resulting
depolarization causes continuous release of glutamate from the
photoreceptor's synaptic terminals.

❖ Absorption of light triggers a hyperpolarizing response in the photoreceptor through a transducin-mediated activation of cGMP
phosphodiesterase and consequent closing of cGMP-activated
cation channels, thereby inhibiting the release of glutamate at
synapses onto bipolar cells.

❖ *On* channel bipolar cells invert inhibitory responses to light to excitatory responses through a metabotropic glutamate receptor that
hyperpolarizes the bipolar cell in the presence of glutamate.
Thus, illumination-induced hyperpolarization of the photoreceptor decreases inhibition of the bipolar cell, and this disinhibition
results in excitation of downstream neurons in the channel that
proceeds through central visual pathways.

❖ The oculomotor system uses ballistic saccades for rapid movements
to explore visual space and smooth pursuit movements to keep a
target image centered on the fovea.

❖ Intrinsic muscles of the eye are controlled by parasympathetic fibers
(ciliary muscle, which regulates accommodation by the lens, and
pupillary constrictor muscles) and by sympathetic fibers (pupillary dilation).

REFERENCES

Connors BW. Sensory transduction. In Boron WF, Boulpaep EL, eds. *Medical Physiology*. Philadelphia, PA: Saunders; 2003: 325-358.

Johnson DA. The visual system. In: Johnson LR, ed. *Essential Medical Physiology*. San Diego, CA: Elsevier Academic Press; 2003: 807-830.

REFERENCES

A 53-year-old man presents to his primary care physician with complaints of feeling like the room is spinning, dizziness, decreased hearing, ringing in the ears, and fullness in both ears. He states that the symptoms have been occurring episodically but increasing in frequency. The ringing in his ears was not present initially but has become more prominent. He denies any recent ear infections or trauma. He is not taking any medications. On examination he is noted to have low-frequency hearing loss. The remainder of the examination is normal. After a complete workup is done, the patient is diagnosed with Ménière disease.

◆ **What part of the vestibular system detects angular acceleration and rotation?**

◆ **What is the effect on the hair cell if the stereocilia are bent away from the kinocilium?**

◆ **Where in the auditory pathway is tonotopic organization first established?**

ANSWERS TO CASE 44: AUDITORY AND VESTIBULAR SYSTEM

Summary: A 53-year-old man has vertigo, tinnitus, and decreased hearing consistent with Ménière disease.

 Angular acceleration and rotation: Semicircular canals.

 Effect of bending stereocilia away from the kinocilium: Hyperpolarization.

 Tonotopic organization initially established in: Organ of Corti.

CLINICAL CORRELATION

Vertigo is a common complaint in the primary care setting. Vertigo can have numerous etiologies, including benign paroxysmal positional vertigo (most common), Ménière disease, toxic damage to labyrinth (medications), tumors (acoustic neuroma), migraine headaches, viral labyrinthitis, vertebrobasilar vascular disease (especially with cerebrovascular disease), head trauma, and multiple sclerosis. Treatment depends on the underlying etiology. Ménière disease is a syndrome of recurrent attacks of vertigo and tinnitus associated with hearing loss. The underlying pathophysiology is a disorder of fluid balance within the endolymphatic system, leading to degeneration of vestibular and cochlear hair cells.

APPROACH TO AUDITORY AND VESTIBULAR SYSTEM PHYSIOLOGY

Objectives

1. Know the physiology of the vestibular system.
2. Describe the physiology of the auditory system.

Definitions

Otolith organs: Vestibular organs (utricle and saccule) which provide tonic information about the position of the head in space as well as linear acceleration, aided by forces exerted by otoliths—dense calcium carbonate particles embedded in the gelatinous cap on the sensory epithelium.

Tonotopic mapping: Encoding of auditory information by the structural features of the cochlear basilar membrane, with higher pitches encoded at the base of the membrane and lower pitches encoded near its apex.

DISCUSSION

Sensory transduction in the vestibular system occurs in **hair cells.** Each hair cell has a hair bundle on the apical end that consists of a large kinocilium and 50 to 100 shorter stereocilia. **Vestibular hair cells** are located in the **otolithic** organs, the **saccule** and **utricle,** which detect gravitational forces during steady head positions. These hair cells project their hair bundles into a gelatinous cap that is encrusted with dense calcium carbonate otoliths. Gravity pulls the otoliths against the gelatinous cap, deflecting the stereocilia. Hair cells in the saccule and utricle are organized so that their polarities cover all directions, allowing these organs to detect changes in linear acceleration in any direction. Hair cells also are located in the three semicircular canals (anterior, posterior, and lateral), which transduce angular acceleration of the head in three dimensions. These organs lack otoliths; bending of stereocilia is produced by inertial forces of the endolymph when the head is rotated.

In all vestibular organs, **bending of the stereocilia toward the kinocilium depolarizes the hair cell,** leading to release of the transmitter **glutamate** from the basal end, whereas deflection away from the kinocilium hyperpolarizes the cell, reducing background release of glutamate. The changes in potential produced by bending involve an unusual mechanism. The tips are bathed in **endolymph,** which has a **remarkably high K$^+$** concentration (150 mM) that exceeds the intracellular K$^+$ concentration (140 mM). Bending toward the kinocilium increases tension on the extracellular filaments ("tip links") that connect the tips of the stereocilia. This opens cation channels in the tips, and the resulting influx of K$^+$ (driven by both the modest concentration gradient and the negative membrane potential) causes depolarization. At rest, a few of the cation channels remain open. When the stereocilia bend away from the kinocilium, these channels are closed, reducing tonic K$^+$ influx and hyperpolarizing the cell.

Release of glutamate from basal ends of hair cells excites peripheral terminals of primary sensory neurons that have their cell bodies in the ipsilateral vestibular ganglion, and the resulting action potentials travel along axons in the vestibular nerve to the vestibular nuclei in the medulla. Postsynaptic neurons in the vestibular nuclei then project to the spinal cord (helping to control posture), to motor nuclei that control eye movement (mediating vestibulo-ocular reflexes), and to the reticular formation (which can produce vertigo and the gag reflex).

Hearing also begins with **sensory transduction in hair cells,** which in this case are located within the **scala media of the cochlea,** in the **organ of Corti.** The inner hair cells, which are less numerous but more richly innervated than the outer hair cells, are primarily responsible for **sensing auditory information.** The primary function of the outer hair cells is to lengthen when depolarized, which increases the distance between the basilar and tectorial membranes, allowing the basilar membrane to bend more and thus produce cochlear amplification of subsequent sound waves. Amplification of the effects of sound waves is also a consequence of the tips of the stereocilia of inner and outer hair cells being embedded in the tectorial membrane. This results in shearing forces being transmitted to the stereocilia during displacements of the basilar membrane by sound waves. Auditory hair cells in adults lack kinocilia, but other properties are the same as in vestibular hair cells. The endolymph has the same high concentration of K^+, and bending of the stereocilia toward the longest stereocilium opens cation channels, permitting an influx of K^+ to depolarize the cell, whereas bending in the opposite direction closes the channels, hyperpolarizing the cell.

Pitch perception is determined primarily, although not exclusively, by the **location in the organ of Corti** that is maximally stimulated. Each tone produces a traveling wave in the cochlea; **high pitches** produce waves that peak **near the base of the cochlea,** and **low pitches** produce waves that peak **near the apex.** This results in a **tonotopic organization** of the hair cells, and this positional relationship is maintained throughout the auditory pathway. The inner hair cells release glutamate at synapses between their basal ends and the terminals of primary afferent neurons that have their cell bodies in the spiral ganglion in the cochlea. The central axons travel in the auditory nerve to make synapses on neurons in the cochlear nuclei, which project successively to the inferior olivary nuclei, the inferior colliculus, the medial geniculate nucleus, and then the primary auditory cortex. At each level, pitch is encoded by tonotopic organization and perhaps some coding by action potential frequency ("phase-lock" code), whereas loudness depends on the total number of active neurons and their firing rates. **Sound localization** depends on processing in the auditory cortex that analyzes differences in both the phase and the loudness of sound waves on the two sides of the head. In addition, directional differences in sound quality resulting from the shape and orientation of the pinna are detected.

COMPREHENSION QUESTIONS

[44.1] Otoliths have which of the following properties?

   A. They contain kinocilia and cation channels that are opened when pulled by extracellular filaments.
   B. They are located only in the saccule and utricle.
   C. They are located only in the semicircular canals.
   D. They bend stereocilia toward but not away from the kinocilium.
   E. They stimulate hair cells, transducing angular acceleration.

[44.2] Depolarization of hair cells during the bending of stereocilia occurs because bending causes which of the following responses?

   A. Closing channels that carry an outward K^+ current
   B. Closing channels that carry an inward Na^+ current
   C. Closing channels that carry an inward Ca^{2+} current
   D. Opening channels that carry an inward Na^+ current
   E. Opening channels that carry an inward K^+ current

[44.3]   A high-pitched tone is associated with which of the following features?

A. Bending of stereocilia toward the kinocilium
B. Encoding primarily by the frequency of firing of primary afferent axons in the cochlear nerve
C. Being detected by maximal activation of hair cells near the apex of the cochlea
D. Encoding by the type of neurotransmitter released by primary afferent neurons in the auditory pathway
E. Being recognized by comparing phase differences between waves detected on the left and right sides of the head

Answers

[44.1]   **B.** Otoliths are located in the otolithic organs, the saccule and utricle, not in the three semicircular canals. They are pulled by gravity against the gelatinous cap containing stereocilia, which can bend either toward or away from the kinocilium. This bending preferentially transduces linear acceleration rather than angular acceleration (which is transduced by hair cells in the semicircular canals).

[44.2]   **E.** Opening of K^+ channels in the stereocilia depolarizes the hair cells because the $[K^+]_o$ in the endolymph surrounding the hair cell exceeds the $[K^+]_i$ in the stereocilia.

[44.3]   **C.** A high-pitched sound maximally excites hair cells near the apex of the cochlea, and those cells provide tonotopically organized input to central components of the auditory system. Hair cells in the organ of Corti in adults lack kinocilia, and they all use glutamate as their primary neurotransmitter. Although lower pitches may be encoded partially by action potential frequency, higher pitches have frequencies that are too high to allow this type of phase-lock code and thus rely solely on tonotopic coding.

PHYSIOLOGY PEARLS

❖ In both the vestibular and auditory systems, sensation depends on transduction of mechanical energy by stereocilia in hair cells.

❖ Modest depolarization of a hair cell under basal conditions is maintained by a continuous influx of K^+ through a fraction of the cation channels in stereocilia. Bending toward the kinocilium (in vestibular organs) or the tallest stereocilium (in the organ of Corti) opens additional channels, producing further depolarization, whereas bending in the opposite direction closes the channels, hyperpolarizing the hair cell.

❖ Depolarization of hair cells increases vesicular release of glutamate, which depolarizes peripheral terminals of primary afferent neurons, initiating action potentials that travel along the vestibular or cochlear nerve into the brainstem.

❖ Hair cells in the saccule and utricle detect the effects of gravity on otoliths, providing information about steady head positions and linear acceleration of the head.

❖ Hair cells in the anterior, posterior, and lateral semicircular canals detect inertial forces exerted by the endolymph when the head is rotated, providing information about angular acceleration in three dimensions.

❖ Hair cells in different regions of the organ of Corti are activated maximally by different pitches because each pitch produces a traveling wave that peaks at a different position along the cochlea, thus providing an initial tonotopic coding of pitch that is propagated throughout the auditory system.

REFERENCES

Connors BW. Sensory transduction. In Boron WF, Boulpaep EL, eds. *Medical Physiology*. Philadelphia, PA: Saunders; 2003: 325-358.

Johnson DA. The vestibular system, The auditory system. In: Johnson LR, ed. *Essential Medical Physiology*. San Diego, CA: Elsevier Academic Press; 2003: 831-847.

A 15-year-old girl is brought to the pediatrician's office because of concern about her development. She has not gone through puberty as have other girls her age. She reports never having had a period or breast development. She also reports that she cannot smell things. She has difficulty recognizing pungent odors such as trash and sweet fragrances such as perfume and flowers. On physical examination, she is sexually infantile without development of axillary or pubic hair or breast tissue and is unable to perceive odors. The remainder of her examination is normal. She has a cervix and uterus on pelvic examination. The patient subsequently is diagnosed with Kallmann syndrome.

◆ **What type of axons constitute the olfactory nerves?**

◆ **Which kinds of chemicals does cranial nerve V detect?**

◆ **What nerve innervates the posterior third of the tongue, and what tastes are detected there?**

ANSWERS TO CASE 45: OLFACTORY/TASTE SYSTEMS

Summary: A 15-year-old girl who is sexually infantile has anosmia consistent with Kallmann syndrome.

◆ **Types of fibers in the olfactory nerves:** Unmyelinated C fibers (slow).

◆ **Chemicals detected by cranial nerve V:** Noxious or toxic substances.

◆ **Innervation of the posterior third of tongue:** Cranial nerve IX (glossopharyngeal) detects sour and bitter tastes.

CLINICAL CORRELATION

Disorders of olfaction are caused by conditions that may interfere with the olfactory epithelium, the receptors in the epithelium, or central neural pathways. Conditions that may interfere with the olfactory epithelium (transport loss) include allergic, viral, and bacterial rhinitis; nasal polyps or tumors; nasal septal deviation; and nasal surgery. Disorders of the receptors can be produced by medications, infections, tumors, toxic chemical exposures, and a history of radiation exposure. The list of central olfactory disorders is more extensive and includes conditions caused by alcoholism, Alzheimer disease, medications, diabetes, hypothyroidism, Kallmann syndrome, malnutrition, trauma, Parkinson disease, vitamin deficiencies, and Huntington chorea. This patient presents with Kallmann syndrome. Kallmann syndrome (hypogonadotropic hypogonadism) is a disorder of both olfactory axonal and gonadotropin-releasing hormone (GnRH) neuronal migration from the olfactory placode in the nose. This is why the patient is sexually infantile and has anosmia. The single gene mutation is on the X chromosome and is responsible for functions necessary for neuronal migration.

APPROACH TO OLFACTORY AND TASTE PHYSIOLOGY

Objectives

1. Describe sensory transduction in the olfactory system.
2. Understand the processing of olfactory information.
3. Describe sensory transduction in the gustatory system.
4. Know the central gustatory pathways.

Definitions

Odorant binding proteins: Proteins secreted into nasal mucus that trap and concentrate odorants, facilitating their interaction with odorant receptor proteins.

Odorant receptor proteins: Members of a superfamily of G protein-coupled receptors expressed in olfactory receptor neurons and encoded by about 1000 genes, with each protein binding a set of different odorants.

Umami taste: The fifth basic taste (in addition to salt, sour, sweet, bitter), stimulated by the binding of glutamate and perhaps other amino acids to ionotropic glutamate receptors expressed in some taste receptor cells.

DISCUSSION

Olfactory receptor cells are **primary afferent neurons** located in **olfactory epithelium** within the **upper levels of the nasal cavities.** They are unusual neurons because they are **replaced continually throughout life, turning over every 4 to 8 weeks.** In addition to the olfactory receptor neurons, the olfactory epithelium contains basal cells (stem cells to replace the receptor neurons) and glial-like support cells. Each olfactory receptor neuron projects a thick dendrite tipped with cilia that end in the mucus layer. The mucus contains odorant-binding proteins that concentrate odorants, as well as enzymes and antibodies. The antibodies provide important protection because olfactory receptor neurons present a direct path into the brain that could be used by viruses and bacteria present in aspirated air.

Each olfactory receptor neuron produces only one of a large family of about 1000 odorant receptor proteins that are localized to the cilia and display a high specificity to particular odorant structures. **Different odors stimulate different combinations of olfactory receptor neurons,** and the **average human can recognize about 10,000 separate odors** (with intensive training that number may go up to about 300,000). Eighty percent of recognizable odors are unpleasant, representing potentially toxic or dangerous substances.

Binding of an odorant to an odorant receptor causes excitation by the same sequence of mechanisms in all olfactory receptor neurons. The odorant receptors are members of the enormous superfamily of **G protein-coupled receptors,** and binding of a specific odorant to a receptor activates the G protein G_{olf}, which in turn activates adenylyl cyclase. The resulting cyclic adenosine monophosphate (cAMP) opens **cAMP-gated cation channels,** permitting the influx of Na^+ and Ca^{2+} (and the efflux of K^+) and depolarizing the cell. The Ca^{2+} (and additional Ca^{2+} that can enter through depolarization-activated Ca^{2+}channels) then activates Ca^{2+}-activated Cl^- channels. Because olfactory receptor neurons have unusually high intracellular Cl^- concentrations, opening these channels causes an efflux of Cl^- and further depolarization, initiating action potentials. The action potentials are conducted relatively slowly along very thin **unmyelinated olfactory receptor neuron axons** a short distance into the overlying olfactory bulb by the olfactory nerve (cranial nerve I). Synapses from a very large number of olfactory receptor neuron axons are made onto a much smaller number of relay neurons (mitral cells and tufted cells) and inhibitory interneurons (periglomerular cells) within **glomeruli in the olfactory bulb.** Information about different odorants is mapped on different glomeruli. The relay cells project directly to the olfactory cortex, which then projects through the thalamus to the orbitofrontal cortex, where odor perception and discrimination occur, and to the amygdala and hypothalamus, where emotional effects are produced.

The **olfactory epithelium is also innervated by the trigeminal nerve** (cranial nerve V), which contains axons of **nociceptive chemoreceptors** that have free nerve endings that detect **noxious chemicals in the air,** such as ammonia and chlorine (as well as components of peppermint and menthol). Activation of these epithelial nociceptors elicits defensive reflexes such as sneezing, lacrimation, and respiratory inhibition. Humans also have a small region of olfactory mucous membrane in the anterior nasal septum that may be homologous to the vomeronasal organ in other mammals. Receptors in this organ transduce olfactory stimuli by mechanisms different from those utilized by other olfactory receptor neurons and project by different pathways to the amygdala and hippocampus. In rodents, and possibly in humans, this accessory olfactory system detects pheromones that can influence sexual function.

Taste receptor cells are **modified epithelial cells that are clustered in taste buds on the tongue** and, to a lesser extent, the palate, pharynx, epiglottis, and part of the upper esophagus. Each **taste bud** contains **50 to 100 receptor cells** as well as basal cells for the generation of new receptor cells (which live only about 10 days). Humans distinguish **five tastes: salt, sour, sweet, bitter, and umami,** although human perception of taste usually involves contributions from olfaction and even texture and temperature. Unlike the olfactory and visual systems, which each utilize a single basic transduction mechanism, transduction in taste receptor cells involves diverse mechanisms. In **salt taste receptors,** transduction occurs when a **rise in Na^+ concentration in the saliva** results in sufficient influx of Na^+ through voltage-insensitive **epithelial Na^+ channels** (ENaCs), which are always open, to depolarize the cell. As in most taste cells, this leads to the opening of depolarization-activated Ca^{2+} channels followed by Ca^{2+}-dependent exocytosis of transmitter onto dendrites of primary afferent neurons. **Sour taste** transduction involves a similar mechanism, with H^+ ions permeating ENaCs to depolarize the cell. In addition, H^+ ions can bind to and block K^+ channels, which also depolarize the cell. **Sweet taste** transduction occurs when sugars bind to specific G protein-coupled surface receptors that stimulate the synthesis of cAMP, ultimately closing K^+ channels.

Other G protein-coupled receptors bound by sugars stimulate the 1,4,5-trisphosphate (IP_3) pathway, which releases Ca^{2+} from intracellular stores, directly enhancing Ca^{2+}-dependent exocytosis of transmitter. **Bitter taste** transduction involves binding of bitter compounds to receptors linked to a G protein, gustducin, which stimulates phosphodiesterase and decreases cAMP and cyclic guanine monophosphate (cGMP) levels. In these cells cAMP and cGMP lead to hyperpolarization, and so their degradation produces depolarization. In addition, other G protein-coupled receptors stimulate the IP$_3$ pathway in bitter taste receptors, causing release of Ca^{2+} from intracellular stores and enhanced transmitter release, as in some of the sweet taste receptors. Finally, as in **sour taste receptors,** some bitter compounds can block K$^+$ channels directly, depolarizing the cell. **Umami taste receptors** are stimulated by certain amino acids, including L-glutamate, which binds to a metabotropic glutamate receptor that activates phosphodiesterase to decrease cAMP and cGMP levels, as in some bitter taste receptor cells.

Primary afferent neurons activated by transmitter released from taste receptor cells project to the gustatory division of the solitary nucleus in the medulla through the facial (cranial nerve VII), glossopharyngeal (cranial nerve IX), and vagus (cranial nerve X) nerves. Information then is relayed through the thalamus to the primary gustatory cortex in the insular and orbitofronal regions. Relatively little is known about central processing of taste.

COMPREHENSION QUESTIONS

[45.1]   Which of the following receptor cells is a primary afferent neuron?

A. Auditory hair cell
B. Bitter taste cell
C. Olfactory receptor cell
D. Photoreceptor cell
E. Vestibular hair cell

[45.2]   Which of the following statements is true of odorant receptors in olfactory receptor cells?

A. Most receptors respond to attractive rather than unpleasant odors.
B. Binding of an odorant stimulates the G protein, gustducin.
C. Odorant receptor proteins are expressed selectively near synaptic active zones.
D. Odorant activation of a G protein–coupled receptor directly leads to the opening of K$^+$ channels.
E. Only one of a family of 10,000 receptor proteins is expressed in each receptor neuron.

[45.3]   Release of transmitter from a salt receptor cell depends primarily on Ca^{2+} accumulation resulting from responses to which of the following?

A. Blockade of K$^+$ channels by Na$^+$
B. Gustducin activating the IP$_3$ pathway
C. Influx of Na$^+$ through voltage-insensitive epithelial Na$^+$ channels
D. Opening of voltage-activated Na$^+$ channels
E. Na$^+$ binding to Ca^{2+} channels

Answers

[45.1]   **C.** Olfactory receptor cells are true primary afferent neurons that conduct action potentials along their axons into the central nervous system (CNS), where they synapse onto second-order neurons in glomeruli within the olfactory bulb. The other receptor cells listed are epithelially derived cells that lack axons. Sensory information from these cells is conveyed by peripheral synapses to axonal terminals of primary afferent neurons that then project (often over long distances) into the CNS.

[45.2]   **E.** Each olfactory receptor neuron expresses only one of 10,000 possible receptor proteins. Odorant binding to its receptor acts through the G protein G_{olf} in peripheral receptor terminals, leading to the synthesis of cAMP, which opens cAMP-gated cation channels that permit diffusion of Na^+, Ca^{2+}, and K^+, producing the net effect of depolarization and initiation of action potentials that travel to central synaptic terminals.

[45.3]   **C.** During a salty meal or drink, Na^+ diffuses into salt taste receptor cells through epithelial Na^+ channels, leading to depolarization of the cell, opening of voltage-gated Ca^{2+} channels, and Ca^{2+}-dependent exocytosis of neurotransmitter at synapses onto terminals of primary afferent neurons in the taste buds.

PHYSIOLOGY PEARLS

❖ Olfactory receptor cells have sensory cilia on an epithelial surface and turn over every few weeks similar to epithelial receptor cells. However, they are true neurons.

❖ Odorants are concentrated and presented to olfactory receptor proteins by odorant-binding proteins in the mucus, which also contains antibodies and enzymes.

❖ Each olfactory receptor neuron produces only one of a large family of about 10,000 odorant receptor proteins.

❖ Binding of an odorant to a receptor activates G_{olf}, which increases the synthesis of cAMP, which opens cAMP-gated cation channels, depolarizing the cell and promoting Ca^{2+} entry, which opens Ca^{2+}-activated Cl^- channels, further depolarizing the cell so that action potentials are initiated.

❖ The major olfactory pathway goes from olfactory sensory neurons to mitral and tufted cells in glomeruli in the olfactory bulb, then to the olfactory cortex, and then to either the orbitofrontal cortex via the thalamus or the amygdala and hypothalamus.

❖ Defensive responses such as sneezing and lacrimation are triggered by noxious chemicals that are detected by chemoreceptors in the olfactory epithelium that send axons to the brainstem in the trigeminal nerve.

❖ Sensory transduction of the five basic tastes—salt, sour, sweet, bitter, and umami—involves many different mechanisms, sometimes for the same substance. In each case, the final step is an increase in intracellular $[Ca^{2+}]$, which triggers Ca^{2+}-dependent exocytosis of transmitter from modified epithelial cells that have become specialized for chemoreception.

REFERENCES

Connors BW. Sensory transduction. In Boron WF, Boulpaep EL, eds. *Medical Physiology*. Philadelphia, PA: Saunders; 2003: 325-358.

Johnson DA. The chemical senses: smell and taste. In: Johnson LR. *Essential Medical Physiology*. San Diego, CA: Elsevier Academic Press; 2003:849-859.

An 18-year-old man is brought to the emergency center by the emergency medical service after being involved in a serious motor vehicle accident. On physical examination, the patient has normal vital signs but he cannot move and has no sensation in either of the lower extremities, which are flaccid and without reflexes. Magnetic resonance imaging (MRI) reveals a fracture of the lower spine with significant swelling of and injury to the spinal cord.

◆ **Which tracts are responsible for direct cortical control of spinal motor systems?**

◆ **What is the muscle response during the reverse myotatic reflex?**

◆ **What do group Ia afferents detect?**

ANSWERS TO CASE 46: LOWER MOTOR SYSTEM

Summary: An 18-year-old man is involved in a motor vehicle accident with resulting lower extremity paralysis.

◆ **Cortical control of motor neurons:** By the lateral and ventral corticospinal tracts.

◆ **Response during reverse myotatic reflex:** Relaxation of muscle that had been strongly contracting.

◆ **Group Ia afferents detect:** Muscle stretch.

CLINICAL CORRELATION

Transections of the central nervous system (CNS) above and within the spinal cord have different effects on motor reflexes. When a transection takes place along the spinal cord, there is loss of voluntary movements and conscious sensation below the level of the transection. The muscles that are innervated below the lesion initially become flaccid and lose reflex responses during spinal shock. Depending on the location of the lesion, various other physical signs may be present, including urinary and/or fecal incontinence, decreased heart rate and pressure, and respiratory failure. Spasticity and hyperreflexia develop later. Lesions of motor pathways above the spinal cord result in muscle rigidity and hyperreflexia without a period of flaccid paralysis. Decerebrate and decorticate posturing may develop with transections above the spinal cord.

Objectives

1. Understand the role of motor neurons and motor units.
2. Know about spinal reflexes.
3. Describe the descending control of spinal motor systems.

Definitions

Motor unit: A single motor neuron plus all of the muscle fibers that it connects synaptically to.

Motor neuron pool: The complete set of all motor neurons innervating a single muscle.

Homonymous muscle: The same muscle as that containing afferents evoking a reflexive contraction of the muscle (eg, reflexive contraction of the same extensor muscle that is stretched).

Muscle tone: The force with which a muscle resists being lengthened, equivalent to stiffness.

Spasticity: Abnormal increase in muscle tone, often associated with enhanced stretch (deep tendon) reflexes.

Spinal interneurons: Spinal neurons which excite or inhibit other neurons in the spinal cord via axons that do not leave the spinal cord.

DISCUSSION

Alpha motor neurons in the **spinal cord** have their **cell bodies in the ventral horn** and **send their axons out the ventral roots to innervate axial, flexor, or extensor muscles in the trunk, limbs, and digits.** Motor neurons that innervate muscles in the head and neck have their cell bodies in motor nuclei in the brainstem and send their axons out the cranial nerves. All the muscle fibers innervated by a single motor neuron constitute a motor unit. Motor units vary in size from two or three fibers in the fingers, where fine control is important, to more than a thousand fibers in antigravity muscles of the leg. **Each action potential in an alpha motor neuron evokes a single twitch** in each fiber in the **motor unit.** Large sustained contractions require the temporal summation of trains of high-frequency twitches. Small motor units are recruited more readily than are large motor units because the size of the motor neuron soma is proportional to the size of the motor unit, and smaller somata are more sensitive to their synaptic inputs than are larger somata (**size principle**). Motor neurons that innervate fast-twitch fibers fire at higher frequencies than do motor neurons that innervate slow-twitch fibers.

Muscle length and tension are monitored by **proprioceptive** sensory (afferent) neurons, whose cell bodies are in dorsal root ganglia and which have peripheral terminals in specialized sensory structures within the muscle. Muscle length properties are sensed by terminals that coil around thin intrafusal fibers in **muscle spindles**. These muscle fibers, which regulate sensory sensitivity, lie in parallel with the thicker extrafusal skeletal muscle fibers that do the effective contractile work. **Group Ia afferents** in the spindle detect both the absolute muscle length and the rate of change in length of the intrafusal fiber. **Group II afferents** monitor static length of the intrafusal fiber. Muscle tension properties are detected in the **Golgi tendon organs**, which lie in series with the muscle fibers and their tendons. **Group Ib afferents** terminate in these organs and monitor the force exerted by extrafusal muscle contraction or passive stretch. By exciting interneurons that inhibit the same or homonymous (synergistic) **alpha motor neurons**, the Ib afferents trigger the **reverse (or inverse) myotatic reflex,** which protects the muscle from excessive contraction. In contrast, the **stretch (also known as the deep tendon or myotatic) reflex** is initiated when Ia afferents detect stretch of the intrafusal fibers. These afferents make monosynaptic excitatory synaptic connections to **alpha motor neurons,** innervating the same or homonymous muscle. The Ia afferent pathway drives a homeostatic system in which imposed stretch automatically elicits a compensatory contraction—an arrangement that contributes to balance, posture, and muscle tone. The sensitivity of this system is maintained during active contraction of surrounding extrafusal fibers by the coactivation of a second type of motor neuron along with the alpha motor neurons. These **gamma motor neurons** excite the intrafusal muscles and prevent them from becoming flaccid when the parallel extrafusal muscles contract. The activity of the gamma motor neurons, and hence the sensitivity of the stretch reflex, can be adjusted by several descending pathways from the brain.

Numerous motor patterns and reflexes are mediated by spinal circuits without the need for input from higher centers. In addition to the stretch and reverse myotatic reflexes, an important reflex is the **withdrawal (flexor) reflex** of a limb triggered by the activation of somatic nociceptor terminals in the limb. These sensory neurons activate excitatory interneurons which in turn activate flexor motor neurons that innervate the ipsilateral limb. In addition, the nociceptors activate inhibitory interneurons that produce **reciprocal inhibition** of the extensor motor neurons which innervate the same limb. Interneurons also activate a second reflex, the **crossed-extensor reflex**, which extends the contralateral leg to provide balance and support during leg flexion. During defensive arm flexion, the crossed-extensor reflex causes a protective extension of the contralateral arm. Another reflex is the **scratch reflex**, which involves repetitive contraction and relaxation of muscles in the arm and hand that are generated by interneuronal circuits within the spinal cord. Groups of interneurons within the spinal cord also generate the complex patterns of motor output responsible for **locomotion.**

The circuits underlying these reflexes and motor patterns are used as building blocks for more complex behaviors that are controlled hierarchically by higher brain structures. Descending input to spinal motor circuits comes by several pathways. One is the **lateral corticospinal tract (pyramidal tract)**, which carries commands for conscious, voluntary movements from upper motor neurons in the primary motor cortex to lower motor neurons in the spinal cord that control distal muscles. Similarly, **lower motor neurons that control proximal muscles** receive commands through the **ventral corticospinal tract.** Upper motor neurons that control muscles in the face and head send their axons into another pyramidal tract, the **corticobulbar tract,** to synapse with lower motor neurons in brainstem motor nuclei. A second major pathway to the spinal cord is the **ventromedial pathway,** which consists of four tracts from brainstem regions that are involved in posture and locomotion: the vestibulospinal, tectospinal, pontine reticulospinal, and medullary reticulospinal tracts. Direct and indirect input to spinal motor neurons also comes from the cerebellum and basal ganglia.

Although **upper motor neurons excite lower motor neurons,** as well as **interneurons, much of the descending input to spinal motor neurons is inhibitory.** Damage to descending pathways at any level above a specific spinal segment (lumped together as upper motor neuron lesions) removes these excitatory and inhibitory influences and thus produces profound effects on reflexes mediated by that segment. These effects include some **weakness** (because of decreased excitation of alpha motor neurons and some interneurons), **increased** muscle tone (rigidity), and prominent spasticity, which is characterized by hyperactive stretch reflexes and increased resistance to rapid muscle stretch. Mechanisms of spasticity are unclear but appear to involve disinhibition of spinal neurons, including interneurons and gamma motor neurons. Transection of the spinal cord causes a period of spinal shock for a few weeks in which all spinal reflexes below the transection are reduced severely or abolished (flaccid paralysis). This probably results from sudden interruption of descending facilitatory influences. Reflexes then gradually recover and eventually become exaggerated, perhaps because of disinhibition, denervation supersensitivity of motor neurons and interneurons, and/or sprouting of additional afferent terminals. Spinal transection also interrupts autonomic pathways, and this can result in urinary and/or fecal incontinence, increased or decreased heart rate and blood pressure, and respiratory failure. Lesions of peripheral nerves that transect motor neuron axons cause flaccid paralysis and a total loss of voluntary and reflex responses from the denervated muscles, spontaneous twitch-like fasciculations, and muscle atrophy. If the entire nerve is not transected, peripheral axons sometimes can regenerate so that many months after nerve injury the reflexes recover partially or (rarely) completely.

COMPREHENSION QUESTIONS

[46.1] A motor unit that innervates only three muscle fibers is likely to innervate muscle in which of the following?

  A. Back
  B. Biceps
  C. Bladder
  D. Thigh
  E. Thumb

[46.2] Which of the following effects is caused by activation of gamma motor neurons during active contraction of extrafusal muscle fibers?

  A. Decreased magnitude of the stretch reflex
  B. Increased force developed by the extrafusal muscle fibers
  C. Increased sensitivity of Ib afferents
  D. Increased summation of motor units
  E. Maintained sensitivity of the Ia afferents during unexpected stretch

[46.3] Which of the following observations would suggest that an upper motor neuron lesion rather than a lower motor neuron lesion is present?

  A. Fasciculations
  B. Hyporeflexia
  C. Profound weakness
  D. Pronounced atrophy
  E. Spasticity

Answers

[46.1] **E.** Motor units are smallest in the parts of the body that have the most precise motor control, such as the thumb, fingers, and tongue.

[46.2] **E.** Coactivation of gamma motor neurons with alpha motor neurons shortens the intrafusal muscle fibers during contraction of extrafusal fibers so that sensitivity of the Ia stretch receptors in the intrafusal fibers is maintained when unexpected stretch occurs during the extrafusal muscle contraction. This would increase rather than decrease the magnitude of any stretch reflex evoked during contraction (answer A) and would have no direct effect on extrafusal force development, the sensitivity of Ib afferents, or the summation of motor units (answers B, C, and D).

[46.3] **E.** Upper motor neuron lesions produce spasticity, involving hyperactive stretch reflexes. Lower motor neuron lesions do not produce spasticity. Fasciculations are not induced by upper motor neuron lesions, and compared with lower motor neuron lesions, there is less dramatic weakness and muscle atrophy.

PHYSIOLOGY PEARLS

❖ Motor units that control fine, precise contractions by distal muscle are much smaller than motor units that control posture or massive contractions by proximal muscle.

❖ Group Ia afferents innervate muscle spindles organized in parallel with extrafusal muscle fibers that, when activated by increased stretch of the muscle, directly excite alpha motor neurons which cause contraction of the same and homonymous muscle fibers, thereby evoking the stretch reflex.

❖ Descending influences can adjust the sensitivity of the stretch reflex by adjusting the background activity of gamma motor neurons to produce contraction of intrafusal muscle and maintain relatively constant tension on Ia afferent terminals in the spindle during extrafusal muscle contractions.

❖ Local circuits composed of spinal afferents, spinal interneurons, and spinal motor neurons mediate a large number of behaviors that can operate relatively independently of the supraspinal circuits. These behaviors include the stretch, reverse myotatic, flexor, crossed-extensor, and scratch reflexes, as well as major components of locomotor patterns.

❖ Conscious, voluntary movements depend on commands to lower motor neurons in the spinal cord and/or brainstem from upper motor neurons in the primary motor cortex that are conveyed by axons in the lateral corticospinal, ventral corticospinal, and corticobulbar tracts.

❖ Descending influences on spinal motor activity related to posture, balance, orientation, and general muscle tone are conveyed from nuclei in the brainstem by axons in the vestibulospinal, tectospinal, pontine reticulospinal, and medullary reticulospinal tracts.

❖ Upper motor neuron lesions are associated with some weakness, increased basal muscle tone, and prominent spasticity and hyperreflexia, whereas lower motor neuron lesions are associated with profound weakness, decreased muscle tone, hyporeflexia, muscle fasciculations, and muscle atrophy.

REFERENCES

Johnson DA. Lower motor neurons of the spinal cord and brain stem. In: Johnson LR, ed. *Essential Medical Physiology*. San Diego, CA: Elsevier Academic Press; 2003: 861-866.

Johnson DA. Sensory and motor pathways controlling lower motor neurons of the spinal cord. In: Johnson LR, ed. *Essential Medical Physiology*. San Diego, CA: Elsevier Academic Press; 2003: 867-876.

❖ **CASE 47**

A 63-year-old man is brought to his primary care physician because of concern on the part of his family that he is acting differently. He has been having a worsening tremor at rest and difficulty walking. His family states that when he walks, he often has difficulty stopping. He has no personal or family medical history. On examination, he has a mask-like facial expression with little blinking. He is noted to have a fine tremor at rest in a "pill-rolling" manner. He has muscular rigidity and a stooped posture. On walking, the patient is noted to have rapid propulsion forward with an inability to stop. He shows no signs of dementia or depression. He subsequently is diagnosed with Parkinson disease.

 Which nuclei compose the basal ganglia?

 Where is the lesion for Parkinson disease located?

 What would be the location of the lesion in a patient with hemiballismus?

ANSWERS TO CASE 47: BASAL GANGLIA

Summary: A 63-year-old man presents with muscle rigidity, resting tremor, and difficulty walking, consistent with Parkinson disease.

 Nuclei composing basal ganglia: Caudate, putamen, globus pallidus, subthalamic, substantia nigra.

◆ **Location of lesion in Parkinson disease:** Substantia nigra.

◆ **Location of lesion in patient with hemiballismus:** Subthalamic nucleus.

CLINICAL CORRELATION

Properly functioning basal ganglia are necessary to control a person's movement. A lesion in any part of the basal ganglia will result in a characteristic movement disorder. Lesions of the striatum result in continuous, quick, and uncontrolled movements, as seen with Huntington disease. Hemiballismus can be seen with lesions of the subthalamic nuclei, and postural support may be lost with lesions of the globus pallidus. A lesion of the substantia nigra will result in Parkinson disease, the symptoms of which are produced by a loss of dopamine-containing nerve cells in the substantia nigra. Patients with Parkinson disease may have a combination of symptoms, including resting tremor, rigidity, bradykinesia, disturbance of gait, and postural problems. The cause of Parkinson disease is unknown.

APPROACH TO BASAL GANGLIA PHYSIOLOGY

Objectives

1. Be able to describe the organization and functions of the basal ganglia.
2. Know the direct and indirect pathways in the basal ganglia motor loop.

Definitions

Disinhibition: Removal of an inhibitory input, resulting in increased excitation of a target.
Hemiballismus: Movement disorder characterized by large, spontaneous, uncontrolled throwing motions of the arm and leg (usually unilateral).
Choreiform: Movements that are dance-like, involving large groups of muscles.

DISCUSSION

The **basal ganglia, located near the thalamus** in the diencephalon, are composed of **five pairs of nuclei:** the **caudate nucleus, putamen, globus pallidus, subthalamic nucleus, and substantia nigra.** The basal ganglia receive synaptic input from motor cortex (as well as from sensory association and prefrontal cortex) and send their output to the thalamus, which then feeds back to the cortex. Although the functions of the basal ganglia are not well understood, strong evidence indicates that through these connections from and back to motor cortical areas, **the basal ganglia provide a motor loop** that contributes to the **planning and programming of voluntary movements.** In addition, the basal ganglia appear to be important for some cognitive processes, such as those involving the organization of behavioral responses and verbal problem solving.

The motor loop comprises two parallel pathways that travel from the cortex through the basal ganglia and then to the thalamus and back to the cortex (Figure 47-1). Each branch has an opposite effect on thalamic targets. The **direct pathway goes through the caudate and putamen** (which together form the neostriatum) to the internal segment of the globus pallidus and the pars reticulata segment of the substantia nigra and then to the ventral anterior and centromedian nuclei of the thalamus. The **indirect pathway** goes **through the external segment of the globus pallidus, then to the subthalamus,** and then (like the direct pathway) to the internal segment of the globus pallidus and substantia nigra. Each pathway is activated by excitatory synapses (releasing glutamate) from cortical regions. Both pathways inhibit neurons in the thalamus via fibers from the globus pallidus and substantia nigra, which release γ-aminobutyric acid (GABA). In the direct pathway, neurons in the neostriatum directly inhibit (via GABA release) the neurons in the globus pallidus and substantia nigra. In the indirect pathway, neurons in the neostriatum inhibit neurons in the external segment of the globus pallidus, which inhibit neurons in the subthalamic nucleus, which then excite neurons in the globus pallidus and substantia nigra. Because the indirect pathway has two inhibitory synapses in series and the direct pathway has only one inhibitory synapse (onto the globus pallidus and substantia nigra), activation of the indirect pathway will increase the activity of the globus pallidus and substantia nigra, whereas activation of the direct pathway will decrease activity in the same nuclei. See Figure 47-1.

The **output neurons for both pathways in the globus pallidus and substantia nigra** are usually **active at high frequency and tonically inhibit target nuclei in the thalamus.** When the direct pathway is activated transiently, the tonically active output neurons are inhibited transiently, and this disinhibition increases activity in the thalamus and thereby in the cortex (the motor loop shows positive feedback). When the indirect pathway is activated transiently, the output neurons are excited, and activity in the thalamus and cortex is inhibited (negative feedback). In the basal ganglia, most of the synapses are inhibitory (releasing GABA), and excitation is produced by inhibiting an inhibitory pathway (disinhibition).

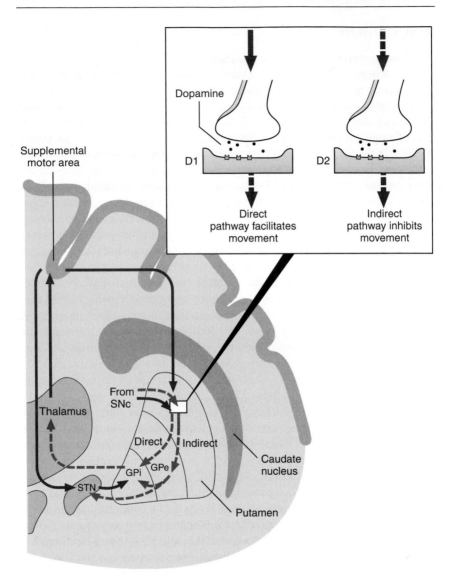

Figure 47-1. Direct and indirect pathways in the motor loop connecting the basal ganglia to the thalamus and cortex. SNc—pars compacta segment of substantia nigra, GPe—external segment of globus pallidus, GPi—internal segment of globus pallidus, STN—subthalamic nucleus, solid lines—excitatory pathways, dashed lines—inhibitory pathways, D1 and D2—classes of dopamine receptors.

Both the **direct and indirect pathways** are **modulated** by the **nigrostriatal pathway** by **neurons in the pars compacta segment of the substantia nigra** that **release dopamine onto neurons in the neostriatum.** Neurons in the neostriatum that mediate the direct pathway have **D1 dopamine receptors that produce excitation.** In contrast, neurons in the **neostriatum that mediate the indirect pathway have D2 dopamine receptors that produce inhibition.**

Thus, dopamine release from pars compacta neurons excites the direct pathway, which inhibits the output neurons, thereby increasing thalamic activity and ultimately facilitating movements initiated in the cortex. Synergistically, dopamine inhibits the indirect pathway, further increasing the inhibition of the output neurons. **Many of the effects of Parkinson disease** can be explained by a **marked reduction in dopamine release** (caused by degeneration and death of neurons in the **substantia nigra**) that results in **less disinhibition of thalamic activity** and thus **decreased facilitation of movements initiated in the cortex.** The substantia nigra is also the source of dopaminergic input to the rest of the brain with the exception of the pituitary gland, which receives dopaminergic fibers from the arcuate nucleus of the hypothalamus. The mesolimbic and mesocortical tracts arising from the substantia nigra contribute to affect, emotion, and motivation and also are involved in schizophrenia.

Basal ganglia disorders also occur after lesions to these nuclei, most commonly caused by **small strokes.** Lesions of the subthalamic nucleus often result in involuntary, sometimes violent movements of the contralateral limbs; this is termed **hemiballism** because of the resemblance to throwing movements. Hemiballism appears to result from **disinhibition of the thalamus** caused by **reduction of activity in the output nuclei of the basal ganglia** (especially the internal pallidal segment) that sometimes is caused by a decrease in excitation from the subthalamic nucleus. **Huntington disease,** a heritable hyperkinetic disorder, is caused by **widespread loss of neurons** that begins in the **striatum** with loss of the neurons that give rise to the **indirect pathway.** This results in inhibition of subthalamic nucleus neurons and choreiform movements and hemiballism-like movements in early stages of the disease. After the disease progresses, rigidity and akinesia develop (as in Parkinson disease) because the neurons that project directly to the internal pallidal segment are lost.

COMPREHENSION QUESTIONS

[47.1]   Which of the following is the major neurotransmitter released by most neurons within the basal ganglia?

    A. Acetylcholine
    B. Dopamine
    C. GABA
    D. Glycine
    E. Glutamate

[47.2] Which of the following provide, respectively, the predominant input
        to, the output from, and the direct synaptic target of the basal ganglia?

    A. Cerebellum, globus pallidus, substantia nigra
    B. Cerebral cortex, globus pallidus, cerebral cortex
    C. Cerebral cortex, globus pallidus, thalamus
    D. Cerebral cortex, putamen, substantia nigra
    E. Thalamus, globus pallidus, cerebral cortex

[47.3] A 62-year-old nursing home patient is brought into the emergency
        department for evaluation of altered mental status. Magnetic resonance
        imaging indicates degeneration of dopamine-containing neurons in the
        substantia nigra. This loss is most likely to do which of the following?

    A. Decrease activity in basal ganglia output nuclei
    B. Produce dyskinesias such as choreiform movements
    C. Produce hemiballism
    D. Suppress activity in the subthalamic nucleus
    E. Suppress the direct pathway and facilitate the indirect pathway
       from the striatum to the basal ganglia output nuclei

Answers

[47.1] **C.** The majority of synapses from neurons in the basal ganglia are
        inhibitory and release GABA. The other major inhibitory neurotrans-
        mitter, glycine, is not important in the basal ganglia and is released
        primarily from inhibitory interneurons in the spinal cord. Dopamine
        is an important neurotransmitter that is released by neurons in the
        substantia nigra, but these neurons account for only a small fraction
        of the total number of neurons in the basal ganglia. In addition, other
        neurotransmitters (eg, acetylcholine, NO, various neuropeptides) are
        released from some neurons in the basal ganglia, but the largest num-
        ber of synapses are GABAergic.

[47.2] **C.** The basal ganglia and thalamus form a motor loop with the cere-
        bral cortex. Input to the basal ganglia comes from prefrontal and sen-
        sory association areas of the cerebral cortex and leaves the basal
        ganglia via the internal segment of the globus pallidus. The immedi-
        ate target of these neurons is the thalamus (ventral anterior, ventral
        lateral, and centromedian nuclei). These thalamic nuclei then project
        to motor areas in the cerebral cortex.

[47.3] **E.** Under normal conditions, dopamine released by neurons in the sub-
        stantia nigra affects both the direct and indirect pathways in the motor
        loop to the cerebral cortex, exciting the direct, stimulatory pathway to
        the thalamus and inhibiting the indirect, inhibitory pathway to the thala-
        mus. Thus, if the dopamine-containing neurons degenerate (as occurs in
        Parkinson disease), the excitatory actions on the thalamus are inhibited

and there is less disinhibition of the inhibitory actions, with the consequence that excitation from the thalamus to motor areas in the cortex is decreased and it becomes more difficult to initiate movements. The other effects listed (answers A–D) would not be produced by selective loss of dopaminergic neurons, but instead by lesions of the subthalamic nucleus or early stages of striatal neuron loss.

PHYSIOLOGY PEARLS

❖ The four principal nuclei of the basal ganglia are the striatum, globus pallidus, substantia nigra, and subthalamic nucleus.

❖ The motor loop comprises two parallel pathways that travel from the cortex through the basal ganglia and then to the thalamus and back to the cortex. In the direct pathway, excitatory input to the basal ganglia excites thalamic neurons by inhibiting the inhibitory output neurons in the internal segment of the globus pallidus. In the indirect pathway, excitatory input to the basal ganglia further inhibits thalamic neurons by disinhibiting the inhibitory output neurons in the internal segment of the globus pallidus.

❖ GABA is the most prominent inhibitory neurotransmitter in most of the brain, although glycine is an important inhibitory neurotransmitter in the spinal cord and brainstem.

❖ Dopamine release from pars compacta neurons in the substantia nigra excites the direct pathway (by D1 receptors), which inhibits the inhibitor output neurons, thereby increasing thalamic activity and ultimately facilitating movements initiated in the cortex, whereas dopamine simultaneously inhibits the indirect pathway (by D2 receptors), further increasing the inhibition of the inhibitory output neurons.

❖ Loss of dopaminergic neurons in Parkinson disease reduces the activation of the direct pathway as well as the inhibition of the indirect pathway, allowing greater inhibition of thalamic neurons and greater suppression of movements initiated in the cortex, resulting in the hypokinetic signs of this disease.

REFERENCES

Johnson DA. The basal ganglia. In: Johnson LR, ed. *Essential Medical Physiology*. San Diego, CA: Elsevier Academic Press; 2003:881-887.

Mahlong RD. The basal ganglia. In: Kandel ER, Schwartz JH, Jessell TM. *Principles of Neuroscience*. New York, NY: McGraw-Hill; 2000: 853-867.

A 34-year-old woman with a long-standing history of seizure disorder presents to her neurologist with difficulty walking and coordination. She has been on phenytoin for several days after having been switched from valproic acid. She states she has had an acute change in gait, unclear speech, blurring of vision, tremor with movement, and loss of hand coordination. She has never had symptoms like this before. She denies headache and vertigo or any other complaints. On examination, she has an unstable gait and poor hand-eye coordination. She is noted to have nystagmus along with a fine tremor of the hand when she is moving it. A urine drug screen is negative. She has a computed tomography (CT) scan and lumbar puncture, which are both normal. Phenytoin levels are slightly elevated. She is diagnosed with cerebellar ataxia, probably as a side effect of phenytoin.

◆ **What part of the cerebellum is responsible for planning and initiation of movement?**

◆ **Is the output of the cerebellar cortex excitatory, inhibitory, or both?**

◆ **What is the neurotransmitter for Purkinje cells?**

ANSWERS TO CASE 48: CEREBELLUM

Summary: A 34-year-old woman has lack of coordination and cerebellar ataxia secondary to the medication phenytoin.

◆ **Part of cerebellum responsible for planning and initiation of movement:** Cerebrocerebellum (neocerebellum).

◆ **Output from cerebellar cortex:** Inhibitory.

◆ **Neurotransmitter for Purkinje cells:** Gamma-aminobutyric acid (GABA).

CLINICAL CORRELATION

Ataxia is defined as a loss of muscle coordination. There are many different etiologies, including inheritable diseases, that can result in ataxia. Signs of ataxia may include gait impairment, nystagmus, tremor with movement, loss of coordination, and inability to perform rapid alternating movements. Cerebellar ataxia is differentiated from vestibular-labyrinthine disease because of a lack of vertigo, dizziness, and light-headedness. Acute and reversible ataxia may be seen during intoxication with alcohol, during gasoline and glue sniffing, and after exposure to mercury. Medications such as phenytoin, lithium, barbiturates, and medications for chemotherapy all may result in a reversible ataxia. Other etiologies of ataxia include infection (AIDS), cerebrovascular disease, vitamin deficiency, multiple sclerosis, malignancies, and thyroid disease. Depending on the etiology, the ataxia may be reversible, and so a search for the underlying cause is of paramount importance.

APPROACH TO CEREBELLAR PHYSIOLOGY

Objectives

1. Understand the general organization of the cerebellum.
2. Know the cerebellar functions.
3. Describe the cellular organization of the cerebellar cortex.

Definitions

Complex spike: Action potential in a cerebellar Purkinje cell occurring simultaneously in its soma and dendrites, which is stimulated by a single, extraordinarily powerful EPSP that is evoked by a single action potential in a single climbing fiber from the inferior olive.

Dysmetria: Abnormal movement characterized by undershoot or overshoot of intended position, associated with an inability to judge distance or scale.

DISCUSSION

The **cerebellum** occupies **10% of the brain volume** but contains **more than 50% of the neurons.** Most of the neurons are in the outer mantle of gray matter, the cerebellar cortex, but nearly all cerebellar output originates from cell bodies in the **four pairs of deep cerebellar nuclei (dentate, emboliform, globose, and fastigial).** Together, the emboliform and globose nuclei are called the interposed nucleus. All the incoming and outgoing axons pass through only three large tracts: the superior, middle, and inferior peduncles. The **vast majority of axons in these tracts** (> 97%) are **afferent** to the **cerebellum.** **Anatomically,** the cerebellar cortex is divided into an **anterior lobe,** a **posterior lobe,** and a **flocculonodular lobe.** Also important, however, are the functional divisions (orthogonal to the lobular divisions) into lateral and intermediate parts of each hemisphere and the central vermis.

The **flocculonodular lobe (vestibulocerebellum)** is the **most primitive part** of the cerebellar cortex, and through its connections from primary vestibular afferents and to the lateral vestibular nuclei, it functions in the **control of balance and eye movements.** The **vermis and intermediate hemispheres** receive somatosensory inputs from the spinal cord and thus are called the **spinocerebellum.** The vermis receives somatic sensory input from proximal parts of the body and head as well as visual, auditory, and vestibular input. It projects via the fastigial nucleus to cortical and brainstem regions that control proximal muscles of the body. It is important for modulating motor programs involved in posture, locomotion, and gaze. The intermediate part of the hemisphere receives somatic sensory input from the limbs and projects by way of the interposed nucleus to lateral corticospinal and rubrospinal systems to control distal muscles. The lateral part of each hemisphere **(cerebrocerebellum or neocerebellum)** evolved most recently and receives input solely from the cerebral cortex. It projects via the dentate nucleus and ventrolateral nucleus of the thalamus to cerebral cortical areas involved in motor control. It functions to help plan complex motor actions and consciously assess errors in movement.

Many parts of the cerebellum are important for motor learning. During the initial stages of much motor learning, conscious effort is required and most of the activity is in the cerebral cortex. However, as learning proceeds, much of the activity is shifted to the cerebellum. Learning in the cerebellum involves temporally precise interactions within Purkinje cells between excitatory input from climbing fibers and excitatory input from parallel fibers. The complex spikes generated by climbing fiber activity result in considerable Ca^{2+} influx, which promotes synaptic plasticity. The **cerebellar synaptic plasticity** allows novel motor patterns to be programmed at least partly in the cerebellum, allowing skilled movements to be executed almost automatically, with little or no conscious effort.

Although the **cerebellar cortex** contains an enormous number of neurons, it is composed of **only three layers** (external molecular, Purkinje cell, and internal granular) and **five types of neurons: Purkinje, granule, basket, stellate, and Golgi.** The two major inputs to the cerebellar cortex are climbing fibers from the inferior olivary nuclei and the mossy fibers, which bring input from the cerebral cortex as well as from proprioceptors all over the body through pontine nuclei and spinocerebellar tracts. Both sets of fibers have collaterals that also excite neurons in the deep cerebellar nuclei. The **climbing fibers** are much less numerous, but each directly and very strongly excites a few (1 to 10) **Purkinje cells.** Indeed, each action potential in a climbing fiber causes each postsynaptic Purkinje cell to reach action potential threshold simultaneously in the soma and dendrites (generating a **complex spike**).

The abundant **mossy fibers** excite **granule cells** in the granular layer, each of which provides weak excitatory input to many Purkinje cells through parallel fibers. Each Purkinje cell is excited by approximately 200,000 parallel fibers but only a single climbing fiber. Basket and stellate cells also are excited by granule cells, but they inhibit the Purkinje cells. Inhibition of the Purkinje cells also comes from the Golgi cells, which are excited directly by mossy fiber collaterals. These inhibitory interneurons release **GABA,** which opens Cl⁻ channels. Because the Cl⁻ equilibrium potential (E_{Cl}) is near the resting potential and opening of these channels tends to clamp the membrane potential close to E_{Cl}, GABA release strongly opposes concomitant excitatory input to the postsynaptic neuron. The Purkinje cells also release GABA, inhibiting neurons in the deep cerebellar nuclei that otherwise are tonically active. Thus, **the entire output of the cerebellar cortex is inhibitory.** In contrast, the neurons in the deep cerebellar nuclei excite neurons in the brainstem and thalamus. The cerebellar cortex provides precisely timed inhibitory control that modulates the excitatory output of the deep cerebellar nuclei and vestibular nuclei. In this regard, the cerebellum acts as an inhibitory modulator of motor activity initiated in the cerebral cortex, similar to the way the basal ganglia inhibit motor activity. Thus, **lesions of the cerebellum,** like lesions of the basal ganglia, **do not produce paralysis or sensory deficits.** Depending on the site of injury, cerebellar lesions disturb **balance** (flocculonodular lobe) or produce **ataxia, slurred speech, dysmetria, and an inability either to stop movements promptly or to alternate opposing movements rapidly** (anterior and posterior lobes).

COMPREHENSION QUESTIONS

[48.1]   Most axons in the superior, middle, and inferior peduncles are which of the following?

A. Afferent to the cerebellum
B. Axons of Golgi cells
C. Axons of Purkinje cells
D. Parallel fibers of granule cells
E. Projections from neurons in the deep cerebellar nuclei

[48.2]   Major functions of cerebellar cortex include which of the following?

A. Directly exciting alpha motor neurons
B. Exciting deep cerebellar nuclei
C. Generating motor patterns that subserve the scratch reflex
D. Learning and controlling novel movement patterns
E. Recognizing emotionally potent stimuli

[48.3]   Activity in climbing fibers will do which of the following?

A. Cause release of GABA from climbing fiber terminals
B. Evoke complex spikes in Purkinje cells
C. Have no effect in the flocculonodular lobe
D. Strongly excite neurons in deep cerebellar nuclei
E. Weakly depolarize Purkinje cells

Answers

[48.1]   **A.** About 97% of the axons in the peduncles connecting the cerebellum to the rest of the brain are afferent to the cerebellum. The output of the cerebellar cortex is conveyed exclusively by the Purkinje cells, which although large and powerful are not numerous.

[48.2]   **D.** One of the most important functions of the cerebellar cortex is to learn and control novel patterns of movement and posture. Cerebellar learning and other cerebellar functions are not implemented by direct actions on motor neurons (answer A) or spinal pattern generators (answer C) but instead modulate activity in the motor cortex by patterned inhibition (not excitation, as in answer B) of deep cerebellar nuclei, which excite thalamic neurons, which in turn excite neurons in motor cortex. The cerebellum is much less important for processing emotional information (answer E) than for controlling the spatial accuracy and temporal coordination of movement.

[48.3]   **B.** A single action potential in a single climbing fiber evokes a complex spike in each of the Purkinje fibers (1–20) on which the climbing fiber synapses. The complex spike, which is activated by glutamate released from the climbing fiber, is an overshooting action potential generated simultaneously in the soma and dendrites. This is the strongest synaptic connection known in the central nervous system (CNS). In contrast, synapses from the climbing fibers to neurons in deep cerebellar nuclei are very weak. Climbing fibers strongly excite Purkinje cells in all regions of the cerebellar cortex.

PHYSIOLOGY PEARLS

❖ The cerebellar surface is divided anatomically into the anterior lobe, posterior lobe, and flocculonodular lobe, but the most important functional divisions are the vermis, intermediate hemispheres, and lateral hemispheres.

❖ Most axons in the peduncles that connect the cerebellum to the brainstem are afferent, and the afferents make excitatory connections in both the deep cerebellar nuclei and the cerebellar cortex.

❖ The cerebellar cortex forms an inhibitory loop, which is excited, along with the deep cerebellar nuclei, by proprioceptive, vestibular, and cerebral cortical input, and which feeds back to inhibit the deep cerebellar nuclei.

❖ Each output neuron of the cerebellar cortex, the Purkinje cell, is weakly excited by each of approximately 200,000 parallel fibers from cerebellar granule cells (which are activated by numerous mossy fibers from brainstem nuclei and the spinal cord) and strongly activated by a single climbing fiber originating in the inferior olivary nucleus.

❖ Purkinje cells, along with the inhibitory interneurons in the cerebellar cortex (basket, stellate, and Golgi), release GABA, which opens postsynaptic Cl⁻ channels to hold the postsynaptic potential close to the resting potential.

❖ Major functions of the cerebellum include modulating intrinsic motor programs involved in posture, locomotion, and gaze as well as motor planning and the unconscious control of novel motor patterns acquired during motor learning.

❖ Lesions of the cerebellum fail to produce paralysis or sensory deficits, but instead can disturb balance and produce ataxia, slurred speech, dysmetria, and an inability to stop movements efficiently or alternate different movements rapidly.

REFERENCES

Ghez C and Thach WT. The cerebellum. In: Kandel ER, Schwartz JH, Jessell TM, eds. *Principles of Neuroscience*. New York, NY: McGraw-Hill; 2000: 832-852.

Johnson DA. The cerebellum In: Johnson LR, ed. *Essential Medical Physiology*. San Diego, CA: Elsevier Academic Press; 2003: 889-895.

A 43-year-old woman is brought to her primary care physician by her family because of concerns about her forgetfulness. The patient has a history of Down syndrome but no other medical problems. She had been living in an assisted living environment for many years. Over the last year, she has become more forgetful. Once-easy-tasks are becoming increasingly difficult such as placing a telephone call, following directions, and housekeeping. She has become lost walking around the grounds and has difficulty naming objects and telling time. She often does not recognize old friends and forgets previous conversations. Physical examination confirms many of the memory and cognitive deficits. After a thorough workup, no specific etiology can be found, and the patient is diagnosed with Alzheimer disease.

◆ **What type of memory is available for conscious retrieval?**

◆ **Which part of the brain stores semantic (factual) memories?**

ANSWERS TO CASE 49: LEARNING AND MEMORY

Summary: A 43-year-old woman has Down syndrome and symptoms consistent with Alzheimer disease.

◆ **Conscious memory:** Explicit (declarative) memory.

◆ **Part of brain that stores semantic memory:** Neocortex.

CLINICAL CORRELATION

Alzheimer disease is a common cause of dementia and memory impairment. Early in the disease the memory losses are gradual, but they eventually increase to the point where daily activities such as driving, following instructions, and shopping are impaired. As the disease progresses, patients require daily supervision and have difficulty remembering names and conversations. Simple tasks such as telling time and changing clothes become extremely difficult. Age and a family history of Alzheimer disease are important risk factors. The pathogenesis is not understood completely, but senile plaques are present and cytoplasmic neurofibrillary tangles occur in increased numbers and frequency in Alzheimer patients. Magnetic resonance imaging (MRI) in the later stages of the disease will show diffuse cortical atrophy, with dramatic loss of neurons in the entorhinal cortex and hippocampus. There has been an association of Down syndrome and Alzheimer disease. The amyloid precursor protein (APP) gene on chromosome 21 is an important membrane-spanning protein that is processed into smaller units, including Abeta amyloid, and is deposited in neuritic plaques in patients with Alzheimer disease. The extra chromosome 21 may lead to excessive production of Abeta amyloid.

APPROACH TO LEARNING AND MEMORY

Objectives

1. Know the types of memory and their general anatomic locations.
2. Know about basic mechanisms of learning and memory.

Definitions

Long-term synaptic potentiation (LTP): A long-lasting (for hours, days, or longer) increase in the effectiveness of a synapse produced by transient, high-frequency activation of the synapse, resulting in an alteration within the brain circuit that can contribute to learning and memory.

Long-term synaptic depression (LTD): A long-lasting decrease in the effectiveness of a synapse produced by low-frequency activation of the synapse, resulting in alterations opposite to those produced by LTP, which can also contribute to learning and memory.

DISCUSSION

Learning is defined **as a process by which information, skills, or habits are acquired,** whereas **memory** is **defined as a phenomenon by which information, skills, or habits are stored.** **Memory** typically is divided into **general categories.** **Explicit** (declarative) **memory** is the storage and retrieval of **information about the world** and **one's personal experiences,** and it generally is recalled by **conscious effort.** Explicit memory is subdivided into **episodic memory** (about **personal experiences**) and **semantic memory** (about facts that have been **learned from others**). All other forms of memory are lumped into the **intrinsic** (nondeclarative) **memory** category. Implicit memory includes **priming** (unconscious facilitation of recognition of previously presented objects) and **memories** acquired by **various forms of learning,** including **procedural learning** (skills and habits), **associative learning** (classical and operant conditioning), and **nonassociative learning** (habituation and sensitization). Orthogonal to these classifications are divisions of memory into **long-term and short-term forms** (including working memory, which briefly keeps information available for immediate processing before being discarded or stored). Learning and memory depend on mechanisms of neural plasticity, especially synaptic plasticity. Such plasticity occurs in nearly all parts of the central nervous system (CNS), including the spinal cord, and plasticity in many parts of the CNS is involved in learning and memory.

By definition, **explicit memory** is the form of memory that people are most conscious of, and the gradual loss of explicit memory caused by conditions such as Alzheimer disease can be devastating to patients and their families. The effects of pathologic lesions in human patients and experimental lesions in animals have shown that the formation of explicit memory **depends critically on the hippocampus** and the rest of the **medial temporal lobe of the cerebral cortex** (ie, the parahippocampal cortex, entorhinal cortex, perirhinal cortex, dentate gyrus, and subiculum). The **earliest pathologic changes detected in Alzheimer disease** are a **marked loss of neurons in the entorhinal cortex,** an observation consistent with the earliest symptoms being impairment of explicit memory formation. Lesions in the hippocampus and medial temporal lobe caused by Alzheimer disease or other insults have little effect on previously established memories, only on the formation of new memories. This and other observations indicate that the hippocampal system controls the initial phases of memory storage, but that long-term storage ultimately takes place in the association areas of neocortex, outside the medial temporal lobe. The hippocampus is particularly important for processing memories involving spatial representation, whereas the other parts of the medial temporal lobe can be more important for processing memories involving other forms of information, such as object recognition. Long-term storage of semantic information is distributed throughout the neocortex, whereas long-term storage of episodic memory is stored in the association areas of the frontal lobes.

There are many forms of **implicit memory,** and different forms are stored in different parts of the CNS. For example, memories with a **strong emotional component** often involve **alterations in the amygdala.** Memories associated with operant conditioning (ie, learning that a particular motor action has a consequence) may involve alterations in the striatum and cerebellar cortex. Some forms of classical conditioning (ie, learning that one stimulus predicts another) involve alterations in both the cerebellar cortex and the deep cerebellar nuclei, and others involve alterations in sensory or motor cortex. The simplest forms of learning—habituation and sensitization of reflex responses—may involve alterations in sensory and motor systems in the spinal cord and brain.

Many different cellular mechanisms contribute to learning and memory. The mechanism that has been studied most intensively and appears to be associated with many forms of learning and memory (both explicit and implicit) is **long-term synaptic potentiation (LTP)** induced by the opening of a class of **glutamate receptors** called **NMDA receptors,** named for the selective agonist N-methyl-D-aspartate. Under normal conditions, NMDA receptor channels are blocked by the binding of Mg^{2+} to a site in the pore even when the channel is opened by glutamate. During strong depolarization caused by intense synaptic input (as occurs in relevant neurons during learning events), electrostatic repulsion expels the Mg^{2+} and permits Na^+, K^+, and, most important, Ca^{2+} to pass through the pore when it is opened by glutamate. Influx of Ca^{2+} leads to the activation of various enzymes, including Ca^{2+}/calmodulin-dependent protein kinase and protein kinase C, as well as protein kinase A, which trigger various plastic changes. The **early phase of LTP (lasting 1-2 hours)** is thought to involve **increases in glutamate release** from the presynaptic terminal and/or **insertion of additional AMPA glutamate receptors** (named for the selective agonist α-amino-3-hydroxy-5-methylisoxazole-4-propionic acid), which are not blocked by Mg^{2+} and thus open fully when bound by glutamate at normal resting potentials. Both of these effects increase the amplitude of subsequently evoked excitatory synaptic potentials (EPSPs) and thus increase the functional strength of the altered synapse. A late phase of LTP also can be induced and may last for weeks or longer. It involves the **growth of new synapses,** which depends on changes in **protein synthesis and gene transcription.** These long-term effects appear to be induced, at least in part, by the ability of protein kinase A and Ca^{2+}/calmodulin-dependent protein kinase to activate transcription factors in the nucleus such as the Ca^{2+}-cyclic AMP response element binding (CREB) protein. An effect opposite to that of LTP, called long-term synaptic depression (LTD), is produced by low-frequency activation of many of the same synapses that exhibit LTP after high-frequency activation. Information storage in a neural network depends upon patterns of expression of LTP and LTD distributed across enormous numbers of synapses throughout the network.

COMPREHENSION QUESTIONS

[49.1]   On mental status examination, a 72-year-old woman is noted to have some difficulty with explicit (declarative) memory. This type of memory includes which of the following?

A. Conscious memory of personal experiences
B. Habituation
C. Memories acquired during operant conditioning
D. Neural alterations underlying new skills
E. Unconscious memory of food-induced illness

[49.2]   An 82-year-old man has been noted by his family to be forgetful and often to get lost. He is diagnosed with very mild Alzheimer disease. Which of the following areas of the brain is likely to be affected by neuronal loss?

A. Basal ganglia
B. Deep cerebellar nuclei
C. Entorhinal cortex
D. Hypothalamus
E. Prefrontal cortex

[49.3]   NMDA-receptor-dependent LTP is induced if which of the following occurs?

A. Ca^{2+} influx during low-frequency synaptic input activates protein phosphatases.
B. γ-Aminobutyric acid (GABA) is released near an NMDA receptor.
C. Glutamate release is inhibited.
D. Strong depolarization expels Mg^{2+} from the pore of the NMDA receptor channel.
E. The equilibrium potential for Ca^{2+} becomes less positive.

Answers

[49.1]   **A.** By definition, explicit or declarative memory is composed of episodic memory about personal experiences and semantic memory of facts learned from others. These memories can be recalled by conscious effort, unlike the other forms of memory listed in this question.

[49.2]   **C.** The earliest signs of neuronal loss during Alzheimer disease have been found in the entorhinal cortex, which is a gateway to the hippocampus. Degeneration is thought to spread to the hippocampus and later appear in other areas of the brain. Intense efforts are under way to develop methods for the early diagnosis of Alzheimer disease (when memory impairment first becomes apparent) by utilizing advanced imaging techniques to compare the relative volumes of the entorhinal cortex and hippocampus with those in other parts of the brain.

[49.3]   **D.** NMDA-receptor-dependent LTP is induced when sufficient depo-
          larization is received postsynaptically, during the release of glutamate
          from the presynaptic terminal, so that Mg^{2+} is expelled from the pore
          of the NMDA receptor channel and substantial amounts of Ca^{2+} can
          then enter through the pore. The surge of Ca^{2+} activates various
          enzymes, including protein kinases, triggering cascades that result in
          a strengthening of that synapse. High-frequency stimulation of mul-
          tiple presynaptic fibers usually is needed to cause enough depolar-
          ization and allow enough Ca^{2+} to enter to activate the protein kinases.
          Low-frequency stimulation allows a much smaller amount of Ca^{2+} to
          enter, which can selectively activate protein phosphatases to produce
          the opposite effect, reducing the strength of the synapse (termed
          long-term depression [LTD]).

PHYSIOLOGY PEARLS

❖   Explicit (declarative) memory includes factual information about
    the world (semantic memory) and recollections of personal expe-
    riences (episodic memory) that can be retrieved consciously.

❖   Implicit (nondeclarative) memory refers to all forms of unconscious
    memory, including memories acquired or expressed during prim-
    ing, procedural learning of skills and habits, classical condition-
    ing, operant conditioning, habituation, and sensitization.

❖   The initial formation of explicit memories depends critically on pro-
    cessing in the medial temporal lobe and especially the hip-
    pocampus and entorhinal cortex.

❖   Long-term storage of semantic information (facts) is distributed in
    the neocortex, whereas long-term storage of episodic memory
    (personal experiences) occurs in the association areas of the
    frontal cortex.

❖   Formation and storage of various forms of implicit memory occur in
    many different parts of the CNS, including the amygdala, stria-
    tum, cerebellum, and spinal cord.

❖   A widespread mechanism that is likely to contribute to many forms
    of learning and memory is NMDA-receptor-dependent LTP, in
    which strong depolarization of NMDA receptors relieves a block
    of the pore by Mg^{2+} and allows Ca^{2+} to enter the cell and trigger
    enzymatic responses that lead to a marked enhancement of sub-
    sequent synaptic transmission.

❖   Long-term memory and persistent synaptic plasticity depend on
    changes in gene transcription and protein synthesis, often involv-
    ing activation of the CREB protein transcription factor in the neu-
    ronal nucleus.

REFERENCES

Byrne JH. Learning and memory. In: Johnson LR, ed. *Essential Medical Physiology*. San Diego, CA: Elsevier Academic Press; 2003: 905-918.

Kandel ER. Cellular mechanisms of learning and the biological basis of individuality. In: Kandel ER, Schwartz JH, Jessell TM. *Principles of Neuroscience*. New York, NY: McGraw-Hill; 2000: 1254-1279.

Kandel ER, Kupfermann I, and Iversen S. Learning and memory. In: Kandel ER, Schwartz JH, Jessell TM. *Principles of Neuroscience*. New York, NY: McGraw-Hill 2000: 1227-1253.

A 16-year-old high school student is brought to the emergency department by the emergency medical service after being found lying in the front yard of a neighbor's house, where he was mowing the lawn. The patient has a regular yard service and has been mowing for several months without problems. The patient was finishing his sixth yard for the day during a summer month with temperatures exceeding 37.8°C. His mowing partner noticed that the patient had been complaining of fatigue, light-headedness, nausea, and profuse sweating in the previous yard. While mowing the last yard, he became very confused and behaved oddly before finally losing consciousness. In the emergency department, he is tachycardic, with a temperature of 40.6°C. He is lethargic, and his skin is dry. He is diagnosed with heat stroke, and therapy is begun immediately.

◆ **What physical processes are used physiologically to dissipate heat from the body?**

◆ **In what part of the brain is the set-point temperature represented?**

◆ **How does aspirin or ibuprofen reduce fever?**

ANSWERS TO CASE 50: REGULATION OF BODY TEMPERATURE

Summary: A 16-year-old boy is brought to the emergency department after having a heat stroke.

◆ **Heat loss mechanisms:** Evaporation, radiation, conduction, and convection.

◆ **Part of brain concerned with set-point temperature:** Hypothalamus.

◆ **Nonsteroidal medications and fever:** Block the production of prostaglandins, which increase the set-point temperature.

CLINICAL CORRELATION

Recognition and early treatment are important when a heat stroke is suspected. Hyperthermia results when the normal heat-reducing mechanisms cannot respond to the heat adequately. A patient's initial response to hyperthermia includes shunting warm blood flow to the surface of the skin to increase heat loss by radiation, conduction, and convection. The most important heat loss mechanism is evaporation. If it is prolonged, copious sweating leads to volume depletion and tissue hypoperfusion. Symptoms of fatigue, light-headedness, nausea and/or vomiting, and hypotension may be present, and the patient will suffer from heat exhaustion. If the hyperthermia is not resolved, heat stroke occurs. This occurs when the temperature exceeds 40°C because the temperature-integrative center in the hypothalamus is inactivated and the normal responses to hyperthermia (most importantly, sweating) cease. Death occurs rapidly unless the body is cooled, for example, by ice water baths or by removing clothing and sponging if an ice water bath is not available. Treatment of a heat stroke includes intravenous (IV) fluid replacement and, because damage may occur in various organs, including the kidneys and liver, close observation of electrolytes and other laboratory values (liver function tests, clotting studies, creatine phosphokinase [CPK], and complete blood count [CBC]). Recognition of heat exhaustion before the development of heat stroke is an important topic to teach workers, athletes, and patients who are at risk of heat exhaustion (eg, from manual labor or intense exercise outdoors during summer months).

APPROACH TO BODY TEMPERATURE PHYSIOLOGY

Objectives

1. Understand heat exchange between the body and its environment.
2. Know about the regulation of heat exchange and heat production.
3. Describe human adaptations to heat and cold.

Definition

Fever: A regulated increase in core temperature caused by elevation of the temperature set-point in the hypothalamus, usually during infection or disease.

DISCUSSION

Maintenance of constant body temperature requires that **heat production** from **metabolism** be **balanced by heat exchange with the environment.** The ability to dissipate heat to the environment is vital because even under resting conditions in a temperate environment, if the heat generated by the body is not dissipated, body temperature will reach lethal levels. **Heat exchange with the environment occurs by three processes: conduction** to or from molecules in contact with the **skin** (or gastrointestinal [GI] or pulmonary epithelia), **radiation** by infrared rays to or from bodies at different temperatures from that of the skin, and **evaporation of sweat or respiratory secretions** from the body. Radiation and conduction can increase or decrease total body heat content, whereas evaporation always decreases body heat content. Both conduction and evaporative heat loss are increased by convection of air around the body.

The **body regulates heat content** by regulating **skin temperature, sweat production, and heat production. Skin temperature** depends on the **insulating properties** of **subcutaneous fat,** which is not subject to rapid regulation, and **cutaneous blood flow.** Through **changes in the diameter of arterioles and precapillary sphincters,** blood flow into **the cutaneous circulation** can be regulated dramatically, from slightly more than 0% up to 30% of cardiac output. **Local heating** (or cutaneous irritation) **dilates the precapillary sphincters,** increasing cutaneous blood flow locally. Cutaneous heating or irritation also triggers spinal reflexes that dilate arterioles across a wider area. **Thermoreceptors** are found not only in the skin but also in the **preoptic anterior hypothalamus,** where the thermoreceptors are much more sensitive to small changes in temperature than the peripheral thermoreceptors are. An **increase in core temperature warms the hypothalamus** and **evokes a reduction in tonic activity in the sympathetic fibers innervating cutaneous arterioles,** permitting the arterioles **to dilate all over the body surface.** The increased blood flow to the skin shifts part of the heat content of the body to the surface, where it can be lost by conduction, convection, evaporation, and radiation. **Cooling has the opposite effects. Local cooling** of the skin causes **precapillary sphincters to constrict,** whereas a drop in core temperature increases sympathetic outflow to cutaneous arterioles, with the resulting constriction reducing cutaneous blood flow and thus heat loss to the environment. **Increased sympathetic activity** also causes **piloerection** (gooseflesh).

The **control of sweat production** is **critical** for survival under conditions in which conduction, convection, and radiation of heat from the skin cannot offset heat absorption and heat production (eg, when the environment is hotter than the body or during intense exercise). **Eccrine sweat glands** are **activated by sympathetic fibers,** which release acetylcholine (ACh) rather than norepinephrine (NE), and **can secrete up to approximately 1.5 L/h in normal adults.** After chronic adaptation to a hot climate, this rate can **increase to 4 L/h.** This is accompanied by **increases in plasma aldosterone levels** to **reduce the loss of Na$^+$ and water.**

Heat production in a normal adult during **maximal exercise** can be **20 times the level at rest.** During extreme heat, behavioral changes (lethargy) that lead to decreased physical activity reduce heat production. During **cold exposure,** behavioral changes such as **stomping the feet and clapping the hands increase heat production.** In addition, **shivering** occurs by involuntary asynchronous contraction of skeletal muscles. This is produced, at least in part, by facilitation of the stretch reflex and can increase heat production fivefold to sixfold. Release of epinephrine and NE from the adrenal medulla also occurs during cold exposure, and this increases metabolic heat production (chemical thermogenesis), especially in brown adipose tissue (in humans this is abundant only in infants). Chronic cold exposure also causes a persistent increase in thyroxin production, which uncouples oxidative phosphorylation and increases the metabolic rate in many tissues (as catecholamines do in brown adipose tissue). If **body temperature falls below 33°C, mental confusion occurs as central nervous system (CNS) function** begins to be impaired. **Below 30°C, thermoregulatory control by the CNS is lost, shivering stops, consciousness is lost, and muscular rigidity and collapse occur.** With further cooling, slow atrial fibrillation and, finally, ventricular fibrillation occur.

Body temperature is regulated by a temperature-integrative center in the **hypothalamus.** The temperature set point varies slightly (by ~0.6°C) each day in a circadian rhythm, with the lowest temperature occurring just before waking in the morning. In women, a small monthly elevation (0.2°C-0.6°C) is associated with ovulation. **Fever,** which can be triggered by infection, dehydration, or thyrotoxicosis, involves an **elevation of the temperature set point in the hypothalamus.** During **infection, exogenous pyrogens** associated with invading microorganisms trigger the release of endogenous pyrogens such as interleukin 1β (IL-1β), IL-6, and tumor necrosis factor (TNF) from leukocytes; this causes the production of prostaglandin E$_2$ and thromboxanes, which elevate the set-point temperature. Heat conservation responses (cutaneous vasoconstriction, inhibition of sweating), increased heat production (shivering), and behavioral responses (eg, pulling on covers) continue until the new set-point temperature is attained.

COMPREHENSION QUESTIONS

[50.1]   An increase in sympathetic activity involving axons going to the skin is noted. Which of the following is most likely to occur?

A. Constriction of capillaries
B. Increased blood flow through the skin
C. Increased release of NE at eccrine sweat glands
D. Inhibition of sweating
E. Piloerection

[50.2]   A 32-year-old man has lived for many years in Death Valley, California, mostly outdoors. Which of the following include adaptations he exhibits to this very hot environment ?

A. A large increase in the maximal rate of sweating
B. Decreases in the mass of brown adipose tissue
C. Decreases in plasma aldosterone levels
D. Facilitation of the stretch reflex
E. Increases in plasma thyroxine levels

[50.3]   A 28-year-old woman has a fever of 40°C as a result of influenza. Which of the following is likely to occur during the fever?

A. Cutaneous vasoconstriction
B. Reduction of hypothalamic set-point temperature
C. Decrease in shivering
D. Increase in sweating
E. Strong subjective sensation of increased heat

Answers

[50.1]   **E.** Some sympathetic fibers going to the skin release NE onto pilo-motor muscles, causing piloerection. Sympathetic activity also decreases blood flow through the skin by releasing NE onto smooth muscles in cutaneous arterioles (not capillaries), which then constrict. Under hot conditions, a separate set of sympathetic axons in the skin stimulates the secretion of sweat from eccrine sweat glands (these sympathetic terminals release ACh rather than NE).

[50.2]   **A.** The rate of sweat production by existing sweat glands increases dramatically after a couple of months in a hot climate. In addition, over longer periods, sweat production increases because the number of sweat ducts increases. Aldosterone production increases (not decreases, as in answer C), and this increases the reabsorption of Na^+ from sweat ducts, conserving Na^+. Brown adipose tissue is not found in adults (answer B), whereas facilitation of the stretch reflex and increases in plasma thyroxin levels (answers D and E) are adaptations to prolonged cold exposure rather than heat exposure.

[50.3] **A.** Fever elevates the hypothalamic set-point temperature, activating heat conservation responses, which include cutaneous vasoconstriction. Sweating is inhibited, and shivering occurs. There is a strong subjective sensation of cold, leading to behavioral efforts to warm the body such as pulling on blankets.

PHYSIOLOGY PEARLS

❖ Heat exchange with the environment occurs by conduction to or from molecules contacting the skin, by radiation via infrared rays to or from bodies at temperatures different from that of the skin, and evaporation of sweat and other secretions from the body surface.

❖ The efficiency of conduction and evaporation from the body surface is increased by convection of air around the body.

❖ Heat exchange across the skin is regulated by controlling the amount of blood flowing (and carrying heat) into the cutaneous circulation.

❖ Cutaneous blood flow is decreased by direct contractile responses of precapillary sphincters to cold as well as by increased sympathetic input to cutaneous arterioles, whereas elevation of local or core temperature produces the opposite effects.

❖ Core temperature is monitored by sensitive thermoreceptors in the hypothalamus, and this temperature is compared to the hypothalamic set point, with any discrepancy triggering appropriate autonomic and behavioral responses to bring the core temperature to the set point.

❖ Evaporation of sweat released by eccrine sweat glands is the only physiological mechanism available for cooling the body when the environmental temperature exceeds body temperature.

❖ Physiologic heat production is decreased during heat stress (primarily by behavioral changes such as lethargy) and increased during cold stress by facilitation of motor activity, shivering, and (in infants) enhancement of metabolic heat production in brown adipose tissue in response to epinephrine and NE release.

❖ Long-term adaptations to hot environments include a large increase in the maximal rate of sweating and increased aldosterone production, whereas adaptations to cold environments include an increase in thyroxine production.

REFERENCES

Nadel E. Regulation of body temperature. In: Boron WF, Boulpaep EL, eds. *Medical Physiology*. Philadelphia, PA: Saunders Elsevier Science; 2003: 1231-1241.

Schafer JA. Body temperature regulation. In: Johnson LR, ed. *Essential Medical Physiology*. San Diego, CA: Elsevier Academic Press; 2003: 921-932.

❖ CASE 51

A 62-year-old man undergoes surgery to correct a herniated disc in his spine. The patient is thought to have an uncomplicated surgery until he complains of extreme abdominal distention and pain about 1 hour after surgery. He is noted to be hypotensive and tachycardic. On examination, his abdomen is distended and tense, with severe rebound pain indicating peritoneal irritation. He is taken back immediately to the operating room, where they find a large amount of blood in his abdomen (2 L) and a small puncture site in the descending aorta with active bleeding. A graft is placed in the aorta to stop the bleeding and repair the injury site. The patient is transfused with blood intraoperatively and is taken to the intensive care unit in critical condition.

◆ **What would be the response of the sympathetic system to this patient's decrease in arterial pressure?**

◆ **What would be the response of the renin-angiotensin-aldosterone system to the decreased arterial pressure?**

◆ **How would antidiuretic hormone (ADH) play a role in this situation?**

ANSWERS TO CASE 51: HEMORRHAGIC SHOCK

Summary: A 62-year-old man presents for back surgery, which is complicated by injury to the aorta with resultant hemorrhagic shock.

 Response of sympathetic system: Increased heart rate and contractility, and increased total peripheral resistance.

 Response of the renin-angiotensin-aldosterone system: Increased angiotensin II causes further vasoconstriction, and aldosterone increases sodium-chloride reabsorption in the kidney to increase blood volume.

 Response of ADH: Causes vasoconstriction and increases water reabsorption in the kidney.

CLINICAL CORRELATION

Circulatory shock can have many different etiologies, including hemorrhage, sepsis, and neurogenic causes. The physiologic response is essentially the same for all the etiologies. All the processes include hypotension, which triggers stimulation of the sympathetic system, increases renin production leading to aldosterone production, and increases ADH secretion. If the circulatory volume is not replaced quickly, the resulting peripheral vasoconstriction, so as to maintain blood supply to the heart, lung, and brain, will result in ischemia to other end organs, such as the kidney and liver. Monitoring urine output is a good way to assess intravascular volume. If the patient is making adequate urine, the kidneys are being perfused and the intravascular volume is probably adequate. After replacement of fluids and/or blood, the underlying cause needs to be addressed and treated.

APPROACH TO PHYSIOLOGIC ADAPTATION TO HEMORRHAGE

Objectives

1. Know the causes of circulatory shock.
2. Understand the body's response to shock (shunt to brain, heart, and lungs).
3. Know the role of blood pressure as an indicator of shock state.
4. Describe the treatment of circulatory shock.

Definitions

Circulatory shock: A condition in which cardiac output is compromised and no longer meets the metabolic demands of the tissues, leading to damage to the peripheral circulation.

Heart failure: A condition in which the ability of the heart to pump blood through the circulation is compromised; the heart tissue has been damaged.

DISCUSSION

Regulation of the cardiovascular system and **blood flow** to the **tissues** constitute a complex process involving the **function of both the heart and the systemic circulation. Circulatory shock** is a condition that can be characterized as **peripheral circulatory failure** in which there is **inadequate perfusion of the peripheral tissues.** The **peripheral circulation no longer meets the metabolic demands of the tissues.** This differs from heart failure, in which the ability of the heart to pump blood is compromised; this, of course, can lead to circulatory shock.

The causes of circulatory shock are varied. Several conditions can lead to circulatory shock, as outlined below:

1. **Inadequate circulatory volume.** The reduced blood volume leads to a reduction in cardiac output as a result of inadequate venous pressure (reduced ventricular filling pressure). This typically occurs with hemorrhage, sepsis, or conditions of hypovolemia.
2. **Impaired ability of the heart to pump blood to the circulation.** In these conditions, the heart tissue is compromised so that it cannot pump adequate blood to the circulation even if the venous pressure is normal or elevated. This is, of course, observed in heart failure (reduced contractility).
3. **A compromise in the autonomic system that controls the vasculature.** Loss of autonomic control leads to reduced vascular tone, causing venous pooling and arteriolar dilation that ultimately result in a reduction in venous and arterial pressure. This can be caused by lesions of the central nervous system.

Conditions leading to shock are normally progressive. A loss of blood volume, by **hemorrhage,** for example, will lead to **sequential decreases in circulating blood volume, venous return, ventricular filling, stroke volume, cardiac output,** and in turn **mean arterial pressure.** If blood loss is greater than 30 percent, or so, or if mean arterial pressure falls much below 70 mm Hg, as may occur in heart failure, progression into circulatory shock can occur if the problem leading to these conditions is not corrected rapidly.

During the initial hypotensive states, a number of **cardiovascular reflexes** are activated in an attempt to **compensate for a fall in mean arterial pressure.** The reduced blood volume and the fall in mean arterial pressure are **sensed by low-pressure receptors** (volume receptors in the atria, pulmonary veins) and **high-pressure baroreceptors** (carotid, aortic, and afferent arteriole baroreceptors), respectively; both types of receptors sense the pressure/volume changes and induce an increase in sympathetic nervous activity. This leads to an **increase in heart rate, cardiac contractility, and venoconstriction** that will serve to elevate mean arterial pressure. Interestingly, this response also leads to **selective arteriolar constriction of the extremities, including the skin, skeletal muscle, kidney, and gastrointestinal tract,** thereby shunting blood away from those tissues. Although local autoregulatory mechanism may respond to this constriction by inducing a subsequent easing of this constriction, partially returning blood flow toward normal, sympathetic-induced vasoconstriction will prevail in severe cases of hypotension. However, the **vasculature serving the brain and heart** and to some extent the lungs is not **markedly vasoconstricted,** and normal autoregulation of blood flow prevails so that blood flow to these tissues is not compromised to the same degree. Hence, the system tries to maintain adequate blood flow to these two vital organs at the expense of other tissues and organs. Further, other systems come into play in an attempt to restore blood volume and mean arterial pressure.

The low blood pressure and the increased sympathetic activity induce the release of renin from the afferent arteriole of the kidney, activating the **renin-angiotensin-aldosterone system** and leading to **aldosterone-induced reabsorption of Na^+ and Cl^- from the cortical collecting duct of the kidney,** along with **water retention.** The hypotension also leads to **secretion of ADH** from the posterior pituitary, leading to enhanced water reabsorption along the entire length of the cortical and medullary collecting ducts of the kidney in an attempt to return extracellular volume toward normal. Other secondary compensatory processes are also active (see the references at the end of this case).

If the compensatory systems noted above do not restore mean arterial pressure adequately, the circulatory system will continue to deteriorate with a further fall in blood pressure in which perfusion of peripheral tissues may be compromised irreversibly, a condition referred to as **irreversible shock.** In these conditions, the fall in arterial pressure will not reverse even if blood volume is restored to normal levels. The reasons underlying irreversible shock are many. **Ischemic tissues release metabolites and other vasodilator molecules that counteract the vasoconstrictor stimuli.** Desensitization of the vascular adrenoceptors or depletion of neurotransmitters may contribute to the loss of vasoconstrictor ability. Compromised perfusion of heart tissue can lead to necrosis of heart muscle, and release of **cardiotoxic molecules** from various organs can lead to reduced contractility. Various other factors may contribute to the decline in the cardiovascular system (see the references at the end of this case). The end result is that the cardiovascular system becomes so compromised that the system will not recover, even with intervention, and the patient eventually will die.

Although the fall in blood pressure would appear to be the defining factor leading to shock, it is really a **fall in cardiac output that is most critical.** During the progression of shock, mean arterial pressure is observed to fall. The body has numerous processes in place to attempt to correct for alterations in low blood pressure, such as baroreceptors, the renin-angiotensin-aldosterone system, and ADH, as outlined above, and so a sudden drop in blood pressure will be defended against. Even so, cardiac output may be reduced so that the underlying problem can be masked partially. Other signs of reduced cardiac output should be apparent, however, such as low urine output caused by reduced blood flow to the kidney, elevated ADH levels, and pale and cold skin resulting from increased sympathetic activity.

The **treatment of circulatory shock** includes only a limited number of options. The primary defect is low cardiac output that arises from a reduced venous pressure or ventricular filling pressure. This has been treated most successfully by **expansion of the blood volume** or **resuscitation.** Three categories of **volume expanders** traditionally have been employed: (1) **whole blood,** (2) **cell-free fluids** with **colloids** (added plasma for oncotic balance), and (3) **colloid-free metabolic fluids.** Good results typically have been observed with the colloid-free fluids, such as lactated Ringer solution, although plasma or whole blood can be more effective in less severe cases. As circulatory shock continues, the capillaries become highly permeable, allowing leakage of macromolecules such as plasma proteins. Normally, the permeability to macromolecules is low so that plasma proteins represent a major osmotic solute (osmotic pressure) in the capillary, and this is critical to osmotic reabsorption of fluid that filtered out of the capillaries. With a highly "leaky" state of the capillaries during shock, the plasma proteins are so permeable across the capillary wall that they do not provide a significant osmotic force. This leads to movement of fluid into the interstitial space, causing pooling or **edema.** Hence, although plasma or whole blood generally is most effective, along with volume expanders in the more severe cases, the **colloid-free fluids, such as lactated Ringer solution, tend to be just as effective** if not more so. Of course, only erythrocytes can provide oxygen-carrying capacity through hemoglobin. Regardless of the volume expander employed, treatment with any volume expander will lead to considerable peripheral edema. However, the benefits of an increased cardiac output far outweigh the problems associated with peripheral edema.

COMPREHENSION QUESTIONS

[51.1]   An individual comes to the emergency room complaining of weakness, dizziness, and fatigue. She states that she has had diarrhea for several days. Examination reveals a low blood pressure and tachycardia consistent with low cardiac output. Plasma bicarbonate is low, and other plasma electrolytes are unremarkable. Urine volume was minimal. The patient most likely has which of the following?

A. Congestive heart failure
B. Edema
C. Excessive fluid loss in the stool
D. Internal hemorrhage
E. Renal failure

[51.2]   An individual was in a car accident and is brought to the emergency room
         in an unconscious state. Examination shows a very low blood pressure
         (80/40 mm Hg), tachycardia, a very weak thready pulse, a distended
         abdomen, and clammy skin. Laboratory values indicate a very low hema-
         tocrit (18%) and hypoalbuminemia. He is diagnosed as having internal
         hemorrhage leading to severe hypovolemia and circulatory shock. To
         avoid having the patient go into irreversible shock, the emergency room
         doctor immediately should initiate which of the following treatments?

         A. Administration of colloid-free volume expanders (eg, normal
             saline or lactated Ringer solution)
         B. Administration of epinephrine to induce vasoconstriction
         C. Administration of oxygen to improve blood oxygenation
         D. Initiation of a platelet transfusion

[51.3]   A 35-year-old man had a tractor accident and lost approximately 1500 mL
         of blood. His initial blood pressure is 90/60 mm Hg, and the heart rate
         is 120 beats per minute. On resuscitation with intravenous lactated
         Ringer solution, his blood pressure increases to 110/70 mm Hg. Two
         hours later, he is noted to have significant peripheral edema of the hands
         and feet. Which of the following is the best explanation for the edema?

         A. Capillary leakage
         B. High-output congestive heart failure
         C. Infiltration of the intravenous line through the vein
         D. Low oncotic pressure

Answers

[51.1]   **C.** Diarrhea over several days can lead to dehydration from loss of fluid
         in the stool. In severe cases, the individual can become volume-
         depleted to the point of circulatory collapse. The reduced blood volume
         and the fall in mean arterial pressure will be sensed by both low-pres-
         sure receptors (volume receptors in the atria, pulmonary veins) and
         high-pressure baroreceptors (carotid, aortic, and afferent arteriole
         baroreceptors), inducing increased sympathetic nervous activity. This
         leads to an increase in heart rate, cardiac contractility, and venocon-
         striction that will serve to elevate mean arterial pressure. In addition,
         the increase in sympathetic nervous activity stimulates the release of
         renin from the afferent arteriole, activating the renin-angiotensin-aldos-
         terone system and leading to aldosterone-induced reabsorption of Na^+
         and Cl^- from the cortical collecting duct; this also stimulates secretion
         of ADH from the posterior pituitary, leading to enhanced water reab-
         sorption along the entire length of the cortical and medullary collecting
         ducts of the kidney. All responses to the hypovolemia represent an
         attempt to return extracellular volume toward normal. To correct the
         problem fully, the cause of the diarrhea must be addressed.

[51.2]   **A.** The best immediate therapy for a person in hemorrhagic shock is usually isotonic crystalloid colloid-free solution such as normal saline, until red blood cells are available. These agents are usually stocked immediately in the emergency center, whereas blood products require the blood bank to ensure matching blood type. The infusion will increase vascular volume and restore hemodynamics to near normal. Crystalloid such as normal saline cannot restore the hematocrit, but a patient normally can withstand a decrease in hematocrit of up to 20% or so without serious consequences. The use of vasoconstrictors and oxygen can be helpful, but again, if the volume depletion is severe, replacement of fluids will be essential to avoid having the patient go into irreversible shock.

[51.3]   **A.** Diffuse capillary leakage is the primary reason for the peripheral edema that occurs regardless of which resuscitation fluid is used.

PHYSIOLOGY PEARLS

❖   Circulatory shock can arise from many causes, such as heart failure, hemorrhage, sepsis, hypovolemia, and lesions of the central nervous system.

❖   The primary defect in circulatory shock is inadequate cardiac output, not just a fall in mean arterial pressure.

❖   The body aggressively defends against a reduction in mean arterial pressure by activating multiple processes, including baroreceptor reflexes and the sympathetic nervous system, carotid bodies, the renin-angiotensin-aldosterone system, and ADH release.

❖   Blood volume expanders can be used to treat circulatory shock, but only if the patient has not reached the irreversible phase of shock.

REFERENCES

Boulpaep EL. Integrated control of the cardiovascular system. In: Boron WF, Boulpaep EL, eds. *Medical Physiology: A Cellular and Molecular Approach.* New York: Saunders; 2003:Chap 24.

Downey JM. Heart failure and circulatory shock. In: Johnson LR, ed. *Essential Medical Physiology.* 3rd ed. San Diego, CA: Elsevier Academic Press; 2003:Chap 64.

Listing of Cases

Listing by Case Number

Listing by Disorder (Alphabetical)

LISTING BY CASE NUMBER

LISTING BY DISORDER (ALPHABETICAL)

❖ INDEX

Note: Page numbers followed by *f* or *t* indicate figures or tables, respectively.